GROWTH AND MATURATION FACTORS

GROWTH AND MATURATION FACTORS

Volume 1

GORDON GUROFF

Editor
Laboratory of Developmental Neurobiology
National Institute of Child Health and Human Development
National Institutes of Health

A Wiley-Interscience Publication

JOHN WILEY & SONS

New York ● Chichester ● Brisbane ● Toronto ● Singapore

Library of Congress Cataloging in Publication Data:

Main entry under title:
  Growth and maturation factors.

  "A Wiley-Interscience publication."
  Includes index.
  1. Growth promoting substances. 2. Nerve growth
factor. I. Guroff, Gordon, 1933–

QP84.G76 1983   612'.6   82-17598
ISBN 0-471-09709-8 (v. 1)

CONTRIBUTORS

Carol Beck, Department of Human Biological Chemistry and Genetics and The Marine Biomedical Institute, The University of Texas Medical Branch, Galveston, Texas

Mariann Blum, Department of Human Biological Chemistry and Genetics and The Marine Biomedical Institute, The University of Texas Medical Branch, Galveston, Texas

Jane E. Bottenstein, The Marine Biomedical Institute and Department of Human Biological Chemistry and Genetics, University of Texas Medical Branch, Galveston, Texas

Ralph A. Bradshaw, Department of Biological Chemistry, Washington University School of Medicine, St. Louis, Missouri

Nicholas V. Costrini, Department of Biological Chemistry, Washington University School of Medicine, St. Louis, Missouri

Joseph E. DeLarco, Laboratory of Viral Carcinogenesis, National Cancer Institute, Frederick Cancer Center, Frederick, Maryland

Bo Ek, Institute of Medical and Physiological Chemistry, University of Uppsala, Uppsala, Sweden

Frederick Grinnell, Department of Cell Biology, University of Texas Health Science Center, Dallas, Texas

Harry T. Haigler, Department of Physiology and Biophysics, University of California, Irvine, California

Carl-Henrik Heldin, Institute of Medical and Physiological Chemistry, University of Uppsala, Uppsala, Sweden

Ann D. Horowitz, Division of Environmental Sciences and Cancer Center, Institute of Cancer Research, Columbia University, New York, New York

Eugene M. Johnson, Jr., Department of Pharmacology, Washington University Medical School, St. Louis, Missouri

Ann Johnsson, Institute of Medical and Physiological Chemistry, University of Uppsala, Uppsala, Sweden

Alan M. Miller, Departments of Medicine, Biochemistry, and Oncology, University of Miami School of Medicine, Miami, Florida

Karin Mellström, The Wallenberg Laboratory, University of Uppsala, Uppsala, Sweden

Monica Nistér, The Wallenberg Laboratory, University of Uppsala, Uppsala, Sweden

J. Regino Perez-Polo, Department of Human Biological Chemistry and Genetics and The Marine Biomedical Institute, The University of Texas Medical Branch, Galveston, Texas

C. Patrick Reynolds, Department of Human Biological Chemistry and Genetics and The Marine Biomedical Institute, The University of Texas Medical Branch, Galveston, Texas

Gary L. Smith, School of Life Sciences, University of Nebraska, Lincoln, Nebraska

Åke Wasteson, Institute of Medical and Physiological Chemistry, University of Uppsala, Uppsala, Sweden

I. Bernard Weinstein, Division of Environmental Sciences and Cancer Center, Institute of Cancer Research, Columbia University, New York, New York

Bengt Westermark, The Wallenberg Laboratory, University of Uppsala, Uppsala, Sweden

Ming-Chi Wu, Departments of Medicine, Biochemistry, and Oncology, University of Miami School of Medicine, Miami, Florida

Adel A. Yunis, Departments of Medicine, Biochemistry, and Oncology, University of Miami School of Medicine, Miami, Florida

To my mother, with love and admiration

PREFACE

Since the first identifiable experiments on growth factors were done more than 30 years ago, the literature on the subject has expanded at a steady pace. Nevertheless, the expansion has been undisciplined. Growth factors appear and many disappear. Conditioned-medium factors and serum factors abound, but the vast majority remain uncharacterized. Of the dozens that have been reported, only a few have been described in any detail. Indeed, despite a large body of work on a few factors, the exact mechanism by which any one of the factors works, in a molecular sense, remains unknown. Even more, there is still a very real question about whether any of these factors, with the possible exception of nerve growth factor, has a role in the normal growth and development of the individual.

Despite the rather primitive state of our current understanding of these materials, the vistas for them are immense. They appear to impinge on the most fundamental processes of life. They influence the rate of cell division, the course of differentiation, and the characteristics of the immune system. They could have roles in clinical problems as diverse as atherosclerosis, sensory deficits, and cancer. Their actions are of concern to scientists in every area of biology.

There is, at present, no continuing source of information about growth factors. Papers appear in all contemporary journals, and reviews are found in virtually every compendium. It would seem useful to have a single set of volumes that would present the unfolding information in this area from several points of view. Reviews of the information concerning specific growth factors should appear, of course, but also there should be discussions of methods applicable to all factors, chapters on growth factors of clinical interest, and coverage of the effects of several factors on specific organs or organ systems. The present series is intended to satisfy this need for a collection of reviews of what appears to be a rapidly expanding field but one still in its infancy.

GORDON GUROFF

Bethesda, Maryland
February 1983

ix

CONTENTS

GROWTH AND
MATURATION FACTORS

1

THE STRUCTURE AND FUNCTION
OF NERVE GROWTH FACTOR

Ralph A. Bradshaw

Nicholas V. Costrini

CONTENTS

Abbreviations

NGF	Nerve growth factor
IGF	Insulin-like growth factor
EGF	Epidermal growth factor
ACTH	Adrenocorticotropic hormone
MSH	Melanocyte-stimulating hormone
SCG	Superior cervical ganglion
anti-NGF	Antiserum to nerve growth factor
TH	Tyrosine hydroxylase
DBcAMP	Dibutyryladenosine 3′,5′-monophosphate
cAMP	Adenosine 3′,5′-monophosphate
SMC	Somatomedin C
MSA	Multiplication-stimulating activity
CNS	Central nervous system

1. INTRODUCTION

Since its discovery some 30 years ago (1,2), nerve growth factor (NGF) has captured the imagination of neurobiologists because it has held the promise that an understanding of its function would reveal fundamental principles of nerve growth that might have broad application, particularly in higher vertebrates. Although the study of NGF has not been without its rewards in this regard, it has probably been more valuable as a model for studying hormones and other growth factors in their various developmental roles. This is true in part because significant aspects of the structure and function of NGF remain to be established. What are the principal sites of synthesis of the substance? What is the exact manner in which it reaches its target tissues? What is the complete spectrum of target tissues? What is the mechanism by which it achieves its effects? Another problem is that there is no clear distinction between biological activities that are bona fide growth responses of physiological significance and those that are the result of *in vitro* manipulations.

The resolution of these uncertainties is of fundamental importance in defining the proper physiological role(s) of NGF. Clearly, the action of the substance on responsive neurons derived from the neural crest (i.e., sympathetic and certain sensory neurons) is of primary importance *in vivo*. It is probable that other neural crest cells early in development also display a responsiveness to the hormone that is subsequently lost (but can at times be manifested in cultured forms of these cells). However, neurons from other parts of the nervous system, most notably the central nervous system (CNS), which maintain a curious but ill-defined responsiveness to NGF, are only of questionable relevance, mainly because it has not been demonstrated that the hormone can reach these tissues *in vivo*. Responses of non-neuronal tissues, such as chondrocytes, are also unlikely to be of significance, although rigorously excluding them is difficult. Although the study of NGF interaction with any responsive cell is likely to be informative, this review focuses only on the action of NGF on sympathetic and dorsal root neurons and the manner in which responses therein are elicited at a molecular level. An account of the molecular properties of NGF, including what is known about its biosynthesis and its overall relationship to other hormones and growth factors, is also presented.

2. MOLECULAR PROPERTIES

As is the case with many hormones and growth factors, an understanding of the functional properties of NGF developed before its detailed molecular characterization. Not surprisingly, this characterization required the identification of a relatively rich source of material. As is evident from the examples of fibroblast growth factor and colony-stimulating factors, characterization proceeds at a very slow rate without such a source (3). The observations that brought about the identification of the submaxillary gland of adult male mice as a rich source of NGF were made by Dr. Stanley Cohen while attempting to purify the factor from sarcoma. In these studies, he used snake venom as a source of phosphodiesterase and discovered that the venom was a far richer source of NGF than the tumor (4). Considering the relationship between the venom-producing gland and the salivary glands of higher vertebrates, he subsequently identified the mouse source (5). With the exception of the tumors, whose production of NGF may reflect a normal process of the tissues from which they are derived, the other sources do not appear at this time to be related to the endocrine functions of NGF in the peripheral nervous system. This is also true of another newly identified source of the factor, the prostate gland of some, but certainly not all, higher vertebrates (6). Nonetheless, there has been a basic assumption, particularly with the mouse submaxillary gland protein, that these proteins are identical in all functional and structural respects with the material produced for interaction with peripheral neurons. In the absence of compelling evidence to the contrary, this is a reasonable hypothesis.

The mouse submaxillary gland protein is synthesized as, and is exported in, a complex containing three unique polypeptide chains (7). These were designated by Varon et al. (8) as α, β, and γ, and the aggregate is known as 7S NGF (representing its sedimentation coefficient). This complex is associated by noncovalent interactions between the three types of polypeptide chains and under certain conditions readily dissociates to its constituent parts. However, under other conditions, the complex is extremely tightly associated, retaining its identity at concentrations below those required for biological activity (9). A key element in the stability of the 7S complex appears to be the 2 gram atoms of zinc that are bound to one or more of the polypeptide subunits (10). Because zinc can inhibit the enzymatic activity of the γ subunit, it is generally held to be associated with the γ subunit in the complex (11). However, this has never been established rigorously and may be a coincidental observation. The complex is assembled from two α chains, two γ chains, and a β dimer, the latter itself containing two chains (12). The complex is a hexamer with at least one twofold axis of symmetry (13). Both the α and the γ chains interact principally with the β subunit, although they appear to derive further stability from interactions with each other when they are complexed with the β dimer (14). Interactions of the γ subunits with the β dimer appear to occur at least in part with the C-terminal arginine residue of the β chain, since its removal prevents the γ–β interaction (15). However, it is likely that interactions between other residues in both polypeptides occur as well. Little is known about the nature of the interactions of the α subunits with the β chains.

The β subunit (βNGF) can be isolated either from the homogeneous 7S complex or directly from gland homogenates (16). The latter preparation, called 2.5S NGF, is distinguished from βNGF in that limited proteolysis has occurred at both the amino and carboxyl termini (9). However, neither modification influences biological and immunological activity. It was this 2.5S form of the hormone that was used for the sequence analysis by Angeletti and Bradshaw (17). These studies showed that the amino acid sequence of the longest constituent chain is 118 residues (Fig. 1). The chain contains three disulfide bonds, which are all intrachain (18); thus the dimer, which is composed of two of these units, is associated by noncovalent forces. The larger chain can be converted to a shorter chain by the removal of the N-terminal octapeptide, which can occur during the preparation of 2.5S NGF. A kallikrein-like enzyme in the submaxillary gland effects this modification by cleaving the peptide bond joining histidine-8 to methionine-9 (19). The octapeptide itself has not yet been shown to possess any biological activity, although the highly specific manner in which it is produced suggests that a role may eventually be found (19,20). The second proteolytic modification occurring in 2.5S preparations is the removal of the C-terminal arginine,

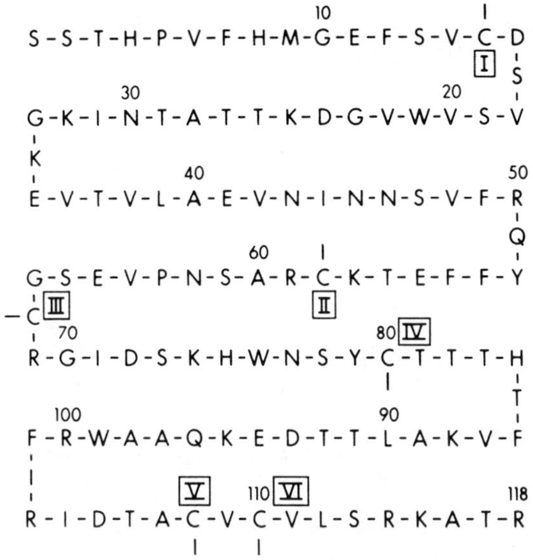

S - S - T - H - P - V - F - H - M - G - E - F - S - V - C - D
                                                        I   S
G - K - I - N - T - A - T - T - K - D - G - V - W - V - S - V
K
E - V - T - V - L - A - E - V - N - I - N - N - S - V - F - R
                                                            Q
G - S - E - V - P - N - S - A - R - C - K - T - E - F - F - Y
- C III   II
R - G - I - D - S - K - H - W - N - S - Y - C - T - T - T - H
                                          IV   T
F - R - W - A - A - Q - K - E - D - T - T - L - A - K - V - F
                    V   VI
R - I - D - T - A - C - V - C - V - L - S - R - K - A - T - R

Figure 1. Sequence of the 2.5S form of NGF.

presumably by the action of a carboxypeptidase-B-like enzyme, and this, as noted above, eliminates γ interactions (14,15).

The γ subunit was originally identified by Greene et al. (21) as an arginine-specific esteropeptidase that shows little activity toward peptide or ester substrates formed by other amino acids including lysine. Silverman (14) demonstrated that this protein is a member of the serine protease family based on diisopropylfluorophosphate (DFP) inhibition and preliminary sequence analysis. The elucidation of the complete structure of the γ subunit by Thomas et al. (22) has confirmed this conclusion. This subunit also undergoes proteolytic modification and is isolated in two principal forms containing two and three polypeptide fragments, respectively. Both forms of the enzyme contain the B1 fragment, which is the N-terminal 82 residues joined by disulfide linkage to the second fragment, designated A. This latter segment comprises the C-terminal two thirds of the molecule. In the γ form containing three polypeptide chains, the A fragment is further cleaved to C and B2 fragments, which contain, respectively, 53 and 98 residues. They are also joined by disulfide bonds. The sequence of the γ chain, given as B1 and A chains, is shown in Fig. 2. The B1 fragment contains one carbohydrate unit N-linked to asparagine-78. The carbohydrate unit is composed solely of mannose and N-acetylglucosamine residues (22). As expected for an enzyme that is a member of the serine protease class, it shows a considerable

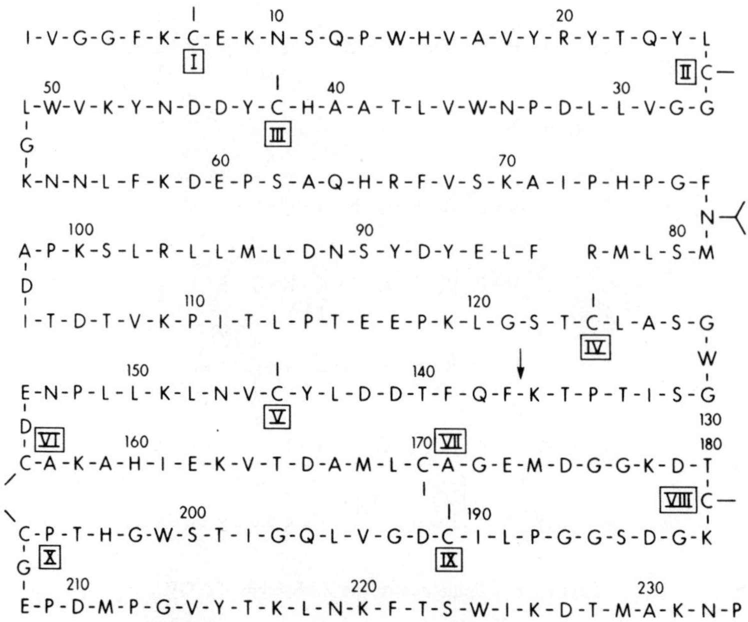

```
                         |         10                                    20
        I - V - G - G - F - K - C - E - K - N - S - Q - P - W - H - V - A - V - Y - R - Y - T - Q - Y - L
                             [I]                                                              [II] C —
          50                              |         40                            30
        L - W - V - K - Y - N - D - D - Y - C - H - A - A - T - L - V - W - N - P - D - L - L - V - G - G
        G                                      [III]
          K - N - N - L - F - K - D - E - P - S - A - Q - H - R - F - V - S - K - A - I - P - H - P - G - F
                    100                                   90                           80   N —<
        A - P - K - S - L - R - L - L - M - L - D - N - S - Y - D - Y - E - L - F       R - M - L - S - M
        D
          110                                  120                  |
        I - T - D - T - V - K - P - I - T - L - P - T - E - E - P - K - L - G - S - T - C - L - A - S - G
                    150                           |        140          ↓              [IV]
                                                                                             W
        E - N - P - L - L - K - L - N - V - C - Y - L - D - D - T - F - Q - F - K - T - P - T - I - S - G
        D [VI]       160                    [V]         170 [VII]                    130
          C - A - K - A - H - I - E - K - V - T - D - A - M - L - C - A - G - E - M - D - G - G - K - D - T  180
                                                              |  190                       [VIII] C —
                    200                                                             190
        C - P - T - H - G - W - S - T - I - G - Q - L - V - G - D - C - I - L - P - G - G - S - D - G - K
        G [IX]                                             [IX]
          210                                  220                                   230
        E - P - D - M - P - G - V - Y - T - K - L - N - K - F - T - S - W - I - K - D - T - M - A - K - N - P
```

Figure 2. Sequence of the γ subunit of 7S NGF.

degree of homology to trypsin, chymotrypsin, thrombin, and so forth. The degree of identity ranges from 41% for bovine trypsin to about 28% for porcine elastase, values that are quite similar to those found with comparisons of other serine proteases. The γ subunit is the first murine serine protease to be sequenced.

Considerably less information is available about the α subunit, the only part of the 7S complex that has not been characterized in great detail. There is also no proven biological activity for this subunit other than the suggestion that it acts to protect the β molecule during incubations with responsive tissues (9). As do the other two subunits, it also undergoes proteolytic modification, producing two principal fragments of 10,000 and 16,000 molecular weight that are joined by one or more disulfide bonds. The sequence analysis of this entity may help to resolve its functionality.

The principal subunit of the 7S complex, with respect to biological activity, is the β subunit. It contains all of the nerve-growth-promoting activity with responsive neurons. The dimeric unit is apparently responsible for these activities since the association of the two constituent polypeptides is extremely tight, with an association constant in the order of $10^{-10} - 10^{-11} M$ (23). This value has been challenged by Young and his colleagues, who concluded that it was about $10^{-7} M$ (24).

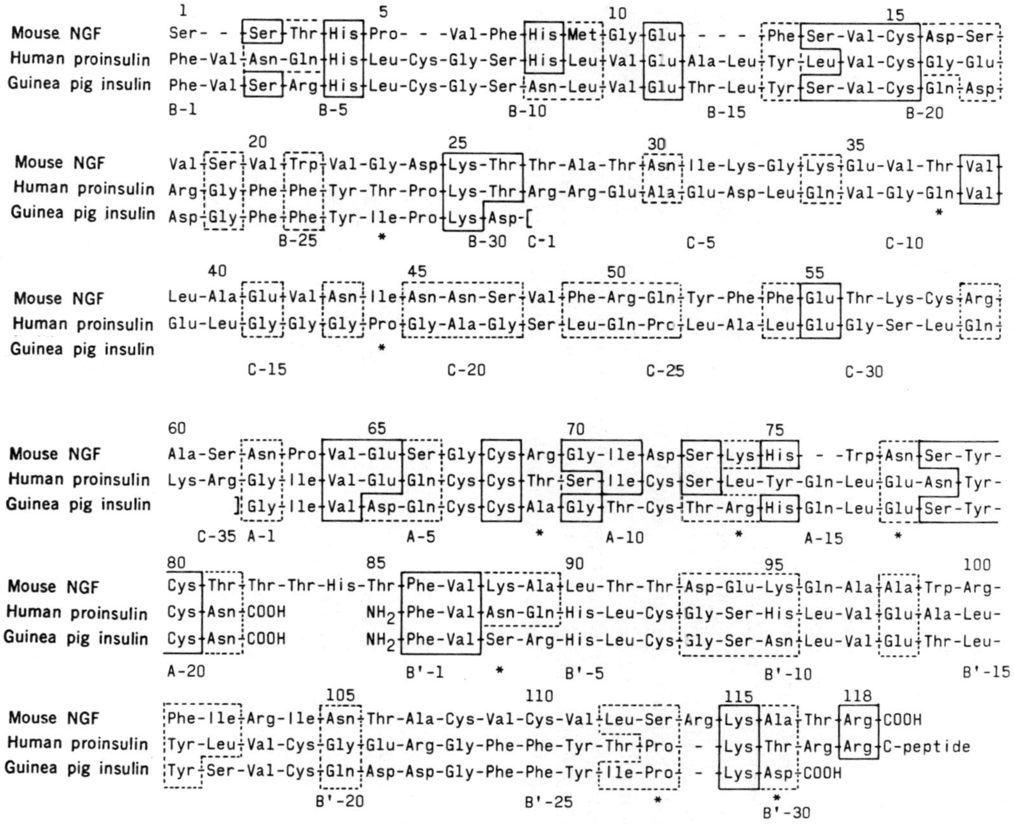

Mouse NGF
Human proinsulin
Guinea pig insulin

```
          1           5                10              15
Mouse NGF           Ser- - -Ser-Thr-His-Pro- - - -Val-Phe-His-Met-Gly-Glu- - - -Phe-Ser-Val-Cys-Asp-Ser
Human proinsulin    Phe-Val-Asn-Gln-His-Leu-Cys-Gly-Ser-His-Leu-Val-Glu-Ala-Leu-Tyr-Leu-Val-Cys-Gly-Glu-
Guinea pig insulin  Phe-Val-Arg-His-Leu-Cys-Gly-Ser-Asn-Leu-Val-Glu-Thr-Leu-Tyr-Leu-Tyr-Ser-Val-Cys-Gln-Asp-
                    B-1       B-5           B-10            B-15        B-20
```

```
          20            25              30              35
Mouse NGF           Val-Ser-Val-Gly-Asp-Lys-Thr-Thr-Ala-Thr-Asn-Ile-Lys-Gly-Lys-Glu-Val-Thr-Val
Human proinsulin    Arg-Gly-Phe-Phe-Tyr-Thr-Pro-Lys-Thr-Arg-Arg-Glu-Ala-Glu-Asp-Leu-Gln-Val-Gly-Gln-Val
Guinea pig insulin  Asp-Gly-Phe-Phe-Tyr-Ile-Pro-Lys-Asp-
                    B-25      B-30  C-1     C-5             C-10
                                                            *
```

```
          40            45              50              55
Mouse NGF           Leu-Ala-Glu-Val-Asn-Ile-Asn-Asn-Ser-Val-Phe-Arg-Gln-Tyr-Phe-Phe-Glu-Thr-Lys-Cys-Arg
Human proinsulin    Glu-Leu-Gly-Gly-Gly-Pro-Gly-Ala-Gly-Ser-Leu-Gln-Pro-Leu-Ala-Leu-Glu-Gly-Ser-Leu-Gln
Guinea pig insulin
                    C-15      C-20            C-25            C-30
                              *
```

```
          60            65              70              75
Mouse NGF           Ala-Ser-Asn-Pro-Val-Glu-Ser-Gly-Cys-Arg-Gly-Ile-Asp-Ser-Lys-His- - -Trp-Asn-Ser-Tyr-
Human proinsulin    Lys-Arg-Gly-Ile-Val-Glu-Gln-Cys-Cys-Thr-Ser-Ile-Cys-Ser-Leu-Tyr-Gln-Leu-Glu-Asn-Tyr-
Guinea pig insulin  Gly-Ile-Val-Asp-Gln-Cys-Cys-Thr-Gly-Thr-Cys-Thr-Arg-His-Gln-Leu-Glu-Ser-Leu-Tyr-
                    C-35 A-1      A-5             A-10            A-15
                              *                   *               *
```

```
          80            85              90              95             100
Mouse NGF           Cys-Thr-Thr-Thr-His-Thr-Phe-Val-Lys-Ala-Leu-Thr-Thr-Asp-Glu-Lys-Gln-Ala-Ala-Trp-Arg-
Human proinsulin    Cys-Asn-COOH          NH2-Phe-Val-Asn-Gln-His-Leu-Cys-Gly-Ser-His-Leu-Val-Glu-Ala-Leu-
Guinea pig insulin  Cys-Asn-COOH          NH2-Phe-Val-Ser-Arg-His-Leu-Cys-Gly-Ser-Asn-Leu-Val-Glu-Thr-Leu-
                    A-20     B'-1     B'-5            B'-10           B'-15
                                       *                *               *
```

```
          105           110             115             118
Mouse NGF           Phe-Ile-Arg-Ile-Asp-Thr-Ala-Cys-Val-Cys-Val-Leu-Ser-Arg-Lys-Ala-Thr-Arg-COOH
Human proinsulin    Tyr-Leu-Val-Cys-Gly-Glu-Arg-Gly-Phe-Phe-Tyr-Thr-Pro- -Lys-Thr-Arg-Arg-C-peptide
Guinea pig insulin  Tyr-Ser-Val-Cys-Gln-Asp-Asp-Gly-Phe-Phe-Tyr-Ile-Pro- -Lys-Asp-COOH
                    B'-20     B'-25           B'-30
                                              *
```

Figure 3. The evolutionary relationship between NGF and insulin.

Upon completion of the sequence analysis, Frazier et al. (25) observed that elements of the primary structure of the β subunit showed statistically significant relatedness to the hormone insulin (proinsulin). Although this proposal has not been without its detractors, it has proved to be a singularly important milestone in the development of research on the function and mechanism of NGF. To wit, it directed attention to the concept that NGF should be considered as a hormone or hormone-like substance in its interaction with target tissues. As will be described, this has certainly proved to be the case.

The original comparison demonstrating an evolutionary relationship between NGF and insulin is shown in Fig. 3. Although some aspects of the comparison are now only superficially important, such as the analysis of conservative replacements and the supposition that the carboxy-terminal extension of NGF represents a gene duplication (*vide infra*), several facets still remain important. First, significant homology exists in sections of the NGF sequence that correspond to the A and B chains of the proinsulin molecule. Second, these clusters of identities are spaced by a segment that corresponds in length to the C bridge that is removed in the conversion of proinsulin to insulin. Third, one of the three disulfide bonds found in both molecules is conserved in exactly the same alignment, allowing for at least

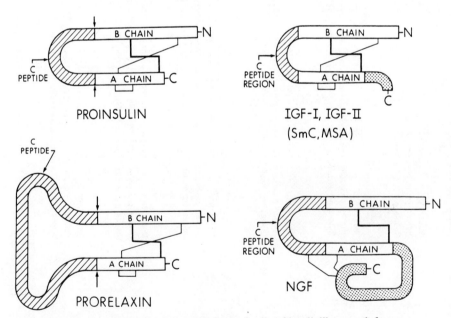

Figure 4.   Structural relationships in the family of insulinlike growth factors.

the surrounding portions of the protein to share three-dimensional homology as well. Although the crystal structure determination of NGF, which is in progress (26,27), may provide further insight into the evolutionary relatedness of these two molecules, additional support has already been provided by the finding that other proteins, such as the insulin-like growth factors (IGF) I and II and relaxin (3,28), are related to this family. In particular, the relaxin molecule, which like insulin is processed to a two-chain structure, contains the same significant extent of homology to insulin in the A- and B-chain regions as is found in NGF. However, the similarity of relaxin to the pancreatic hormone is greatly enhanced by the complete conservation of the disulfide-bonding pattern. On the other hand, NGF is not related either to IGF I, IGF II, or relaxin more than it is to insulin. As shown in Fig. 4, which illustrates the relationship of all five of these substances schematically, NGF appears to be the most altered form of this subset if insulin is taken to be the "parent." These changes almost certainly reflect the alterations accompanying the evolution of the new function represented by the present-day form.

3. BIOSYNTHESIS

The 7S NGF complex represents the principal and probably the only form of the hormone stored in the mouse submaxillary gland. Furthermore, it appears to be the predominant form exuded into the saliva, a phenomenon apparently regulated by α-adrenergic substances (29). However, some processing in the form of limited proteolysis of at least two, and probably all three, of the constituent polypeptide chains from precursor molecules is required for complex formation. Detailed description of these precursors, the processing events, and the sequence in which they occur are not yet available. However, the information that has been determined has provided considerable insight into the main features of the pathway.

Not surprisingly, the molecular properties of the immediate precursor to the β subunit are best understood. Berger and Shooter (30) have demonstrated that a polypeptide chain of about 22,000 molecular weight (22K), recognized by antibodies directed against the β subunit, is made by adult male mouse submaxillary glands. This material can be converted to a 13,000 molecular weight entity by the γ subunit of 7S NGF as well as by trypsin and the arginine esteropeptidase associated with epidermal growth factor (EGF). Experiments utilizing [^{35}S]cystine incorporation either *in vivo* or *in vitro* demonstrated that all of the tryptic peptides found in the 13,000 molecular weight entity of the β subunit are present in the 22K species. Although these data clearly demonstrate the existence of pro-NGF species, they still leave unanswered the important question of whether or not the 22K precursor is the sole high molecular weight form containing the βNGF sequence. In this regard, the synthesis of a 46,000 molecular weight precursor to NGF by a cell-free system derived from rat glioma C6 cells has been reported, but this material was characterized only by immunological means, and the identification must be viewed as preliminary (31).

There are other important questions that also require clarification. Is the 22K molecule biologically active or is the conversion to the 13,000 molecular weight form a prerequisite for activation? What is the nature of the 9000 molecular weight unit removed? Is the removal accomplished by a single cleavage? Does it occur solely at the carboxyl terminus or are both termini involved? And finally, is the γ subunit the only enzyme necessary (if it is used at all), and if so, why is the process apparently not specific for it? The resolution of most of these questions awaits the isolation and translation of the appropriate mRNA. To date, this has proved to be a difficult task, perhaps because of its lability or low concentration.

Similar studies with EGF, also synthesized in the adult male mouse submaxillary gland, have proved equally challenging. Frey et al. (32) have demonstrated a precursor (9000 molecular weight; 9K) that is converted to the 6000 molecular weight active peptide by the binding protein that is analogous to the γ subunit of NGF. In this case, the processing appears to be specific and is accomplished solely at the carboxyl end. By implication, these results suggest a similar role for the γ subunit.

It is possible that βNGF and EGF are synthesized as part of a single precursor polypeptide. This idea is supported by the observation that parallel synthesis of NGF and EGF, in terms of amount, occurs in the guinea pig prostate as well as the mouse submaxillary gland (33). Further, the unidentified 9K unit in the NGF precursor, removed by a proteolytic event, is the correct molecular size to accommodate the pro-EGF molecule. Despite the many attractive features of such a model, it is at present only one possibility.

Preliminary evidence for the presence of a precursor species for the α subunit of 7S NGF has also been obtained (P. Isackson and R. A. Bradshaw, unpublished observation). The molecular weight of this species, determined from cell-free synthesis experiments with mouse submaxillary gland mRNA, has been tentatively identified as 35,000–40,000. Its conversion to the 26,000 molecular weight form has not yet been studied. In a similar fashion, a precursor of the γ subunit of approximately 31,000 molecular weight has also been tentatively identified. It probably represents a zymogen form of this serine protease. If this is correct, then there must be at least one other enzyme involved in the formation of 7S NGF, namely the enzyme required to activate the γ subunit. The α subunit could be processed by the same enzyme, by the activated γ subunit, or by another, as yet unidentified, enzyme. It is also unclear whether the α and γ subunits can bind to the 22K (or larger) βNGF precursor or only associate with the mature form (13K). Although it seems probable that this binding occurs only after the α and γ subunits are processed, this also remains to be established.

The question why such a cascade of events is necessary for the preparation of the 7S complex is also intriguing. The formation of 7S NGF may be part of the processing of a larger species to yield other hormones or growth factors (such as EGF), a species analogous to the 31K precursor, synthesized in the pituitary, that yields such hormones as adrenocorticotropic hormone (ACTH), melanocyte-stimulating hormone (MSH), β-lipotropin, and so forth (34). However, if this is the case, it is uncertain why the γ subunit (or the EGF arginine esteropeptidase) is required in stoichiometric amounts as a processing enzyme. There is no compelling evidence that either the α or the γ subunit has any material effect on the hormonal action of βNGF on responsive neurons, and 7S NGF itself has been shown to be biologically inactive. It may also be that the elaborate pathway for the production of 7S NGF is related to an exocrine role, since the 7S has only been well characterized in the submaxillary gland. However, a subunit containing arginine esteropeptidase activity has not been found associated with guinea pig prostate NGF, a finding that further confounds the role of the γ subunit in the biosynthetic process (35). The final resolution of this important question will require definitive characterization of the NGF produced by tissues that prepare the hormone for delivery to the peripheral neuron targets.

4. RELATIONSHIP OF NGF TO OTHER ENDOCRINE SUBSTANCES

4.1. Polypeptide Growth Factors

As the name suggests, the hormone-like polypeptide growth factors regulate the phenomena of growth, that is, the increase in cell number (hyperplastic effects) and/or cell size (hypertrophic effects). Most elicit both effects on their respective target cells. In terms of development and survival of the organism, these cellular events underlie the processes of normal growth, as well as regeneration following traumatic injury, and the routine turnover of cells that characterizes tissues after development is complete (3). One activity, not normally thought of as a growth process, that is particularly germane to NGF, is the maintenance of viability. Some cells require, even in the mature state, a constant supply of hormone, the interruption of which can result in severe damage and even death. In embryonic cells, this situation can be far more acute. Since the molecular basis for such activity is difficult to distinguish from that involved in the other growth-related events, it is convenient to consider them together.

The role of NGF as a survival or maintenance factor appears to substitute for any hyperplastic activity. Despite earlier reports to the contrary, it now seems clear that all cells of the peripheral nervous system responsive to NGF are postmitotic and do not divide under the influence of NGF or anything else (36). It is important to realize, however, that the lack of mitogenic activity of NGF on peripheral neurons is not a distinguishing feature of the factor, but rather of the cells themselves. In most other respects, the behavior of the hormone (*vide infra*) resembles that of the other members of this family, particularly those of the insulin-related subset (3). Thus there is no apparent reason why NGF should be viewed any differently because of its lack of mitogenic activity than the other hormones of this type.

4.2.   The Secondary Hormones

The larger group in which NGF can be classed includes other protein growth factors and several "classical" polypeptide hormones (3). This grouping is based on overall functional similarities that clearly distinguish the secondary hormones from other polypeptide messengers by a number of criteria. This subdivision, which was suggested by Robison et al. (37), is based primarily on the observation that some hormones directly stimulate membrane-bound adenyl cyclase through complexation with a receptor entity, and others do not. The resulting production of intracellular cyclic adenosine monophosphate (cAMP) by the one group stimulates the remainder of the cellular apparatuses to yield the various hormonal effects. These responses are rather rapid and are generally proportional to the amount of time the receptor is occupied by the hormone. The other group, which includes growth factors, is not so easily described. Of those for which cell-surface receptors exist (mainly polypeptides), most show a variety of rapid responses following complex formation that are only, at best, transiently related to the production of cAMP. Changes in membrane permeability are common. Of equal importance, these substances also produce several long-term effects that seem to be generally manifested by modulation of the protein-synthesis machinery. These occur at either the transcriptional or the translational level (or in between) and result in the amplification or deamplification of the expression of specific genes. It is these long-term or secondary effects (hence the name *secondary hormones*) that clearly distinguish the members of this group from the cAMP-dependent hormones. It is important to note that no classification that encompasses such a broad range of substances can possibly be inclusive. Therefore, it is not surprising, as anticipated by

Robison et al. (37), that there are clear exceptions to this classification scheme. However, these exceptions do not detract from the main purpose of this organization, which is to emphasize the similarities between growth factors and some of the classical hormones.

Although such a diverse group of substances will certainly not have a single mechanism of action, several functional features of different members of the group, as they have been elucidated, have often been found to be instructive with respect to others. The observation that NGF is internalized and transported to cell bodies by retrograde axonal transport, which provided one of the earliest clues that receptor-mediated endocytosis might be a common event resulting from the interaction of secondary hormones with their target cells, illustrates the point. It may be anticipated that other mechanistic features will have some commonality as well.

5.   NEURAL CREST CELL DEVELOPMENT AND THE ROLE OF NGF

5.1.   NGF Effects on the Survival of Sensory and Sympathetic Neurons

Over the past several years it has become apparent that the specific nature and extent of the NGF responsiveness and dependency for survival vary among neural crest derivatives. Sympathetic neurons respond to NGF from midgestation through life. They appear to require NGF for survival continuously from midgestation until at least the late neonatal period (38); thereafter, short-term NGF deprivation, although impairing neuronal function, does not cause cell death (39). In spite of this apparently decreased need for NGF, the finding that NGF can prevent synaptic depression subsequent to axotomy of adult sympathetic neurons (40) supports the concept that sympathetic neurons require NGF throughout life. Sensory neurons overtly seem to require NGF for only a limited period of time during embryologic development (41). However, this conclusion is tentative since adult sensory neurons still bind and transport NGF (42). In contrast, adrenal medullary chromaffin cells, although modestly responsive to NGF (43), have not been shown to have an absolute requirement for it at any time during ontogenic development or thereafter (44). In the following section the data that support an essential role for NGF in sympathetic and sensory neuron development from the primitive neural crest cells are discussed. Emphasis has been placed on the sympathetic nervous system, since much more is known about the events occurring during autonomic neuron development and the numerous factors that modulate this process. NGF is considered a potential participant in the currently recognized processes effecting sympathetic neuron maturation.

5.2.   Modulating Factors Acting on Sympathetic Neuron Development

The neural crest is a transient embryonic structure that arises in a junctional zone between the neuroectoderm of the neural plate and the ectoderm that makes up the remainder of the embryonic disc. As the neural folds meet and fuse to form the neural tube, the neural crest cells may be seen in the angle between the dorsal wall of the neural tube and the surface ectoderm. From a dorsolateral and symmetrical position, these clusters of primitive cells of the neural crest begin migration and differentiation into diverse populations of cell types. There are two major migratory routes of the neural crest cells: dorsolaterally into the epithelial area or ventrally into the mesenchyme. Cells taking the former path may disperse as melanocytes, whereas those taking the latter route become segmentally oriented and develop into a variety of neural crest derivatives, including postganglionic neurons comprising the sympathetic ganglia, sensory neurons of dorsal root ganglia, and adrenal medullary chromaffin cells. Mesenchymal derivatives of the cephalic region are also derived from precursors in the neural crest. Although the relative times for accomplishing these migratory and differentiative events vary, the patterns are similar in most animal species. For example, in the chick embryo the earliest time of recognition of specific sympathetic ganglia is 3.5 days, whereas in the rat, rabbit, and mouse the comparable recognition interval is approximately 13 days. Establishment of adult levels of sympathetic innervation is not complete by birth, and anatomic and functional maturation continues for various times into the neonatal period for each species.

There are numerous factors that influence the course and success of the development of the precursor neural crest cells. Although only partially understood, they have been the subject of several excellent reviews (38,45,46). The recognized modulators of sympathetic neuron development include (1) premigratory *programming*, (2) the *cellular environment* during migration and that of the axial level at which differentiation proceeds, (3) *support cells* within ganglia and associated with neuronal axons, (4) *anterograde transsynaptic communications* in ganglia, and, more remotely, the higher CNS influences, (5) the influences of the *peripheral target* itself, and (6) *humoral influences* such as thyroxine and glucocorticoids. The demonstration that NGF may participate in several of these currently recognized general control mechanisms will serve to dramatize the potential for multiple and strategic influences of the hormone and provide some perspective for its place in sympathetic neuron development.

5.3.   Possible Roles of NGF in Sympathetic Neuron Development

There is very little evidence to suggest that NGF is involved in the earliest neural crest activities that program cells for future development.

This process occurs prior to cell migration into the dorsal and ventral planes. There is, however, some evidence that the peptide contributes as an *environmental factor* during migration to the survival of the early differentiated adrenergic neuron. Norr (47) has shown that the ventral neural tube interacts with adjacent mesenchyme through which migration occurs and that this interaction endows mesenchyme with the capacity to induce neural crest differentiation into early sympathoblasts. It has also been shown that the ventral neural tube promotes cell survival after differentiation. In the same report (47) it was also shown that NGF can replace this survival function of the ventral neural tube, which can be taken as evidence that NGF influences events during the migration period prior to ganglion formation. Bjerre and Bjorklund (48) noted that NGF increases, and anti-NGF serum decreases, the catecholamine content, which is a marker of differentiation or survival, in explants of cranial neural tissue from early chick embryos. These observations suggest that NGF may function in early neuronal development.

The importance of NGF in adrenergic neuronal survival and differentiation increases, or at least becomes progressively easier to demonstrate, as embryonic development continues (49). Levi-Montalcini and Hamburger (2) noted that chick sympathetic ganglia respond to NGF-producing tumors only after the seventh day *in ovo*. The critical work of Coughlin et al. (50), using superior cervial ganglia (SCG) from embryonic mice, indicated that whereas such ganglia are responsive to NGF at days 13–15, the NGF requirement for survival does not become manifest until day 18. The authors suggested that although it appears that the sympathetic neurons of the SCG acquire NGF dependence, there are other possible explanations for the data. Since antibodies against NGF were employed to define NGF-dependent processes (i.e., the induction of tyrosine hydroxylase (TH) activity), one of the alternate explanations is that support cells within the SCG may be capable of providing NGF to neurons directly and in a manner that may preclude interference by anti-NGF early (day 13) in development, but not at the later time (day 18).

The participation by *non-neuronal support cells* in the development and survival of adrenergic neurons as well as the survival of sensory neurons is supported by the following observations: (1) survival in culture of adrenergic and sensory neurons (51) increases progressively as increasing numbers of non-neuronal cells are supplied, (2) ganglionic non-neurons allow full NGF effects at a 1000-fold lower NGF concentration than do control mesenchymal cells, and (3) the survival-promoting (NGF-like) effects of ganglion support cells are not observed with heterologous support cells such as fibroblasts (52). Although the ganglionic populations of non-neuronal cells have NGF-like effects, the effects of exogenous NGF are certainly not synonymous with those of non-neurons. In this regard it has been observed that non-neuronal sympathetic ganglion cells do not display an NGF-like effect upon sensory neurons, but do so when cocultured with their own homologous neurons. To what extent, then, if any, do the neurotrophic influences of support cells involve or depend upon NGF? Varon et al. (53) provided evidence that NGF is responsible in part for the effects of homologous glial cells on embryonic sensory neurons by showing that antibodies to βNGF depress attachment and survival of sensory neurons in culture when neuronal support is exclusively provided by ganglionic glia. Additional circumstantial support is provided by the observation that glial cells can produce an NGF-like protein (54,55). Such a model has considerable mechanistic appeal since the maturing neuron would be provided with a source of NGF prior to and during the period of establishment of communication of terminal neurons with their peripheral target tissues.

Within the past 10 years it has become clear that NGF is present in at least minute amounts in many tissues. This has led to the general concept that functionally important NGF is derived from the non-neuronal support cells in ganglia and/or from cells in the *peripheral field of innervation* (45,50). These latter cells represent another major factor modulating adrenergic neuron development in which NGF may be involved. During normal development in the rat, adrenergic innervation is present in various organs at 19–21 days of gestation, but adult levels of endogenous norepinephrine are not reached until the third to the fifth postnatal week. The reduction of neurons in the autonomic ganglia that normally occurs in late development is determined in part by the peripheral field, since removal of the target leads to an increase in the proportion of neurons that die during the neonatal period of development (56). In contrast with the effects of limiting the field of innervation, expansion results in less cell death (57). Indeed, the original experiments of Bueker (1) with a mouse sarcoma tumor were carried out to assess the influences of an expanded peripheral field on embryonic neurons in the process of establishing contact with the periphery; that NGF is the humoral mediator of neuronal hypertrophy and survival was the critical observation that resulted.

Results of axotomy experiments also indicate that a peripheral source of NGF may be important in regulating these events. If surgical transection of postganglionic nerve fibers is performed during the postnatal development period, adrenergic neuronal death occurs; if NGF is administered, the destructive effects of axotomy are prevented (58). Similarly, if the end organ of sympathetic innervation is removed during the neonatal period, the subsequent neuronal death can be prevented by supplying a local source of NGF (59).

Our understanding of the role of the periphery and the relationship of NGF to target-organ-mediated effects upon neuronal survival was materially improved by the demonstration of axonal transport of NGF by Hendry et al. (60) in 1974. Radiolabeled NGF injected into the anterior chamber of the eye is taken up by adrenergic nerve terminals in the iris and transported intact to the cell bodies in the ipsilateral superior cervical ganglion. In neonatal animals, conditions that interfere with the process of retrograde transport of NGF result in cell death; survival can be maintained if NGF is provided (61,62). In this regard, it has been proposed (63) that some neurotoxic drugs as well as anti-NGF antibodies and axonal ligation are neuropathic because they deprive the cell body of NGF located in the peripheral field.

There is some direct evidence supporting the concept that NGF located in the region of the distal neurite has a preferential significance for neuronal growth. Campenot (64) has cultured dissociated sympathetic neurons of the newborn rat in a multichamber vessel in which the soma and the distal neurites were separated by fluid-impermeable barriers. Extension of neurites into the distal compartment required the presence of NGF in both somal and distal compartments. Subsequent removal of NGF from the chamber occupied by the soma had no effect upon survival of the soma or the distal neurite. In contrast, removal of NGF from the distal compartment caused eventual degeneration of the corresponding neurite. This study provides evidence for the role of NGF in the periphery as a *tropic* agent, since neurite growth from the soma chamber into the distal chamber occurred only into those chambers containing NGF. It is important to note that the somata of neurons deprived only of distal NGF did not die when their distal neurites degenerated. Since surgical (58), chemical (62,63), or immunological (65,66) methods for removing peripheral NGF in the intact neonate animal leads to neuronal loss, it is reasonable to infer that in the neonatal stage of development, the major source of NGF is in the periphery, that is, from the target organ or from Schwann cells along the axon rather than from the region of the soma. This inference is consistent with the concept that glial sources of NGF may be essential for neuron survival during ganglion formation and that such proximal sources are replaced by peripheral sources during and after the period of innervation of the periphery.

In contrast with the case of the other influences on the development of neural crest cells, there is no evidence for the involvement of NGF in anterograde transsynaptic effects. These result from the interaction of the preganglionic neurons from the spinal cord on the neuronal cell bodies in adrenergic ganglia. Transection of the preganglionic cholinergic trunk in neonatal mice or rats prevents the normal postnatal sixfold–10-fold increase in postsynaptic TH activity. Whether the failure of the TH activity to rise is due to cell death or to loss of a positive modulating factor is uncertain. In either case, NGF cannot prevent or reverse this effect (67). Also, NGF exerts its effects on decentralized ganglia, and anti-NGF action does not

Table 1.   Major Factors Regulating Adrenergic Neuron Ontogeny and the Probability of NGF Participation

FACTOR	NGF PARTICIPATION
Premigratory programming	Unknown
Cellular environment during transit from neural crest	Possible
Support cells (glia, satellite)	Likely
Peripheral target tissue	Likely
Anterograde transsynaptic regulation	No

require intact preganglionic innervation (68). Thus anterograde transsynaptic regulation appears to be quite independent of NGF.

The major factors influencing adrenergic neuron development and the possible involvement of NGF are summarized in Table 1. From these observations one can formulate a scheme of neuronal development and NGF participation as follows. The role of NGF in early development before ganglion formation is uncertain. After formation of the ganglion, NGF, which may be present in the support cells, acts by limiting the number of neurons that die as well as by serving as a stimulator of anabolic activity. In this way NGF may ensure the survival of required neurons, promote neurite extension by immature ganglion cells, and regulate the synthesis of key enzymes required for neurotransmitter synthesis. Peripheral NGF reaching the cell body by retrograde transport performs similar functions during the critical neonatal period and after maturation. Although the dependence upon NGF of sympathetic neurons in adult animals markedly diminishes, the sum of experimental data indicates that NGF continues to be important for sympathetic neuron function. The retrograde transport of the peptide from the periphery to the cell body is a lifelong characteristic of both sympathetic and sensory neurons even though the latter have thus far not displayed a need for NGF for survival in the adult animal.

6.   MOLECULAR BASIS OF THE NGF RESPONSE

The intense research efforts into the role of NGF in the development of selected neural crest derivatives have been matched by equally aggressive efforts to determine how NGF functions to produce its multiplicity of cellular and subcellular effects, which ultimately participate in processes of neural survival, growth, and differentiation. The specific mechanism by which

Table 2.   Physiological Influences of NGF

Morphological
    Neurite proliferation
    Cytoskeletal polymerization
    Organelle augmentation
    Nuclear-membrane alterations
General trophic
    Metabolic-precursor uptake
    Maintenance of anabolic activity
Specific anabolic
    Tyrosine hydroxylase synthesis
    Dopamine-β-hydroxylase synthesis
    Ornithine decarboxylase synthesis
Neurotropic
    Directional orientation for growth
Cell surface
    Cell–cell, cell–substratum adhesion
    Surface-glycoprotein alterations

NGF may induce selected physiological events, such as the production of enzymes that regulate neurite outgrowth and the synthesis of neurotransmitters, is overshadowed by the more general question of whether NGF acts at one locus in the cell to trigger a set of cascading, coordinated metabolic events leading ultimately to these functional expressions. It is equally possible that NGF interacts with the cell at more than one location to stimulate location-specific cellular responses. In the following sections the variety of physiological consequences attending exposure to NGF (Table 2) are described, and the progress toward defining their molecular mechanisms outlined.

6.1.   Physiological Responses to NGF

The physiological effects of NGF have been extensively reviewed (36,69) and are therefore summarized here only as a prerequisite for mechanistic considerations. These effects can be categorized for purposes of discussion as morphological, general trophic, selected anabolic, tropic, and cell-surface effects.

The initial appreciation of the striking morphological effects of NGF was actually the basis for the discovery and subsequent isolation of the hormone. Based on the augmentation of local neurite production observed by Bueker (1) in transplantation experiments of mouse sarcoma tumors into chick embryos, the humoral factor promoting nerve growth was sought and defined (2,65,70). The transfer of the growth factor to an *in vitro* culture using chick embryo ganglia provided the basis for the bioassay still used today (71). When sensory or sympathetic ganglia from 8–12-day chick embryos are placed in an *in vitro* culture system, NGF is required to maintain neuron viability beyond 6 hours. In the presence of increasing amounts of NGF in concentrations of 0.1–10 ng/ml, neurite outgrowth in a radial fashion occurs in a dose-related fashion. The extent of outgrowth is usually graded on a relative scale of 1 to 4. One biological unit is defined as the lowest concentration of NGF providing the maximal neurite proliferative response after 12–24 hours; this dose is approximately 10 ng/ml. The neurite proliferative response is accompanied by (1) an increase in cell volume, (2) proliferation of preformed tubulin into microtubules (72,73), and (3) changes in cellular organelles including enlargement of the Golgi complex, increase in the number of ribosomes, and changes in the nucleus, with deep infoldings of the nuclear membrane and an increase in the electron density of the chromatin (74).

These ultrastructural consequences of exposure to NGF are accompanied by a general trophic stimulation of metabolic processes including (1) uridine uptake, (2) RNA synthesis, (3) glucose uptake and utilization, (4) amino acid uptake and protein synthesis, and (5) lipid synthesis (75,76). NGF has been referred to as a positive "pleiotypic" agent because it promotes or maintains such a constellation of metabolic events that allow survival and growth of its target cells (77). In recent years it has been clearly shown that not all of these responses are required for, but may only accompany, selected phenotypic expression of NGF exposure. For example, although RNA synthesis accompanies neurite outgrowth by dorsal root ganglia explants, it is not essential for that process (72,78). Similarly, although NGF promotes microtubule polymerization during the process of neurite outgrowth, *de novo* protein synthesis of the specific microtubule subunit, tubulin, is not required (72,73).

In addition to the general neurotrophic influences on immature sensory and sympathetic neurons, NGF has a number of specific anabolic effects. Among them is the induction of an increase in the synthesis of TH, the rate-limiting enzyme in the synthesis of norepinephrine in sympathetic neurons (38,79). Dopamine-β-hydroxylase synthesis is also increased (79). NGF may also participate in controlling the synthesis and activity of the enzyme that is important in the production of polyamines, ornithine decarboxylase (80). The ability of NGF to influence the synthesis of selected enzymes suggests that NGF acts directly or indirectly upon transcriptional processes.

Effects of NGF on phosphorylation of nuclear proteins (81) and RNA polymerase (82) lend support to this concept.

One question that arose very early in NGF research was whether or not local NGF served not only a trophic role but also acted as a tropic factor that directed the axonal growth of proliferating neurons. This has been a very difficult problem to resolve, but two major observations have led to the current belief that NGF does indeed act tropically as well as trophically. One observation comes from the *in vitro* experiments of Campenot (64), detailed in Section 5.3, and the other is the observation of Levi-Montalcini (83), who demonstrated that intracerebral injection of NGF into newborn rats and mice causes the sympathetic neurons to grow aberrantly into the CNS. Thus in development the local source of NGF in peripheral tissue may not only support the metabolic requirements for growth of axons, but also provide directional information to aid in successful innervation.

The directional influence exerted by NGF on growing axons may be related to a number of cell-surface influences of the hormone including its ability to promote neuronal cell adhesion (84–87) by altering the interaction of leading growth cones to the substratum. Thus NGF may provide the necessary condition that guides the growing axon, rather than the growth cone following a substratum-associated gradient of NGF. Preliminary investigations of NGF-induced specific changes in cell-surface composition (88) or functional responses to lectin probes (85) suggest that cell-surface glycoproteins may participate in expression of NGF-induced neuronal adhesion. Discrimination between these alternatives cannot be made at present.

6.2. Molecular Mechanisms for Induction of the NGF Response

The first demonstration of the presence of a cell-surface receptor for NGF was provided by the observations of Frazier et al. (89), who coupled NGF to Sepharose beads and observed neurite outgrowth by only those explanted embryonic chick sensory and sympathetic ganglia that were in contact with the beads. These results supported the concept that NGF interacts in some specific fashion with the plasma membrane of target cells and that it need not enter the cell in order to induce neurite outgrowth. Subsequently these workers (90) and others (91,92) demonstrated the presence of specific NGF receptors on the surfaces of numerous cells of neural crest origin by using NGF labeled with ^{125}I.

The evidence that supports the existence of a physiologically relevant receptor on the surface of NGF-responsive cells is as follows. First, the binding of [^{125}I]NGF to embryonic dorsal root ganglia is maximal on day 8 of development and less on earlier or later days (41). This specific binding pattern parallels that seen for the ability of NGF to induce neurite outgrowth by ganglia and the development of the target sensory mediodorsal cells in the ganglia. In embryonic sympathetic ganglia, where NGF responsiveness evolves to become a continuous property of the neurons, [^{125}I]NGF binding can be demonstrated in embryonic (90) and mature neurons (92). Second, the binding of chemically modified [^{125}I]NGF derivatives parallels the ability of these compounds to evoke neurite outgrowth (91,92). Third, the concentration of [^{125}I]NGF at which specific binding can be readily demonstrated is similar to, or is lower than, that required to elicit neurite outgrowth (89–94).

The kinetic aspects of the association between [^{125}I]NGF and the plasma membrane receptor of various preparations of embryonic sensory (90,91) and sympathetic (90) neurons, mature sympathetic neurons (92), and responsive neoplastic cells in culture (95) have been reported. Although the qualities of binding of NGF to the variety of tissues studied have similarities, they are not entirely identical. Frazier et al. (90), using [^{125}I]NGF (2.5S) prepared by a solid-phase chloramine-T method and homogenates of embryonic chick sensory or sympathetic ganglia, observed (1) nonsaturable binding, (2) a curvilinear Scatchard plot with multiple equilibrium binding constants (K_A) between 10^{-10} and 10^{-6} M, and (3) accelerated dissociation of bound [^{125}I]NGF by unlabeled NGF, which suggests negatively cooperative interactions between NGF and its receptor. In contrast, Banerjee et al. (92), using a similar preparation of [^{125}I]NGF and a microsomal fraction from mature rabbit superior cervical ganglia, reported a pattern of saturable binding with a maximum K_A of 10^{-10} M. Herrup and Shooter observed similar results (91). More recently, Sutter et al. (93) have reassessed binding of [^{125}I]NGF to dissociated embryonic sensory neurons; they observed saturable binding and a curvilinear Scatchard plot consistent with two receptor types possessing affinities of 10^{-11} and 10^{-9} M. Tait et al. (94) have also reexamined this issue and concluded that neither a two-site nor a negatively cooperative model adequately fit the binding data. As with other studies of this type, the principal complicating factors appear to be the underlying assumptions upon which such studies are usually based, that is, simple mass-action conditions. The multiple aggregation states of cell-surface receptors and the probable changes in affinity associated with these different conditions probably account for the problems encountered (94).

Physical characterization of the NGF receptor has shown that it is trypsin sensitive but unaffected by neuraminidase (96). Although binding to microsomes is phospholipase sensitive (96), it has been found that the receptor is probably not destroyed by the enzyme but simply released from the membrane. In fact, receptor binding activity can be recovered from the supernatant fraction of phospholipase-treated microsomes (M. Kogan, N. V. Costrini, and R. A. Bradshaw, unpublished observations). The receptor behaves as an intrinsic membrane protein in that detergents are required to extract it from the membranes of sympathetic ganglia (97,98). It is important to note that receptor binding activity is not affected by Triton X-100 (1–2%) detergent extraction (97,98). Using Sepharose 6B chromatography and sucrose density centrifugation in H_2O and D_2O, which allows assessment of detergent binding, it has been shown that the ligand–receptor–detergent complex has an apparent Stokes radius of 71 Å, has an $s_{20,w}$ of 4.3S, and is minimally hydrophobic by virtue of a partial specific volume of 0.74 ml/g (97,99). The receptor–hormone complex binds less than 0.3 mg of Triton X-100 per milligram of receptor protein, is highly asymmetrical, and has a molecular weight of 135,000 ± 15,000. These properties of the NGF receptor from rabbit superior cervical ganglia are summarized in Table 3. Such characteristics are of interest because they imply that since the receptor is minimally hydrophobic, only a minor portion of the molecule is in contact with the lipid bilayer. Similar values for these physical parameters have been noted for other membrane proteins, such as rat kidney adenyl cyclase (100).

The NGF receptor has also been characterized by sodium dodecyl sulfate (SDS) gel electrophoresis and autoradiography following covalent attachment of [125I]NGF to the receptor by reaction with N-hydroxysuccimidyl-p-azidobenzoate (101). The complex was formed before either the active ester or the photoactivated azido function was reacted. Productive complexes presumably resulted from insertion of the nitrene into appropriate bonds in

Table 3.   Physical Characteristics of the Triton X-100 Solubilized NGF Receptor[a]

PARAMETER	VALUE[b]
Stokes radius (Å)	71 ± 2.2 (5)
Sedimentation coefficient ($s°_{20,w}$)	4.3 ± 0.1 (11)
Partial specific volume (ml/g)	0.74 ± 0.03 (2)[c]
Molecular weight (M_r)	135,000
Detergent bound (mg/mg protein)	<0.31
Frictional ratio, f/f_0	1.8[d]

[a] From Costrini et al. (99).
[b] Values are mean ± SE for the number of determinations shown in parentheses.
[c] Two separate experiments, each of which consisted of parallel sucrose density gradients prepared in H_2O and D_2O. Mean value based on 11 gradient analyses.
[d] The value of the solvation factor was taken to be 0.2 g of solvent per gram of protein.

the NGF moiety, since reaction of NGF with the active ester before photoactivation did not result in labeling.

Two species of labeled receptors were observed, with apparent molecular weights of 143,000 and 112,000. Both species were specifically labeled with an affinity consistent with previously determined association constants. Only NGF displaced the [^{125}I]NGF (prior to reaction); insulin, IGF, multiplication-stimulating activity, and EGF were ineffective. Proteolytic mapping of both species suggested that the smaller entity was derived from the larger one by limited proteolysis.

These results support the hydrodynamic measurements (99). Both studies suggest that the receptor exists on the external surface of the cell membrane and is minimally associated with the lipid bilayer. However, it should be noted that neither set of results excludes the presence of additional non-covalently attached subunits that could function in nonrecognitive capacities.

The intracellular events following the binding of NGF to its receptor are still a subject of active investigation. The observation that dibutyryladenosine 3′,5′-monophosphate (DBcAMP) could promote neurite outgrowth by embryonic dorsal root ganglia led to the suggestion that cAMP might by the second messenger for NGF (65). Frazier et al. (102) systematically investigated the possibility by assessing the now-classical criteria of cAMP involvement as a second messenger. These criteria are as follows: (1) the hormone response should be mimicked by cAMP or a derivative, (2) the intracellular level of cAMP should change appropriately in response to hormone stimulation, (3) the hormone response should be potentiated by agents that inhibit phosphodiesterase activity, and (4) the hormone should be able to stimulate adenyl cyclase activity in broken-cell preparations (37). When explanted embryonic chick sensory ganglia were used, only the first criterion was partially fulfilled by NGF (102). In this regard, the DBcAMP-induced neurite outgrowth was qualitatively and quantitatively different from the NGF response; it was pH dependent, and similar effects could be seen with sodium butyrate alone. From these results, it was concluded that cAMP is not involved in the process of NGF-induced neurite outgrowth. Hier et al. (103) reached a similar conclusion.

In contrast with these findings, Narumi and Fujita (104) have reported a threefold rise in ganglionic cAMP within 10 minutes of exposure to 2 ng/ml of NGF and a dose-related neurite outgrowth response to DBcAMP (10^{-5} –10^{-3} M). Skaper et al. (105) have reported that NGF produces a rapid and transient fivefold rise in cAMP in embryonic sensory ganglia and that under their experimental conditions the rate of increase of cAMP is related to the concentration of NGF. They have also noted a temporal relationship between the NGF-associated rate of rise of cAMP and deoxyglucose uptake.

In the sympathetic system, the status of cAMP as a mediator of NGF action is similarly unsettled. Recklies et al. (106) reported that DBcAMP could cause some neurite outgrowth by embryonic sympathetic ganglia *in vitro*; they also noted the lack of other evidence and the qualitative differences that led them to conclude that NGF did not act via cAMP modulation. In 1975, Nikodijevic et al. (107) examined this question using organ cultures of superior cervical ganglia obtained from neonatal rats. They observed an increase in ganglionic cAMP content from 0.8 pmol/ganglion to approximately 2 pmol/ganglion within 5 minutes of exposure to 3 μg/ml of 2.5S NGF. The lowest concentration of NGF that produced a significant rise in ganglionic cAMP was 40 ng/ml. Subsequently (108) these workers reported that both NGF and DBcAMP could cause an increase in TH activity, but that DBcAMP did not potentiate this effect of NGF nor did theophylline cause a rise in TH activity. Because of these and other reservations, it was concluded that the role of cAMP as the mediator of NGF-induced increases in the activity of TH was questionable. This conclusion was in agreement with that of Otten et al. (109), who showed that only a small portion of total ganglionic cAMP was present within adrenergic neurons, and that although isoproterenol *in vivo* caused a rapid and short-lived increase in the adrenergic pool of cAMP [similar to that seen *in vitro* with NGF by Nikodijevic et al. (107)], it did not lead to a rise in TH activity. Also, in the rat adrenal medulla, reserpine-induced rises in cAMP and TH were not causally related. Most recently, Otten et al. (110) have repeated the organ-culture studies using mature rats and have found that NGF induces only an insignificant, short-lived rise (30%) in cAMP while causing a significant rise in TH. Thus the weight of evidence from both neuron types argues against a critical role of cAMP in NGF-associated responses. However, minor or secondary roles for cAMP are certainly not eliminated.

The effects of NGF on membrane permeability are reflected in a number of experimental observations. Nerve growth factor has been shown in a variety of systems to promote incorporation of uridine and amino acids into RNA and protein, respectively (111,112). It has been shown (76,113) that (1) NGF deprivation is associated with a decline in substrate incorporation into cellular macromolecules, (2) NGF, if supplied within a period of 6 hours, can fully restore substrate incorporation, and (3) these effects of NGF are due to NGF-induced changes in membrane permeability to substrates. The effects of NGF on membrane permeation are rapid; that is, they occur within minutes of exposure of initially NGF-deprived sensory neurons to the growth factor. NGF-induced permeation changes are not relevant to all exogenous substrates; although permeability to uridine, cytidine, guanosine, probably adenosine, 2-deoxyglucose, and α-aminoisobutyric acid increases on exposure to NGF, free leucine accumulation is not sensitive to NGF deprivation nor is it augmented upon NGF exposure. It was postulated that regulation of selected membrane permeation properties could be the primary process through which NGF exerts its trophic role. This hypothesis has merit because the events are rapid and easy to relate to the general neurotrophic character of the growth factor. However, when this permeation effect is related to subsequent events such as neurite outgrowth and enzyme induction, as-yet-undefined specifying influences, either intracellular or extracellular, are also necessary.

Investigations of postreceptor events in the mechanism of action of NGF dealing with the role of cAMP and with the role of substrate permeation have led to a common postulate, namely that the essential immediate post-receptor event may involve transmembrane mobilization of cations (85,114). Skaper and Varon (115) have shown that NGF-induced substrate permeation changes are dependent upon extracellular sodium, are energy dependent, and are inhibited by ouabain and veratridine. They have also shown, using $^{22}Na^+$, that NGF deprivation leads to sodium accumulation, and NGF exposure promotes its efflux (115,116). This loss of sodium in response to NGF is specific, occurs within minutes, is dose related, and occurs at appropriate concentrations of the growth factor. These recent studies indicate an intimate temporal relationship between receptor binding and a neuronal sodium-pump mechanism such as Na^+-K^+-ATPase. Since the receptor and the membrane pump are both integral membrane proteins, a physical relationship between the two may exist. It is also possible that sodium may move in association with other ions, such as calcium or potassium, and that one of these ions may be the actual trigger for subsequent permeation changes as well as other effects. Correlative observations by Sisken and Lafferty (117) that direct current has NGF-like effects on embryonic sensory ganglia support the concept that a transmembrane cation-exchange process is at least a part of NGF action.

It can be suggested that NGF acts at multiple loci to cause its multiplicity of effects. This would account for the failure to find a second messenger. The demonstration of retrograde transport of NGF (60) and the presence of apparently distinct NGF binding sites in the nuclear fractions of NGF-responsive cells (118) also supports the concept. That binding of NGF to nuclear receptors occurs normally and results in an NGF-associated event remains to be demonstrated, however.

The spectrum of NGF actions can be organized by separating those due to interaction of NGF at the cell surface from those that occur as a consequence of NGF that has been internalized and transported to the cell body. The major influences of NGF on adrenergic neurons are survival, hypertrophy, neurite extension, and induction of synthesis of selected enzymes involved in neurotransmitter synthesis. Conceptually, NGF acting at the neuronal plasma membrane may lead to early postreceptor events such as anabolic-precursor uptake, changes in cell-surface properties that promote neuronal adhesion, and microtubule polymerization. These plasma-membrane events may explain NGF-associated hypertrophy and neurite extension. To the extent that anabolism and adhesion support neuronal survival, these effects also could occur as a consequence of, or be promoted by, interaction of NGF with its plasma-membrane receptor. These postreceptor events may have a currently undefined second messenger mediating their occurrence. The induction of the synthesis of TH and dopamine-β-hydroxylase may depend upon NGF or its receptor, which reaches the cell body by retrograde transport. In fact, these receptors may in part become the sites identified in the nuclear fraction (118). Thus although the exact purpose for retrograde transport of NGF is undefined, the sum of the experimental evidence seems to indicate that internalized NGF is functional and important. The fundamental data required are those demonstrating that some critical intracellular effect of NGF occurs as a result of internalization. The locus-specific model of NGF action requires a role for internalized NGF in any hypothesis for the mechanism of expression of the physiological effects of the growth factor.

REFERENCES

1. Bueker, E. D., *Anat. Rec.*, **102**, 369 (1948).
2. Levi-Montalcini, R., and Hamburger, V., *J. Exp. Zool.*, **116**, 321 (1951).
3. Bradshaw, R. A., and Rubin, J. S., *J. Supramol. Struct.*, **14**, 183 (1980).
4. Cohen, S., and Levi-Montalcini, R., *Proc. Natl. Acad. Sci. USA*, **42**, 571 (1956).
5. Cohen, S., *Proc. Natl. Acad. Sci. USA*, **46**, 302 (1960).
6. Harper, G. P., Barde, Y. A., Burnstock, G., and Carstairs, J. R., *Nature*, **279**, 160 (1979).
7. Burton, L. E., Wilson, W. H., and Shooter, E. M., *J. Biol. Chem.*, **253**, 7807 (1978).
8. Varon, S., Nomura, J., and Shooter, E. M., *Biochemistry*, **7**, 1296 (1968).
9. Server, A. C., and Shooter, E. M., *Adv. Prot. Chem.*, **31**, 339 (1977).
10. Pattison, S. E., and Dunn, M. F., *Biochemistry*, **14**, 2733 (1975).
11. Bothwell, M. A., and Shooter, E. M., *J. Biol. Chem.*, **254**, 8458 (1978).
12. Angeletti, R. A., Bradshaw, R. A., and Wade, R. D., *Biochemistry*, **10**, 463 (1971).
13. Thomas, K. A., and Bradshaw, R. A., in R. A. Bradshaw and D. M. Schneider, Eds. *Proteins of the Nervous System*, Raven, New York, 1980, pp. 213–230.
14. Silverman, R. E., Ph.D. thesis, Washington University, St. Louis, Mo. (1977).
15. Moore, J. B., Mobley, W. C., and Shooter, E. M., *Biochemistry*, **13**, 833 (1974).
16. Bocchini, V., and Angeletti, P. U., *Proc. Natl. Acad. Sci. USA*, **64**, 787 (1969).
17. Angeletti, R., and Bradshaw, R. A., *Proc. Natl. Acad. Sci. USA*, **68**, 2417 (1971).
18. Hogue-Angeletti, R., Hermodson, M. A., and Bradshaw, R. A., *Biochemistry*, **12**, 100 (1973).
19. Bothwell, M. A., Wilson, W. H., and Shooter, E. M., *J. Biol. Chem.*, **254**, 7287 (1979).
20. Hogue-Angeletti, R. A., Bradshaw, R. A., and Marshall, G. R., *Int. J. Pept. Protein*

Res., **6**, 321 (1974).

21. Greene, L. A., Shooter, E. M., and Varon, S., *Biochemistry*, **8**, 3735 (1969).
22. Thomas, K. A., Baglan, N. C., and Bradshaw, R. A., *J. Biol. Chem.*, **256**, 9156 (1981).
23. Bothwell, M. A., and Shooter, E. M., *J. Biol. Chem.*, **252**, 8532 (1977).
24. Young, M., Saide, J. D., Murphy, R. A., and Arnason, B. G. W., *J. Biol. Chem.*, **251**, 459 (1976).
25. Frazier, W. A., Hogue-Angeletti, R., and Bradshaw, R. A., *Science*, **176**, 482 (1972).
26. Wlodawer, A., Hodgson, K. D., and Shooter, E. M., *Proc. Natl. Acad. Sci. USA*, **72**, 777 (1975).
27. Gunning, J. and Blundell, T., in E. Gross and J. Meienhofer, Eds. *The Peptides*, Academic, New York, 1981, Vol. 4, pp. 55–84.
28. Bradshaw, R. A., and Niall, H. D., *Trends Biochem. Sci.*, **3**, 274 (1978).
29. Wallace, L. J., and Partlow, L. M., *Proc. Natl. Acad. Sci. USA*, **73**, 4210 (1976).
30. Berger, E. A., and Shooter, E. M., *J. Biol. Chem.*, **253**, 804 (1978).
31. Wiche, G., *Biochem. Biophys. Res. Commun.*, **89**, 620 (1979).
32. Frey, P., Forand, R., Maciag, T., and Shooter, E. M., *Proc. Nqtl. Acad. Sci. USA*, **76**, 6294 (1979).
33. Rubin, J. S., Ph.D. thesis, Washington University, St. Louis, Mo. (1982).
34. Roberts, J. L., and Herbert, E., *Proc. Natl. Acad. Sci. USA*, **74**, 5300 (1977).
35. Rubin, J. S., and Bradshaw, R. A., *J. Neurosci. Res.*, **6**, 451 (1981).
36. Hendry, I. A., *J. Neurocytol.*, **6**, 299 (1977).
37. Robison, G. A., Butcher, R. W., and Sutherland, E. W., *Cyclic AMP*, Academic, New York, 1971.
38. Hendry, I. A. in S. Ehrenpreis and I. J. Kopin, Eds., *Review of Neurosciences*, Raven, New York, 1976, Vol. 2, pp. 149–194.
39. Angeletti, P. U., Levi-Montalcini, R., and Caramia, F., *Brain Res.*, **27**, 343 (1971).
40. Purves, D., and Nja, A., *Nature*, **260**, 535 (1976).
41. Herrup, K., and Shooter, E. M., *J. Cell Biol.*, **67**, 118 (1975).
42. Stoeckel, K. and Thoenen, H., *Brain Res.*, **85**, 337 (1975).
43. Unsicker, K., Krisch, B., Otten, U., and Thoenen, H., *Proc. Natl. Acad. Sci. USA*, **75**, 3498 (1978).
44. Klingman, G. I. and Klingman, J. D., in G. Steiner and F. Schonbaum, Eds. *Immunosympathectomy*, Elsevier, Amsterdam, 1972, pp. 111–130.
45. Black, I. B., *Annu. Rev. Neurosci.*, **1**, 183 (1978).
46. Patterson, P. H., *Annu. Rev. Neurosci.*, **1**, 1 (1978).
47. Norr, S. C., *Dev. Biol.*, **34**, 16 (1973).
48. Bjerre, B., and Bjorklund, A., *Neurobiology*, **3**, 140 (1973).
49. Varon, S., and Bunge, R., *Annu. Rev. Neurosci.*, **1**, 327 (1978).
50. Coughlin, M. D., Boyer, D. M., and Black, I. B., *Proc. Natl. Acad. Sci. USA*, **74**, 3438 (1977).
51. Burnham, P., Raiborn, C., and Varon, S., *Proc. Natl. Acad. Sci. USA*, **69**, 3556 (1972).
52. Varon, S., Raiborn, C., and Burnham, P., *Neurobiology*, **4**, 231 (1974).
53. Varon, S., Raiborn, C., and Burnham, P., *Neurobiology*, **4**, 317 (1974).
54. Longo, A. M., and Penhoet, E. E., *Proc. Natl. Acad. Sci. USA*, **71**, 2347 (1974).

55. Arnason, B. G. W., Oger, J., Pantazis, N. J., and Young, M., *J. Clin. Invest.*, **53**, 2a (1974).

56. Cowan, W. M., and Wenger, E., *J. Exp. Zool.*, **168**, 105 (1968).

57. Dibner, M. D., and Black, I. B., *J. Neurochem.*, **30**, 1479 (1978).

58. Hendry, I. A., *Brain Res.*, **94**, 87 (1975).

59. Hendry, I. A., and Iversen, L. L., *Nature*, **243**, 500 (1973).

60. Hendry, I. A., Stoeckel, K., Thoenen, H., and Iversen, L. L., *Brain Res.* **68**, 103 (1974).

61. Levi-Montalcini, R., Aloe, L., and Johnson, E. M., in E. Usdin and S. H. Snyder, Eds., *Frontiers in Catecholamine Research*, Pergamon, New York, 1973, pp. 267–276.

62. Menesini, V., Chen, M. E., Chen, I. S., Calissano, P., and Levi-Montalcini, R., *Proc. Natl. Acad. Sci. USA*, **74**, 5559 (1977).

63. Johnson, E. M., *Brain Res.*, **141**, 105 (1978).

64. Campenot, R. B., *Proc. Natl. Acad. Sci. USA*, **74**, 4516 (1977).

65. Levi-Montalcini, R., and Angeletti, P. U., *Physiol. Rev.*, **48**, 534 (1968).

66. Gorin, P. D., and Johnson, E. M., *Proc. Natl. Acad. Sci. USA*, **76**, 5382 (1979).

67. Black, I. B., Hendry, I. A., and Iversen, L. L., *J. Neurochem.*, **19**, 1367 (1972).

68. Hendry, I. A., *Brain Res.*, **56**, 313 (1973).

69. Mobley, W. C., Server, A. C., Ishii, D. N., Riopelle, R. J., and Shooter, E. M., *N. Engl. J. Med.*, **297**, 1097, 1149, and 1211 (1977).

70. Levi-Montalcini, R., and Booker, B., *Proc. Natl. Acad. Sci. USA*, **46**, 373 (1960).

71. Levi-Montalcini, R., Meyer, H., and Hamburger, V., *Cancer Res.*, **14**, 49 (1954).

72. Yamada, K. M., and Wessells, N. K., *Exp. Cell Res.* **66**, 346 (1971).

73. Stoeckel, K., Solomon, F., Paravicini, U., and Thoenen, H., *Nature*, **250**, 150 (1974).

74. Levi-Montalcini, R., Caramia, F., Luse, S. A., and Angeletti, P. U., *Brain Res.* **8**, 347 (1968).

75. Larrabee, M. G., *Fed. Proc.* **29**, 1919 (1970).

76. Horii, Z.-I. and Varon, S., *Brain Res.* **124**, 121 (1977).

77. Hershko, A., Mamont, P., Shields, R., and Tomkins, G. M., *Nature*, **232**, 206 (1971).

78. Burnham, P. A., and Varon, S., *Neurobiology*, **4**, 57 (1974).

79. Thoenen, H., Angeletti, P. U., Levi-Montalcini, R., and Kettler, R., *Proc. Natl. Acad. Sci. USA*, **68**, 1598 (1971).

80. MacDonnell, P. C., Nagaiah, K., Lakshmanan, J., and Guroff, G., *Proc. Natl. Acad. Sci. USA*, **74**, 4681 (1977).

81. Yu, M. W., Tolson, N., and Guroff, G., *J. Biol. Chem.*, **255**, 10481 (1980).

82. Huff, K., Lakshmanan, J., and Guroff, G., *J. Neurochem.*, **31**, 599 (1978).

83. Levi-Montalcini, R., in M. A. Corner and D. F. Swaab, Eds., *Progress in Brain Research*, Elsevier, Amsterdam, **45**, 1976, pp. 235–256.

84. Merrell, R., Pulliam, M. W., Randano, L., Boyd, L. F., Bradshaw, R. A., and Glaser, L., *Proc. Natl. Acad. Sci. USA*, **72**, 4270 (1975).

85. Schubert, D., LaCorbiere, M., Whitlock, C., and Stallcup, W., *Nature*, **273**, 718 (1978).

86. Letourneau, P. C., *Dev. Biol.*, **44**, 77 (1975).

87. Glaser, L., Merrell, R., Gottlieb, D. I., Littman, D., Pulliam, M. W., and Bradshaw, R. A., in R. A. Bradshaw, W. A. Frazier, R. C. Merrell, D. I. Gottlieb, and R. A.

Hogue-Angeletti, Eds., *Surface Membrane Receptors, Interface Between Cells and Environment* Plenum, New York, 1976, pp. 133–145.

88. McGuire, J. C., and Greene, L. A., *Cell*, **15**, 357 (1978).

89. Frazier, W. A., Boyd, L. F., and Bradshaw, R. A., *Proc. Natl. Acad. Sci. USA*, **70**, 2931 (1973).

90. Frazier, W. A., Boyd, L. F., and Bradshaw, R. A., *J. Biol. Chem.*, **249**, 5513 (1974).

91. Herrup, K., and Shooter, E. M., *Proc. Natl. Acad. Sci. USA*, **70**, 3884 (1973).

92. Banerjee, S. P., Snyder, S., Cuatrecasas, P., and Greene, L. A., *Proc. Natl. Acad. Sci. USA*, **70**, 2519 (1973).

93. Sutter, A., Riopelle, R. J., Harris-Warrick, R. M., and Shooter, E. M., *J. Biol. Chem.*, **254**, 5972 (1979).

94. Tait, J. F., Weinman, S. A., and Bradshaw, R. A., *J. Biol. Chem.*, **256**, 11086 (1981).

95. Fabricant, R. N., DeLarco, J. E., and Todaro, G. J., *Proc. Natl. Acad. Sci. USA*, **74**, 565 (1977).

96. Banerjee, S. P., Cuatrecasas, P., and Snyder, S. H., *J. Biol. Chem.*, **250**, 1427 (1975).

97. Costrini, N. V., and Bradshaw, R. A., *Proc. Natl. Acad. Sci. USA*, **76**, 3242 (1979).

98. Banerjee, S. P., Cuatrecasas, P., and Snyder, S. H., *J. Biol. Chem.*, **251**, 5680 (1976).

99. Costrini, N. V., Kogan, M., Kukreja, K., and Bradshaw, R. A., *J. Biol. Chem.*, **254**, 11242 (1979).

100. Neer, E. J., *J. Biol. Chem.*, **249**, 6527 (1974).

101. Massague, J., Guillette, B. J., Czech, M. P., Morgan, C. J., and Bradshaw, R. A., *J. Biol. Chem.*, **256**, 9419 (1981).

102. Frazier, W. A., Ohlendorf, C. E., Boyd, L. F., Aloe, L., and Bradshaw, R. A., *Proc. Natl. Acad. Sci. USA*, **70**, 2448 (1973).

103. Hier, D. B., Arnason, B. G., and Young, M., *Science*, **182**, 79 (1973).

104. Narumi, S., and Fujita, T., *Neuropharmacology*, **17**, 73 (1978).

105. Skaper, S. D., Bottenstein, J. E., and Varon, S., *J. Neurochem.*, **32**, 1845 (1979).

106. Recklies, A. D., Rathbone, M. P., and Hale, R. H., *Can J. Physiol. Pharmacol.*, **52**, 840 (1974).

107. Nikodijevic, B., Nikodijevic, O., Yu, M., Pollard, H., and Guroff, G., *Proc. Natl. Acad. Sci. USA*, **72**, 4769 (1975).

108. Yu, M. W., Nikodijevic, B., Lakshmanan, J., Rowe, V., MacDonnell, P., and Guroff, G., *J. Neurochem.*, **28**, 835 (1977).

109. Otten, U., Mueller, R. A., Oesch, F., and Thoenen, H., *Proc. Natl. Acad. Sci. USA*, **71**, 2217 (1974).

110. Otten, U., Hatanaka, H., and Thoenen, H., *Brain Res.*, **140**, 385 (1978).

111. Schubert, D., and Whitlock, C., *Proc. Natl. Acad. Sci. USA*, **74**, 4055 (1977).

112. Burnham, P. A., and Varon, S., *Neurobiology*, **4**, 57 (1974).

113. Partlow, L. M., and Larrabee, M. G., *J. Neurochem.*, **18**, 2101 (1971).

114. Horii, Z.-I., and Varon, S., *J. Neurosci. Res.*, **1**, 361 (1975).

115. Skaper, S. D., and Varon, S., *Brain Res.*, **172**, 303 (1979).

116. Skaper, S. D., and Varon, S., *Biochem. Biophys. Res. Commun.*, **88**, 563 (1979).

117. Sisken, B., and Lafferty, J. F., *Bioelectrochem. Bioenergetics*, **5**, 459 (1978).

118. Andres, R. Y., Jeng, I., and Bradshaw, R. A., *Proc. Natl. Acad. Sci. USA*, **74**, 2785 (1977).

2

HUMAN NERVE GROWTH FACTOR: COMPARATIVE ASPECTS

J. Regino Perez-Polo
Carol Beck
C. Patrick Reynolds
Mariann Blum

CONTENTS

Abbreviations

NGF	Nerve growth factor
MSG	Mouse submaxillary gland
RIA	Radioimmunoassay
SDS	Sodium dodecyl sulfate
EGF	Epidermal growth factor
BU	Biological unit
gp-NGF	Guinea pig nerve growth factor
IEF	Isoelectric focusing
PEGG	Preparative flat-bed electrofocusing in a granulated gel

1. INTRODUCTION

As early as 1913 it had been suggested that specific substances in the microenvironment of neurons were likely to have potent trophic effects (1). However, it remained for Rita Levi-Montalcini, Victor Hamburger, and Stanley Cohen to develop a suitable assay system for one such factor and subsequently to isolate from mouse submaxillary gland (MSG) and snake venom the active subunit of what has come to be known as the nerve growth factor (NGF) (2–4). Since that time, it has been established that NGF plays a central role in the development of vertebrate sympathetic and sensory ganglia, both of neural crest origin (5). It has further been suggested that nodose ganglia of mesodermal origin respond to NGF (6).

It has been proposed that NGF acts as a neuronotrophic factor in mammalian peripheral nervous systems (5). Neuronotrophic or permissive factors are extracellular substances that quantitatively regulate the anabolic machinery of a particular class of cells as compared with specifying or instructive factors that determine which genetic programs are expressed (7). The mechanism of action of NGF (5) and the detailed biochemistry of MSG-NGF (8,9) have been reviewed in Chapter 1. Possible roles for NGF in the central nervous system (10,11) as well as its putative involvement in a number of neuropathies (12–14) remain controversial issues at this time. This review discusses features of NGF isolated from tissues from a variety of species compared with NGF of human origin.

Nerve growth factor has recently also been isolated from guinea pig prostate (15) and from human placenta at term (16). In all instances, NGF activity has been defined in terms of the neurite-promoting effects of the substance on embryonic chicken sensory ganglia in organ culture (4). As early as 1954, it became useful to use the profuse outgrowth of neurites induced by NGF in explanted chicken embryonic dorsal root ganglia as a way of measuring levels of NGF activity (4). The early inverted plasma clot assay has been modified in several ways (17–19). Assays using dissociated ganglia, as opposed to whole excised ganglia, have also been developed. These have increased sensitivity, whether neurite outgrowth (20), attachment (21), or survival (22) are measured. For pure murine NGF, whole-ganglia assays yield an optimal response at 10 ng of NGF per milliliter (17). Thus, the amount of protein that when tested in such a bioassay elicits optimal neurite outgrowth is called a biological unit (BU). It is this response that is meant when speaking of NGF activity, NGF-like activity, or NGF biological activity, as shown in Fig 1. Two established cell lines (PC12 rat pheochromocytoma, SK-N-SH-SY5Y human neuroblastoma) that respond to NGF by exhibiting neurite elongation but do not require NGF for survival have also been adapted to assay for NGF activity (23,24).

Some basic problems are encountered in making determinations of NGF activity in serum or tissues. The first is that the assay depends on the response of a heterogenous group of cells devoid of their normal surroundings, and thus the assay is affected by the degree of clotting of the matrix in the

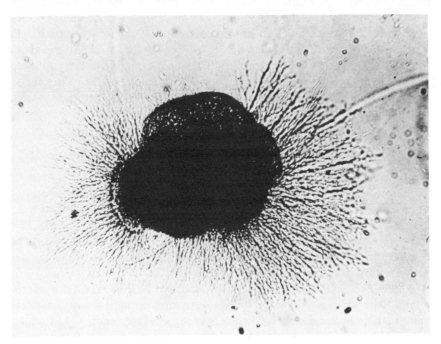

Figure 1. Nine-day-old embryonic chicken dorsal root ganglia explanted for 24 hours in the presence of 10 ng of MSG-NGF per milliliter.

whole-ganglia assay or by the degree of cell damage during ganglion disruption in the dissociated-cell assay. Other problems not easily overcome are the sensitivity of responsive neurons to other endogenous inhibitors or effectors present, in addition to NGF, in the sample being assayed, the very "sticky" nature of NGF due to its positive charge at neutral pH, and the high error of the assay. Finally, chick sensory ganglia respond differently to NGF at different stages of their development *in ovo* (25). These problems become more significant in discussing levels of NGF activity in partially purified preparations, in accounting for yields of NGF during purification, or in describing levels of NGF in serum or other tissues (26).

Almost all of the biological experiments that have been carried out to date on the mechanism of action of NGF have been carried out with preparations of NGF isolated from MSG and antibodies directed against MSG-NGF. As the number of NGF-like activities in the literature has proliferated, it has been suggested that the name NGF should be reserved for those substances that elicit a bioassay response that can be successfully blocked by antibodies to MSG-NGF (27). Unfortunately, this description of NGF is severely dependent on the immunological responses of the species used to raise antibodies to those species used for the isolation of NGF. A more biological approach would be to reserve the term NGF for those substances isolated from a species that, when injected into animals of the same species yield hypertrophied sympathetic or sensory ganglia, and for when treatment of these animals with antibodies to this NGF results in immunosympathectomized animals. However, these criteria would be impossible to apply to NGF of human origin. Another approach is to characterize the NGF species in question structurally and compare it to the NGF isolated from MSG and snake venom, both well characterized.

2. NGF AND DISEASE

Many attempts have been made to relate NGF to pathological conditions in man. Several studies are available that show elevation of levels of NGF activity in the peripheral circulation of neuroblastoma patients (28,29), although other studies have found no differences from controls (30). The response of neuroblastoma tumor tissue to NGF has been used in the development of a diagnostic assay (31).

Another clinical state that might be related to NGF is familial dysautonomia. Although several early studies were unable to show any consistent abnormality in circulating NGF levels (32), a recent report (33) found a threefold increase of material related immunologically to NGF in the sera of dysautonomic patients when compared with controls. It was suggested that elevation of MSG-NGF cross-reacting material was secondary to some other lesion and that the origin of familial dysautonomia was within the scope of functions influenced by NGF (33).

Neurofibromatosis, a relatively common condition, is one of a group of dysgenetic syndromes associated with tumors or tumor-like malformations of the nervous system. It manifests itself clinically in one of four presentations: peripheral, central, visceral, or *formes frustes*. A few reports are available in which an attempt to study NGF in neurofibromatosis was made. Schenkein et al. (34) studied the sera of a group of 24 patients with "disseminated neurofibromatosis" and 55 controls. It was observed that 79% of patients had NGF "activity values" greater than 1.0, whereas only 5.6% of controls had such levels. Although Siggers et al. (35) made no attempt to equate bioassay results with NGF levels present in a group of five patients with "disseminated neurofibromatosis" (peripheral form) and 17 controls, data obtained by a radioimmunoassay (RIA) technique for NGF were presented. The difference between patients and controls was not statistically significant. Siggers suggested that the NGF-like activity noted by Schenkein was not NGF itself, but a different molecular species. Using the same RIA, Siggers also examined three patients with central neurofibromatosis. In contrast with patients with disseminated disease, two out of three had elevated serum levels of a material immunologically similar to NGF, suggesting the presence of two distinct species of molecules with NGF-like activity, one antigenically related to mouse NGF, the other not so related. In more recent reports on the central form of the disease (36), nine patients with this disease and 22 at risk were examined; NGF antigenic activity was significantly elevated in the former group. In the latter, two subgroups evolved, one with normal and another with elevated antigenic levels. Receptor-binding activity in the sera of all groups was normal or low, contrasting with Siggers' report, wherein receptor binding was elevated and antigenic activity normal or low. Although assay problems may play a role in the variability of results, a potential metabolic aberration of NGF in this important disorder of neural development is still worthy of serious consideration and further investigation. Other neuroplastic processes in man have been associated with the production of NGF or an NGF-like material (37,38). In addition, there are reports of *in vivo* regulatory effects of MSG-NGF on neural-specific carcinogenic induction in mice and rats (39–41).

3. NGF IN SERUM

Analysis of reports of NGF levels in the sera of controls compared with sera of patients with several diseases potentially related to NGF reveals a striking lack of consistency and reproducibility, whether the disease is neuroblastoma, neurofibromatosis, familial dysautonomia, or schizophrenia.

Table 1.   Detection of NGF in Serum

SOURCE	BIOASSAY (DRG)	ONE-SITE RIA	TWO-SITE RIA	ROCKET IMMUNO-ELECTROPHORESIS
Human serum	+	++	−	−
Human serum + anti-MSG-β-NGF	+	+	ND[a]	ND
Amniotic fluid	−	ND	−	ND

[a] ND = not determined.

The NGF levels reported in control human sera have ranged from 0.40 to 40.0 ng/ml. Although internally consistent assay results are easily obtainable with NGF dissolved in buffers, such is not the case when human serum samples have been analyzed (26,42), and the same has been reported for mouse and rat sera (27). At least part of the problem appears to be the presence of a binding protein for NGF in human and mouse serum (26). It has been possible to utilize marked differences between the molecular weights and isoelectric points of NGF and the binding protein to separate them by gel-filtration chromatography at pH 4.0. This technique was used in one study (36) that demonstrated a difference between the apparent amounts of NGF present in the sera of patients with neurofibromatosis measured by an RIA and those measured with a radioreceptor assay. Unfortunately, no absolute values were given for the quantity of NGF present in patients or controls measured by either assay, and no bioassay results were presented.

All of these reports rely on measurement of NGF by bioassay, receptor assay, or RIA. Although receptor assays lack some of the disadvantages of bioassays, receptor-assay results can be influenced by the presence of NGF-binding proteins (Hübner, K. and J. R. Perez-Polo, unpublished observations) and down-regulation of receptor binding by other peptide hormones. Attempts to quantitate NGF levels in human serum, body fluids, and tissues using non-species-specific antisera yield conflicting results. We have used a number of RIAs to test if there is significant cross-reaction between antibodies directed toward murine NGF when challenged with human NGF in human biological fluids of interest (43). The use of a two-site RIA procedure reduces problems associated with NGF-binding proteins found in sera (27), but results in false values when the total protein concentrations are not comparable in all samples tested (43,44). At detectable levels of 500 pg of NGF per milliliter of serum, using this RIA technique, we have been unable to demonstrate human NGF reproducibly in either normal adult sera or in amniotic fluid samples collected at varying times during pregnancy (Table 1). We feel that this failure to detect human NGF could be due to the low cross-reactivity we have observed between monospecific antibodies to murine NGF and human NGF isolated from human placenta at term.

4. EXOCRINE SOURCES: MOUSE

The best-characterized forms of NGF are those isolated from exocrine glands such as the male MSG (8,9), a number of snake venoms (8), and the guinea pig prostate (15) (Table 2). In all these species, biological activity is associated exclusively with a basic dipeptide called βNGF. In the male MSG, βNGF is associated into an oligomer called 7S NGF (45). 7S NGF is a pentamer with a subunit composition of $\alpha_2\beta\gamma_2$ and containing 2 moles of Zn^{2+} per mole of NGF (8) (Fig. 2).

The βNGF isolated from male MSG (MSG-βNGF) is a highly basic protein (pI 9.4, Fig. 3) made up of two identical polypeptides of 118 residues each with arginine residues at the carboxyl terminus (8,9). These two polypeptides are strongly held together by noncovalent forces and dissociate when treated with sodium dodecyl sulfate (SDS), a strongly ionic detergent known to denature proteins (46). If the arginine residues at the carboxyl terminus of βNGF are removed enzymatically, there is no loss of biological activity. However, the modified βNGF molecule, called 2.5S NGF, is not able to recombine with α and γ to form a 7S complex (47,48). Although the *other subunits*, α and γ, have no biological activity, their acidic nature is likely to give the 7S form a less basic net charge (pI 5.5), which may make the molecule more stable *in vivo*. In addition, the γ subunit is a highly specific

Table 2. NGF Protein Structure

Source	Biologically Active Basic Protein	NGF Subunit Containing Complex
Mouse		
Submaxillary gland	+	+
Saliva	+	+
S-180 Mouse sarcoma cell line	+	+
Snake		
Crotalus adamenteus	+	+
Vipera russelli	+	−
Naja naja	−	−
Guinea pig prostate	+	+
Human		
Placenta	+	+
Fibroblast primary cultures	+	?

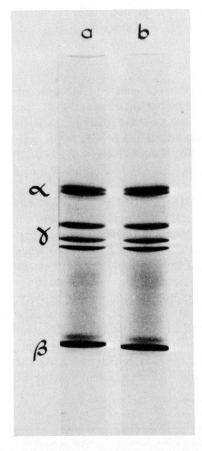

Figure 2. Isoelectric-focusing development of MSG-NGF in polyacrylamide disc gels. (*a*) Purified 7S NGF. (*b*) Dissociated and reconstituted 7S NGF in MSG crude homogenate.

and potent arginyl endopeptidase (49) and arginyl esterase (50). It has been proposed that in a manner akin to that of insulin, βNGF is made as a pro-β form that is not active but can be specifically cleaved into an active form, βNGF, by the γ subunit, which removes a polypeptide segment from the carboxyl terminus (51). Following this activation, the γ remains bound to the β and with both the α and β subunit forms a stable complex in equilibrium with the free β subunit (51). In the male MSG, βNGF is synthesized as a 22,000-dalton peptide, pro-βNGF, which can be immunoprecipitated with antibodies directed against the 13,500-dalton peptide known as βNGF (51). Pulse-chase experiments and incubation with peptidase suggest that the precursor form is processed to the active species (51). Whether the precursor is biologically active is not known at this time.

That NGF is synthesized and processed in the submaxillary gland for subsequent retrograde transport to the superior cervical ganglion is consistent

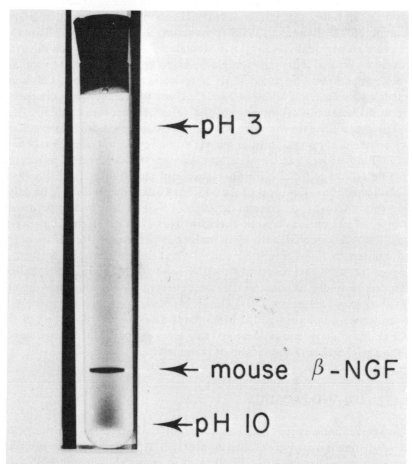

←pH 3

← mouse β-NGF

←pH 10

Isoelectric focusing on 7½%
disc polyacrylamide gels with
3-10 pH gradient of 150 μg
purified mouse β-NGF.

Figure 3. Isoelectric-focusing development of MSG-βNGF in a polyacrylamide disc gel.

with the role of NGF in maintaining a differentiated state in its target neurons. It is thus surprising that immunocytolocalization studies show that NGF is secreted into the glandular lumen of the submaxillary gland for release (52) and eventual degradation (53). Levi-Montalcini has suggested that this NGF activity associated with saliva might be taken up in the gut and eventually affect sympathetic structures (54). It is interesting that both saliva and mother's milk have low levels of NGF (55), and this might play an important role in mammalian development of the peripheral nervous system. Alternatively, as is the case for other peptide hormones, NGF from saliva might play different hormonal roles in gut via down-regulation of EGF receptors and EGF-dependent gastric secretion. Whether this is pertinent to recently reported effects of MSG-NGF on gastric acid secretion in dogs remains to be confirmed (56). Removal of the MSG has either no effect (57) or only a temporary effect (58) on circulating levels of NGF in mice and no permanent adverse effects on sympathetic function. However, given the controversy about the levels of NGF activity or antigen in peripheral circulation of rats and humans, perhaps this issue should be examined anew. A problem in the past has been that blood was usually collected following decapitation, a procedure likely to contaminate the collected blood samples with submaxillary gland fragments (59). Thus it is not clear whether the processing of pro-βNGF demonstrated for MSG plays a role in the regulation of that NGF activity endogenous to neuronal structures and pertinent to development of the peripheral nervous system of mammals.

5.   VENOM AND PROSTATE

Snake venom was found to be a rich source of nerve-growth-promoting activity before it was discovered in the MSG (2). Although *Bothrops jararaca*, *Brotalus atrox*, *Vipera russelli*, *Naja naja*, and *Crotalus adamenteus* all have snake venoms with NGF activity, only *V. russelli*, *C. adamenteus*, and *N. naja* have large enough amounts to be suitable for biochemical analysis (Table 3). The presence of protease activity in most snake venoms investigated might be the reason why no αβγ-like NGF complexes have been purified to date. The *N. naja* venom contains an active, although degraded NGF molecule (60,61). The *N. naja* NGF has been isolated as a low-molecular-weight protein, 25,000 daltons, with an isoelectric point of 6.6 (60). This species has a high degree of sequence homology to mouse βNGF, although it is less biologically active, and will not recombine with mouse αNGF and mouse γNGF subunits to form a complex (62). This is not surprising insofar as it appears that *N. naja* NGF is isolated in a degraded form because of the action of proteolytic enzymes endogenous to that par-

Table 3.   Nerve Growth Factor and Esterase Activity in Snake Venom

SAMPLE	BIOLOGICAL UNIT (ng)	ESTERASE ACTIVITY[a] (μmol/min/mg)
Mouse gland supernatant	400	4.11
NGF (mouse)	10	39.0
Snake venom		
Vipera russelli	729	0.14
Crotalus adamenteus	2000	0.28
Bothrops jararaca	2860	0.61
Naja naja	707	0.024

[a] The substrate used for the esterase assay was 5×10^{-4} _M_ TAME in phosphate buffer at pH 7.0, I = 0.2.

ticular snake venom (61). The _V. russelli_ NGF can be isolated as a basic (pI 9.3) polypeptide dimer (25,800 daltons) with a specific biological activity of 25–40 ng/biological unit and does not recombine with mouse α- and γNGF subunits since it lacks two arginine residues at the carboxyl terminus (61) (Fig. 4, Table 4).

From _C. adamenteus_ venom, NGF can be isolated as a $\gamma\beta$ complex or alternatively as a basic (pI 9.5) polypeptide dimer (βNGF) (Fig. 5) (63). The $\gamma\beta$ complex has a molecular weight of about 55,000, whereas the βNGF is 28,600 daltons. The presence of arginyl esterase activity in snake venom NGF is not surprising given that the tissue of origin is homologous to the mammalian submaxillary gland. Comparison of the amino acid composition and specific biological activity of the _C. adamenteus_ βNGF with murine βNGF from submaxillary gland shows them to be very similar (Table 5). This also is true of the γNGF from _C. adamenteus_, which is very similar to its murine counterpart. It has not been possible to construct hybrid NGF molecules (62,63), suggesting that there is a high degree of specificity among NGF subunits in their association as a complex (64).

In guinea pig prostate, NGF can also be isolated as a basic protein (30–60 ng/BU) or a high-molecular-weight complex (15). The βNGF-like dimer has a pI of 8.5 ± 0.5 and a molecular weight of 29,000 (15). Although NGF activity has been detected in the prostate glands of rabbit and bull, it is present there at lower concentrations and is not detectable in the male sex organs of the mouse, rat, hamster, or human (65). Guinea pig βNGF (gp-NGF) has a similar amino acid composition (Table 5) and sequence

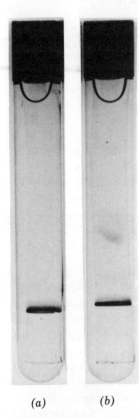

(a)   (b)

Figure 4. Isoelectric-focusing development of MSG-βNGF (A) and *Vipera russelli* NGF (B) in polyacrylamide disc gels.

to MSG-βNGF (87). Although antibodies directed against MSG-βNGF cross-react with both gp-NGF and rabbit prostate NGF (34% and 23% relative to MSG-βNGF, respectively), there is a much lower cross-reaction (less than 1%) to bovine prostate NGF (65). Since gp-NGF has an amino acid composition and partial sequence that is very similar to that of MSG-βNGF, it can be concluded that the active sites of NGF-like molecules from different species are highly conserved, although there are regions of high variability as demonstrated by immunological analysis.

6. HIGH-MOLECULAR-WEIGHT NGF

Although it was established early on that NGF activity could be detected associated with high-molecular-weight forms in MSG (45), various snake venoms (63,67), guinea pig prostate (15,66), and human placenta at term

Table 4. Purification of *Vipera russelli* NGF

Step	Protein (mg)	BU × 10⁻³	ng/BU
Snake venom	616	875	730
G 100	143	675	210
DEAE 11	44	205	215
G 150	3.7	87	90
CM 52	2.8	102	25

(16), the characterization of the oligomeric forms has lagged behind that of the active subunit often identified as β. The NGF γ MSG subunit, the arginyl endopeptidase, has recently been well characterized and sequenced (68,69) and found to be typical of the trypsin family of esterases. A similar subunit can be isolated in *C. adamenteus* NGF (63) with similar properties of size and charge and specific activity to its murine counterpart (Fig. 5).

Table 5. Amino Acid Compositions of NGFs from Various Sources

Amino Acid	Mouse Submaxillary (77)	Crotalus Adamenteus (63)	Guinea Pig Prostate (66)
Aspartic acid	11	14	16
Threonine	14	14	13
Serine	11	10	10
Glutamic acid	8	7	8
Proline	2	6	3
Glycine	5	13	6
Alanine	8	7	10
Half-cystine	6	6	6
Valine	13	10	14
Methionine	1	1	1
Isoleucine	5	5	3
Leucine	3	8	3
Tyrosine	2	2	2
Phenylalanine	7	4	7
Histidine	4	5	4
Lysine	8	8	9
Arginine	7	7	5
Tryptophan	3	3	4
Total	118	130	124

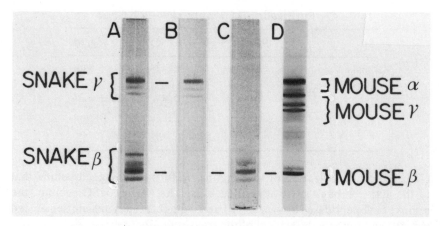

Figure 5.   Subunit composition of *Crotalus adamenteus* NGF. The subunit composition of *C. adamenteus* NGF was determined by isoelectric-focusing analysis in a linear 3.5–10 pH range in 7.5% polyacrylamide disc gels. (*A*) 50 μg of *C. adamenteus* NGF (γβ); (*B*) 25 μg of *C. adamenteus* γNGF isolated by flat-bed electrofocusing in a Sephadex G-75 granulated gel; (*C*) 25 μg of *C. adamenteus* βNGF isolated by flat-bed electrofocusing in a Sephadex G-75 granulated gel; (*D*) 50 μg of mouse 7S NGF.

The high-molecular-weight form of guinea pig NGF can also be dissociated and a β subunit isolated (15). However, there is no arginyl esterase activity in the oligomeric form of any of the subunits isolated to date (66), although such activity is present in the crude homogenates made from the gland (15).

Epidermal growth factor (EGF) isolated from MSG (70), a peptide with mitogenic action on many cell types, can be isolated bound to another subunit, the EGF-binding protein, which has arginyl esterase activity (71) and has been implicated in processing of pro-EGF forms (72). Again, no NGF-EGF (71) hybrids can be formed, illustrating the high degree of specificity of the oligomeric interactions.

7.   NONEXOCRINE SOURCE: HUMAN PLACENTA

Nerve growth factor can be isolated from human placenta using one of several protocols (Fig. 6). It can be isolated as a basic dimer with NGF-like activity (16,73) or can be copurified with an 80,000–140,000 dalton fraction similar to that isolated from MSG by Sephadex chromatography (16). From this high-molecular-weight fraction, a basic protein (pI 9.3) can be isolated by preparative isoelectric focusing in a sucrose gradient (Fig. 7). This basic protein, called human βNGF, has a specific biological activity of 1–3 ng/BU in the chick-embryo sensory-ganglia clot assay (16) as well

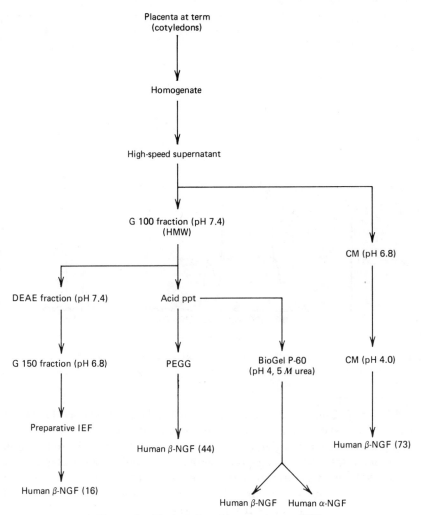

Figure 6.   The isolation of human placenta NGF.

as markedly stimulating differentiation of two different MSG-NGF-responsive human neuroblastoma clones (74). Analysis of human βNGF by dynamic isoelectric focusing yields a single protein band (Fig. 8). Analysis of pure human βNGF by electrophoresis in the presence of SDS yields a molecular weight of $14,260 \pm 700$ (44,73). Since gel-filtration experiments suggest that human βNGF has a molecular weight of about 30,000 daltons, human βNGF, like its murine counterpart, is a dimer held together by noncovalent bonds.

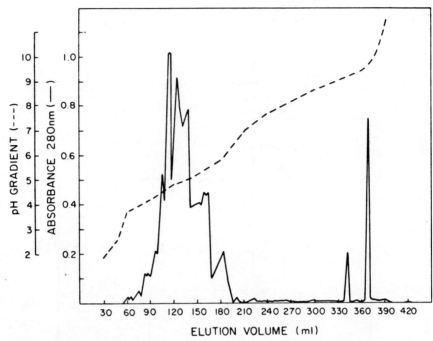

Figure 7.   Preparative isoelectric focusing in a sucrose-gradient column of 33 mg of the Sephadex G-150 human NGF fraction.

When rabbit antisera directed against purified human βNGF is challenged with mouse βNGF by immunodiffusion, there is no detectable cross-reaction (43). Similarly, when different preparations of human βNGF are tested in a two-site RIA for NGF using monospecific rabbit antibodies directed against MSG-βNGF, there is little cross-reaction (Table 6) (43,73). However, there are reports that by competition RIA using monoclonal antibodies against MSG-βNGF, there is a cross-reaction (75).

The isolation of β-like species from the high-molecular-weight human NGF requires not only a pH shift, but also the addition of 5 M urea, suggesting that, as is the case for guinea pig NGF, the NGF complex from human sources is more tightly bound than that from MSG or snake venom (15,44). It is curious and there may be a relationship between these differences in the affinity of the subunits for each other and the difficulty in identifying γ-like activity with NGF in both guinea pig prostate and human placenta at term.

In MSG-NGF, the γ endopeptidase is not active when in the 7S form, and activity is best detected in the free γ subunit (50). Thus activity can be used as an index of dissociation (48). Treatment of the complex of human NGF in a manner that would have caused dissociation and hence expression of arginyl esterase activity for mouse 7S NGF did not yield any esterase activity (44). Analytical isoelectric focusing of complexed human NGF supports the hypothesis that there are molecular species with size and charge properties similar to those of MSG-βNGF. However, since neither enzymatic activity nor cross-reaction to antisera directed against murine γNGF could be detected, it is reasonable to assume that only for salivary structures (mouse, snake), is NGF activity associated with an endopeptidase that plays a role in processing of pro-NGF forms. In guinea pig prostate and human placenta then, there is no evidence for either the existence of γ-like components or for processing of pro-βNGF forms.

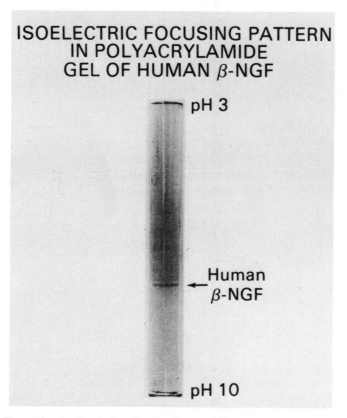

Figure 8.   Isoelectric-focusing development of human placenta βNGF in a polyacrylamide disc gel.

Table 6. Cross-Reactivity of Human Placental βNGF with Rabbit Anti-Mouse βNGF in the Two-Site RIA

Placenta Identification Code (n)	Method of Preparation of Human βNGF[a]	pI	mg/ml	Cross-Reactivity (%)
8 (6)	Sliced from IEF gels	—	0.094	0.027
8 (3)	Sliced from IEF gels	—	0.450	0.025
14-29 (2)	PEGG	—	0.505	0.006
14-30 (3)	PEGG	—	0.568	0.007
15CD-29 (3)	PEGG	9.32	0.509	0.008
15CD-29 (3)	PEGG	9.32	0.509	0.010
15CD-30 (3)	PEGG	9.55	0.485	0.014
15CD-30 (3)	PEGG	9.55	0.485	0.019
16AB-29 (2)	PEGG	9.26	0.575	0.049
16AB-29 (3)	PEGG	9.26	0.575	0.061
16AB-30 (3)	PEGG	9.45	0.690	0.043
16AB-30 (3)	PEGG	9.45	0.690	0.049

16CD-29 (3)	PEGG	9.21	0.433	0.012
16CD-29 (3)	PEGG	9.21	0.433	0.012
16CD-30 (3)	PEGG	9.46	0.442	0.013
16CD-30 (3)	PEGG	9.46	0.442	0.016
17AB-29 (3)	PEGG	9.10	0.337	0.080
17AB-29 (3)	PEGG	9.10	0.337	0.057
17AB-30 (3)	PEGG	9.41	0.409	0.016
17AB-30 (3)	PEGG	9.41	0.409	0.013
17CD-29 (3)	PEGG	—	0.804	0.002
17CD-29 (3)	PEGG	—	0.804	0.003
17CD-30 (3)	PEGG	—	0.609	0.007
17CD-30 (3)	PEGG	—	0.609	0.011
Average		9.34 ± 0.15		0.022 ± 0.020

[a] Fractions 29 and 30 of each PEGG preparation were tested at differing protein concentrations. Also tested for cross-reactivity were samples of human βNGF from slices of disc IEF gels.

Alternatively, there may be an arginyl esteropeptidase that processes human βNGF, but rather than remaining bound to the prohormone, the enzyme dissociates from the β after processing. Whether there is a different processing mechanism for putative pro-NGF forms in exocrine (MSG, snake venom glands) as opposed to endocrine NGF stores (human placenta) remains to be seen. The observations made on gp-NGF are too preliminary to provide any clues. It cannot be ruled out that there is a subunit associated with the human high-molecular-weight NGF complex with enzyme activity other than arginine esteropeptidase activity. However, analysis of the primary structure of several prohormones has revealed that processing usually occurs at basic amino acid residues, namely arginine or lysine residues. Further characterization is needed in order to determine if there are other similarities between the various high-molecular-weight forms of NGF.

Until recently the only NGF species having α-like subunits was MSG-NGF. Although there is no evidence that αNGF has biological or enzymatic properties, it has been suggested that αNGF stabilizes the 7S MSG-NGF complex (9). MSG-αNGF consists of a heterogeneous group of four 26,500-dalton polypeptides. Each of the α subunits is made up of two peptide chains of dissimilar sizes held together by disulfide bridges (76). Although there is evidence that a high-molecular-weight form of NGF similar in size to MSG-NGF is present in C. adamenteus and V. russelli (61), because of ongoing proteolytic events during purification, only a γβ complex can be isolated from C. adamenteus snake venom (63). It was therefore of great interest that in human placenta at term, preparative isoelectric focusing of oligomeric NGF yields, in addition to the basic peptide with which all nerve-growth-promoting activity is associated, βNGF, other more acidic proteins (Fig. 7). Analysis of these acidic proteins by immunodiffusion against antibodies directed against mouse-αNGF gave positive results (44). Comparison of the range of isoelectric points of the human α subunits compared with their murine counterparts and the high degree of immunological cross-reaction suggests that these α-like peptides are very similar. Since not much is known about the role of α in MSG-NGF, it is difficult to speculate about the significance of these findings.

Perhaps of more importance, these results suggest a possible explanation for the many conflicting reports about the levels of NGF in human serum. That is, values obtained for NGF levels would depend on the degree of anti-α present in the antisera used. This in turn would depend on the amount of α present in the MSG-NGF used as antigen. Studies using bioassays have also given contradictory results. There are studies showing no NGF activity in mouse or rat serum (27) or in human serum (42). There are many reports of detectable levels of NGF activity in human serum, although in some instances it is reported that a proportion of samples showed no activity whatsoever (10). In all instances, when activity was detected, it was only after various manipulations of the serum (10). Also, the assays used were not always equivalent, and in some instances actual photographs are not provided, making evaluation of results difficult. Thus it might be necessary to wait for results based on RIAs using antibodies directed against human β-NGF before making definitive conclusions.

8. SUMMARY

In most instances, NGF can be isolated as a stable subunit-containing protein complex that can be reversibly dissociated through pH shifts. Although a basic protein (βNGF, the biologically active subunit) is structurally similar in all species investigated to date, it is not definite whether the processing of pro-βNGF forms, as demonstrated in the MSG, is relevant to nonsalivary tissues and/or the ambient levels of NGF in neural structures. The association of subunits into a high-molecular-weight complex is highly specific and does not allow for interspecies hybrids. Both biological and enzymatic activities of subunits are suppressed in the high-molecular-weight species, suggesting an *in vivo* regulatory role for the NGF quaternary structure. The regulation of NGF activity via dissociation/association phenomena *in vivo* may have different properties in different tissues. This may be significant in understanding the role that NGF plays in the normal development of the sensory and sympathetic system of mammals.

Although it has been suggested that a number of neuropathies result in altered levels of NGF in human sera, reports are difficult to evaluate at this time because there are components in human sera that interfere with both competitive binding and two-site RIAs for NGF. When monospecific affinity-purified antibodies to mouse βNGF are used, it is not possible to demonstrate the presence of βNGF antigen in human sera, although there is evidence for NGF activity. However, since there is no significant level of immuno-logical cross-reaction between mouse βNGF and human βNGF, the conclusion that there is no endogenous NGF in human sera must remain tentative.

Human NGF can be isolated as a high-molecular-weight complex of ~140,000 daltons that can be dissociated by a shift in pH and the addition of 5 M urea. The biological activity resides in a basic subunit, βNGF. The molecular weight of the βNGF monomer is 14,260 $\pm$ 700. Oligomeric human NGF contains a subunit whose pH and antigenic recognition by anti-MSG-αNGF has prompted us to call it human αNGF. All evidence to date indicates that there is no arginine esteropeptidase activity associated with a subunit in the human NGF complex. Thus further studies on human NGF will be useful in elucidating regulatory features pertinent to both normal and abnormal neural development.

ACKNOWLEDGMENTS

Supported by NINCDS Grants NS14034 and NS15324 and Robert A. Welch Foundation Grant H698 and RCDA NS00213 to J.R.P-P. The authors wish to thank Barbara Dzambo for manuscript preparation.

REFERENCES

1. Ramón y Cajal, S. *Degeneration and Regeneration of the Nervous System.* London: Oxford Univ. Press (1928).
2. Cohen, S. *J. Biol. Chem.*, **234**, 1129 (1959).
3. Cohen, S. *Proc. Natl. Acad. Sci. USA*, **46**, 302 (1960).
4. Levi-Montalcini, R., Meyer, H., and Hamburger, V., *Cancer Res.*, **14**, 49 (1954).
5. Greene, L. A., and Shooter, E. M., *Annu. Rev. Neurosci.*, **3**, 353 (1980).
6. Hedlund, K.-O., and Ebendal, T., *J. Neurocytol.*, **9**, 665 (1980).
7. Varon, S., *Annu. Rev. Neurosci.*, **1**, 327 (1978).
8. Bradshaw, R. A., *Annu. Rev. Biochem.*, **47**, 191 (1978).
9. Server, A. C., and Shooter, E. M., *Adv. Protein Chem.*, **31**, 339 (1977).
10. Freed, W. J., *Brain Res. Bull.*, **1**, 393 (1976).
11. Kimble, D. P., Bremiller, R., and Perez-Polo, J. R., *Physiol. Behav.*, **23**, 653 (1979).
12. Mobley, W. C., Server, A. C., Ishii, D. N., Riopelle, R. J., and Shooter, E. M., *N. Engl. J. Med.*, **297**, 1096, 1149, and 1211 (1977).
13. Perez-Polo, J. R., Dy, P., Westlund, K., Hall, K., and Livingston, K., *Birth Defects: Orig. Art. Ser.*, **14**, 311 (1978).
14. Rosenberg, R. N., *N. Engl. J. Med.*, **305**, 1181 (1981).
15. Chapman, C. A., Banks, B. E. C., Carstairs, J. R., Pearce, F. L., and Vernon, C. A., *FEBS Lett.*, **105**, 341 (1979).
16. Goldstein, L. D., Reynolds, C. P., and Perez-Polo, J. R., *Neurochem Res.*, **3**, 175 (1978).
17. Varon, S., Nomura, J., Perez-Polo, J. R., and Shooter, E. M., in R. Fried, Ed., *Methods in Neurochemistry*, Dekker, New York, 1972, vol. 3, p. 203.
18. Ebendal, T., Olson, L., Seiger, Å., and Hedlund, K.-O., *Nature*, **286**, 25 (1980).
19. Mizel, S. B., and Bamburg, J. R., *Dev. Biol.*, **49**, 11 (1976).
20. Greene, L. A., *Neurobiology*, **4**, 286 (1974).
21. Schulze, I., and Perez-Polo, J. R., *J. Neurosci. Res.*, in press.
22. Manthorpe, M., Skaper, S. D., and Varon, S., *Brain Res.*, **230**, 295 (1981).
23. Greene, L. A., *Brain Res.*, **133**, 350 (1977).
24. Reynolds, C. P., and Perez-Polo, J. R., *J. Neurosci. Res.*, **6**, 319 (1981).
25. Edgar, D., Barde, Y-A., and Thoenen, H., *Nature*, **289**, 294 (1981).
26. Perez-Polo, J. R., Beck, C. E., and Blum, M., in C. Baxter and T. Melnechuk, Eds., *Perspective in Schizophrenia Research*, Raven, New York, 1980, p. 237.
27. Suda, K., Barde, Y.-A., and Thoenen, H., *Proc. Natl. Acad. Sci. USA*, **75**, 4042 (1978).
28. Burdman, J. A., and Goldstein, M. N., *J. Natl. Cancer Inst.*, **33**, 123 (1964).

29. Meyer, W. J., Schochet, S. S., Perez-Polo, J. R., Werrbach-Perez, K., Davis, A., and Haggard, M. E., *Bull. Cancer*, **67**, 333 (1980).

30. Hill, A. H., Seibert, E. S., Beckwith, J. B., and Hartmann, J. R., *J. Natl. Cancer Inst.*, **43**, 1121 (1969).

31. Reynolds, C. P., Perez-Polo, J. R., and Smith, R. G., *Clin. Res.*, **26**, 796a (1978).

32. Siggers, D. C., Rogers, J. G., Boyer, S. H., Margolet, L., Dorkin, H., Banerjee, S. P., and Shooter, E. M., *N. Engl. J. Med.*, **295**, 629 (1976).

33. Schwartz, J. P., and Breakefield, X. O., *Proc. Natl. Acad. Sci. USA*, **77**, 1154 (1980).

34. Schenkein, I. Bueker, E. D., and Helson, L., *N. Engl. J. Med.*, **290**, 613 (1974).

35. Siggers, D. C., Boyer, S. H., and Eldridge, R., *N. Engl. J. Med.*, **292**, 1134 (1975).

36. Fabricant, R. N., and Todaro, G. J., *Arch. Neurol.*, **38**, 401 (1981).

37. Waddell, W. R., Goldstein, M. N., Bradshaw, R. A., and Kirsch, W. M., *Lancet*, **1**, 1365 (1972).

38. Cramer, S. F., Bradshaw, R. A., Baglan, N. C., and Meyers, J. A., *Hum. Pathol.*, **10**, 731 (1979).

39. Stahn, R., Rose, R., Sanborn, S., West, G., and Herschman, H., *Brain Res.*, **96**, 287 (1975).

40. Vinores, S. A., and Perez-Polo, J. R., *J. Neurosci. Res.*, **5**, 351 (1980).

41. Vinores, S. A., and Perez-Polo, J. R., *J. Cancer Res.*, **98**, 59 (1980).

42. Skaper, S. D., and Varon, S., *Dev. Neurosci.*, in press.

43. Beck, C. E., Blum, M., Turpin, K., Jacque, C., and Perez-Polo, J. R., *Soc. Neurosci. Abstr.*, **7**, 552 (1981).

44. Blum, M., Beck, C. E., and Perez-Polo, J. R., *Soc. Neurosci. Abstr.* **7**, 145 (1981).

45. Varon, S., Nomura, J., and Shooter, E. M., *Biochemistry*, **6**, 2202 (1967).

46. Greene, L. A., Varon, S., Piltch, A., and Shooter, E. M., *Neurobiology*, **1**, 37 (1971).

47. Moore, J. B., Jr., Mobley, W. C., and Shooter, E. M., *Biochemistry*, **13**, 833 (1974).

48. Perez-Polo, J. R., and Shooter, E. M., *Neurobiology*, **5**, 329 (1975).

49. Perez-Polo, J. R., and Shooter, E. M., *Neurobiology*, **4**, 197 (1974).

50. Greene, L. A., Shooter, E. M., and Varon, S., *Proc. Natl. Acad. Sci. USA*, **60**, 1383 (1968).

51. Berger, E. A., and Shooter, E. M., *J. Biol. Chem.*, **253**, 804 (1978).

52. Schwab, M. E., Stöckel, K., and Thoenen, H., *Cell Tiss. Res.*, **169**, 289 (1976).

53. Wallace, L. J., and Partlow, L. M., *Proc. Natl. Acad. Sci. USA*, **73**, 4210 (1976).

54. Stach, R., personal communication.

55. Aloe, L., Calissano, P., and Levi-Montalcini, R., in preparation.

56. Watson, L. C., Townsend, C. M., Jr., Perez-Polo, J. R., and Thompson, J. C., Proceedings of 1981 Meeting of Surgical Forum at San Francisco, Calif.

57. Murphy, R. A., Saide, J. D., Blanchard, M. H., and Young, M., *Proc. Natl. Acad. Sci. USA*, **74**, 2330 (1977).

58. Hendry, I. A., and Iversen, L. L., *Nature*, **243**, 500 (1973).

59. Harper, G. P., and Thoenen, H., *J. Neurochem.*, **34**, 5 (1980).

60. Hogue-Angeletti, R. A., Frazier, W. A., Jacobs, J. W., Niall, H. D., and Bradshaw, R. A., *Biochemistry*, **15**, 26 (1976).

61. Morton, M. E., and Perez-Polo, J. R., *Trans. Am. Soc. Neurochem.* **5**, 75 (1974).

62. Server, A. C., Herrup, K., Shooter, E. M., Hogue-Angeletti, R. A., Frazier, W. A., and Bradshaw, R. A., *Biochemistry*, **15**, 35 (1976).

63. Perez-Polo, J. R., Bomer, H., Beck, C., and Hall, K., *J. Biol. Chem.*, **253**, 6140 (1978).

64. Shine, H. D., and Perez-Polo, J. R., *J. Neurochem.*, **26**, 513 (1976).

65. Harper, G. P., and Thoenen, H., *J. Neurochem.*, **34**, 893 (1980).

66. Rubin, J., and Bradshaw, R. A., *J. Neurosci. Res.*, **6**, 451 (1981).

67. Angeletti, P., Calissano, P., Chen, J. S., and Levi-Montalcini, R., *Biochim. Biophys. Acta*, **147**, 180 (1967).

68. Thomas, K. A., Silverman, R. E., Jeng, I., Baglan, N. C., and Bradshaw, R. A., *J. Biol. Chem.*, **256**, 9147 (1981).

69. Thomas, K. A., Baglan, N. C., and Bradshaw, R. A., *J. Biol. Chem.*, **256**, 9156 (1981).

70. Carpenter, G., and Cohen, S., *Annu. Rev. Biochem.*, **48**, 193 (1979).

71. Server, A. C., and Shooter, E. M., *J. Biol. Chem.*, **251**, 165 (1976).

72. Frey, P., Forand, R., Maciag, T., and Shooter, E. M., *Proc. Natl. Acad. Sci. USA*, **76**, 6294 (1979).

73. Walker, P., Weichsel, M. E., and Fisher, D. A., *Life Sci.*, **26**, 195 (1980).

74. Perez-Polo, J. R., Reynolds, C. P., Tiffany-Castiglioni, E., Ziegler, M., Schulze, I., and Werrbach-Perez, K., in B. Haber, J. R. Perez-Polo and J. D. Coulter, Eds., *Proteins in the Nervous System*, Alan R. Liss, New York, 1982.

75. Warren, S. L., Fanger, M., and Neet, K. E., *Science*, **210**, 910 (1980).

76. Stach, R. W., Pignatti, P. F., Baker, M. E., and Shooter, E. M., *J. Neurochem.*, **34**, 850 (1980).

3

THE AUTOIMMUNE APPROACH TO THE STUDY OF NERVE GROWTH FACTOR AND OTHER GROWTH FACTORS

Eugene M. Johnson, Jr.

CONTENTS

Abbreviations

NGF	Nerve growth factor
anti-NGF	Antibodies to nerve growth factor
DRG	Dorsal root ganglion
SCG	Superior cervical ganglion
CNS	Central nervous system
TH	Tyrosine hydroxylase

Nerve growth factor (NGF) is one of the most thoroughly studied of the "growth factors." It is probably the factor that has been most studied *in vivo*, and it is the only factor whose physiological role has been clarified to even a modest extent. The state of our understanding of the biology of NGF is reviewed in Chapters 1 and 2 of this volume and in several recent reviews. The purpose of this chapter is to describe an experimental approach that we have developed in this laboratory to attempt to better understand the role of NGF in the development and maintenance of NGF-responsive cell types.

1. STUDIES WITH HETEROLOGOUS ANTI-NGF

In vivo studies of NGF have involved one of two approaches. In the first approach, exogenous NGF is administered to animals and the effects of this administration on various tissues are examined. The experiments provide demonstrations of *pharmacological* effects of exogenous NGF. They can only be suggestive of a physiological role for NGF.

A second approach to the study of the role of a hormone or "factor" is to deprive the animal of the factor and observe the adverse effects of the deprivation on the whole animal. In cases where the hormone or factor has a discrete biological source (e.g., insulin), surgical ablation or chemical destruction of the tissue that produces the hormone may be carried out to produce deprivation. Antagonists of the hormone, when available, may be chronically administered, and the effects of denying the hormone access to its receptor can be assessed.

Neither of these approaches is applicable to the study of the physiological role of NGF. There is no single discrete source of physiologically active NGF since it presumably is elaborated by all tissues that are innervated by NGF-responsive or dependent neuronal types. Likewise, no antagonists of NGF have been developed. However, NGF deprivation has been produced by the administration of heterologous antibodies to mouse NGF (anti-NGF), thus providing a second approach to the study of the physiological role of

NGF. Original studies by Levi-Montalcini, Cohen, and co-workers demonstrated that administration of antisera against mouse NGF to newborn of several species results in the destruction of the peripheral sympathetic nervous system (immunosympathectomy) (1–3). Over the ensuing two decades, many studies have been carried out to assess the range of effects caused by the administration of anti-NGF. These studies, mostly conducted in neonatal animals, demonstrated that paravertebral and prevertebral sympathetic ganglia are destroyed by administration of anti-NGF. Destruction of other neural crest derivatives, such as dorsal root ganglion neurons, adrenal medullary cells, and short adrenergic neurons of the male genitalia, does not occur, despite the fact that these cell types may respond to NGF in a variety of ways *in vitro* or *in vivo* (4). In contrast with the massive destruction of sympathetic neurons caused by even a few injections of anti-NGF in the neonate, injection of anti-NGF up to 5 days in adult mice does not result in destruction of neurons even though there is atrophy of the cells (5,6).

The ability to equate the effects of anti-NGF with those of NGF deprivation depends upon the assumption that anti-NGF does not produce a toxic effect on the cell (e.g., complement-mediated lysis). Considerable evidence now supports this assumption. Anti-NGF produces sympathectomy in complement-deficient animals (7,8), the effects of anti-NGF are reversible in neonates for up to 48 hours by compensatory doses of NGF (8), and anti-mouse NGF from avian source produces sympathectomy in neonatal rats (unpublished observations), although it cannot fix mammalian complement. These observations, coupled with the demonstration that sympathetic neurons require NGF for survival *in vitro*, argue strongly that NGF deprivation is the mechanism by which cell death occurs *in vivo*.

It is much more difficult to induce NGF deprivation by administration of heterologous anti-NGF at times other than the neonatal period. In the adult animal, administration of anti-NGF for 5 days produces biochemical and morphological atrophy, but not death, of sympathetic neurons. Hence mature sympathetic neurons are clearly not as acutely dependent on NGF for survival as are immature sympathetic neurons. Whether longer-term NGF deprivation would result in cell death cannot be determined by this approach, since it is not practical to continue to give heterologous antisera for long periods because of the immunological response in the recipient to the sera (e.g., serum sickness).

Administration of anti-NGF to neonates does not, of course, provide any information about the role of NGF prenatally, during which many critical events in neuronal development occur. One approach that has been used is to inject anti-NGF directly into the fetus (9,10). This approach is technically difficult and traumatic and does not allow repeated administration and, therefore, a continuous supply of antisera to the fetus. It does, however, have the advantage of allowing a precise determination of when the fetus is first exposed to antibody.

2.   RATIONALE FOR AN AUTOIMMUNE APPROACH

In an effort to overcome these inherent limitations in the use of heterologous anti-NGF as a means of producing NGF deprivation, Pamela Gorin and I examined the possibility that an animal immunized with mouse NGF would produce antibodies that would cross-react with its own NGF and would thus produce an "autoimmune NGF deprivation." In our initial experiments (11) we demonstrated that sera from rats immunized with mouse NGF produce an immunosympathectomy when injected into neonatal rats. The ability of rat anti-mouse NGF to destroy the sympathetic nervous system of neonatal rats confirmed the similar observation, made in the original work on immunosympathectomy (1), that rabbit anti-mouse NGF destroys the sympathetic ganglia of newborn rabbits.

These data indicate that both the rat and the rabbit make antibodies directed against mouse NGF that cross-react with their own NGF. We could not test this supposition directly *in vitro*, since authentic rat or rabbit NGF's were not available. Subsequently, with the availability of guinea pig (12) NGF, we demonstrated that the guinea pig anti-mouse NGF neutralized guinea pig NGF *in vitro* in the classical dorsal root ganglion (DRG) bioassay system (13,14).

Satisfied that the autoimmune approach to NGF deprivation was feasible, we asked two general questions:

1.   What effects are seen in an adult mouse-NGF-immunized animal that is making antibodies against its own NGF?
2.   What effects are seen in the offspring of such an animal when exposed to maternal anti-NGF prenatally and/or postnatally?

Using this approach, we hoped to study the effects of NGF deprivation both much earlier and later than had been done by the use of heterologous anti-NGF. I describe below many of the observations we have made in these animals and also some of the problems we have encountered with respect to variability of responses, and our attempts to resolve these problems. Finally, I speculate on possible implications relative to human birth defects and on the potential that this experimental approach may have in the study of other "growth factors."

3.   EFFECTS IN ADULT ANIMAL IMMUNIZED WITH NGF

Our initial objective was to use the autoimmune approach as a means of producing long-term NGF deprivation to determine whether the mature sympathetic neuron requires NGF for *survival* as well as for normal function. As previously mentioned, the administration of heterologous anti-NGF for 5 days to adult mice results in atrophy, but not death, of sympathetic neurons as would be seen in the neonate. Although these experiments demonstrated that the mature neuron is less acutely dependent on NGF for survival than the immature neuron, they could not determine whether long-term NGF deprivation would or would not affect neuronal survival. In order to determine the effects of long-term NGF deprivation, we (15) immunized adult outbred Sprague-Dawley rats with mouse NGF (100 μg of 2.5S mouse NGF in complete Freund's adjuvant, boosting monthly with 10–15 μg of NGF in the same adjuvant). These rats developed highly variable titers against mouse NGF as assessed in the DRG bioassay. Rarely were titers greater than 1000 observed. The titer of antibody against *rat* NGF was not known since authentic rat NGF was not and is not yet available. The animals were assessed after about 6 months. We observed marked decreases in norepinephrine levels in peripheral tissues (heart, spleen, brown fat) and decreases in the enzymes involved in norepinephrine biosynthesis in sympathetic ganglia (superior cervical and celiac). Decreases in these parameters ranged from 60 to 90% in animals with titers >500. A general correlation existed between the decreases in these parameters and the titers against mouse NGF. Examination of superior cervical ganglia (SCG) from these animals at the light microscope level showed obvious atrophy of sympathetic neurons and an apparent decrease in neuronal number (photomicrographs shown in reference 15).

Table 1. Neuronal Counts, Protein Content, and Tyrosine Hydroxylase Activity in the SCG of Adult Rats Immunized With NGF

EXPERIMENTAL GROUP[a]	NEURONAL NUMBER IN SCG	PROTEIN CONTENT (mg/SCG)	TYROSINE HYDROXYLASE ACTIVITY (nmol tyrosine/ SCG/hour)
Control (n = 4)	28,180 ± 1277	0.22 ± 0.02	3.50 ± 0.36
NGF-immunized (n = 4)	18,598 ± 922	0.13 ± 0.03	0.31 ± 0.09

Source: Data taken from and methods detailed in reference 15.
[a] Rats were immunized with 100 μg of NGF in complete Freund's adjuvant and boosted with 10–20 μg of NGF in complete Freund's adjuvant at 4–6-week intervals for 5 months. Serum titers of anti-NGF were ≥500<1000. Controls were age-matched rats that were either immunized with cytochrome c or were unimmunized.

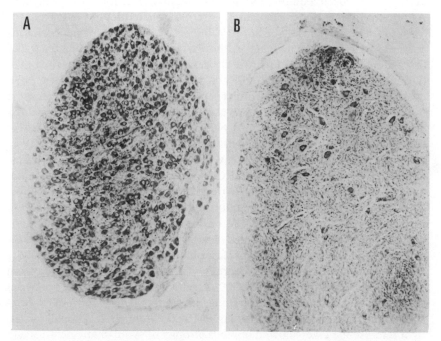

Figure 1. Photomicrographs of toluidine-blue-stained sections of SCGs of adult female rabbits. (*A*) Control rabbit immunized with cytochrome *c*. (*B*) Rabbit immunized for >10 months against NGF. Sections are from midpoint of ganglia. The larger size of the section from the NGF-immunized rabbit is due to the angle of section and not to an enlargement of the ganglion. Taken from reference 16.

In order to quantitate these changes, Gorin performed a morphometric analysis to determine the number of neurons in the SCGs of control and NGF-immunized rats. Results of the analysis are shown in Table 1. Chronic immunization with NGF resulted in a 35% decrease in the number of neurons in the SCG.

The chronically-immunized rabbit presented more impressive evidence for neuronal death (16). Rabbits generated much higher titers of antibody against mouse NGF, usually >2000, although, as in the rat, we could not determine titers against *rabbit* NGF. A much more profound destruction of sympathetic neurons in the SCG occurred in rabbits with high titers. Light micrographs of cross-sections of the SCG taken from a normal rabbit (Fig. 1*A*) and from an age-matched rabbit immunized for over 10 months (Fig. 1*B*) show the marked neuronal loss. The number of neurons in this affected ganglion was 9700 compared with 75,900 ± 5000 (*n* = 3) in SCGs from normal animals. The SCGs from guinea pigs immunized in a similar manner also showed massive destruction of neurons.

The most straightforward interpretation of our results is that the NGF deprivation induced by antibody directed against NGF causes the neuronal death, thus arguing that the mature sympathetic neuron continues to require NGF for *survival* throughout the entire life of the animal. Other mechanisms of neuronal destruction, although unlikely for a variety of reasons, cannot be absolutely excluded. It is possible that some immunological mechanism (e.g., cytotoxic T cells, antibody-dependent cell-mediated cytotoxicity, delayed hypersensitivity, complement-mediated cytotoxicity) is responsible for the cell death.

We have not yet performed detailed analysis of other cell types. In the Sprague-Dawley rat we observed no adverse effects on short adrenergic neurons or on the adrenal medulla. We observed no obvious light microscopic changes in DRG sensory neurons. A more detailed analysis of these tissues in the species that generate higher titers or that have been immunized for longer periods of time should be conducted.

4. ADVERSE EFFECTS OF MATERNAL ANTI-NGF ON THE DEVELOPING OFFSPRING

Over the last few years we have carried out a partial analysis of the effects of maternal anti-NGF on the developing rat, rabbit, and guinea pig (11,16,17,18, and unpublished data). Female Sprague-Dawley rats when immunized with mouse NGF developed variable titers of antibody to mouse NGF. Some, but not all, of these animals that had titers of $>500<1000$ produced offspring that *at birth* showed clear evidence of adverse effects of maternal anti-NGF. The SCGs of these newborn rats were markedly reduced in size and had very low levels of tyrosine hydroxylase (TH) activity. More interestingly, the DRGs of these animals were moderately reduced in size (about a 30% decrease in protein content). Anti-NGF-producing female rats produced litters of normal size, and the offspring grew normally. Titers of antibody in the sera of newborn rats (prior to suckling) were $>10<25$. In cross-fostering experiments, offspring *born to* a normal rat but *nursed by* an anti-NGF rat had higher titers of antibody at 2 weeks of age than the offspring born to the anti-NGF rat had at birth. The offspring born to a normal rat but suckled by an anti-NGF-producing rat showed a marked decrease in the size and TH activity of the SCG, but no decrease in the size of the DRG. The offspring grew normally, had no gross sensory deficits, but were ptotic, indicating sympathetic denervation of the eye. A summary of some effects in sympathetic and dorsal root ganglia of animals allowed

Table 2.   Permanent Changes in Rats Born to and/or Nursed by Anti-NGF-Producing Mothers

	EXPOSURE TO MATERNAL ANTI-NGF			
PARAMETER[a]	NONE	IN UTERO	IN MILK	BOTH
Tyrosine hydroxylase in SCG	100	8 ± 3	11 ± 2	1.5 ± 0.5
Neurons in SCG	100	7 ± 1	9 ± 1	ND[b]
Protein content of DRG (C8)	100	71 ± 8	93 ± 6	77 ± 13
Retrograde transport of NGF in DRG (C5–C8)	100	24 ± 3	78 ± 6	15 ± 5
Neurons in DRG (C8)	100	31 ± 2	104 ± 4	ND
Substance P in DRG (per mg protein)	100	ND	ND	44 ± 3

[a] All values expressed as percentage of control. Data taken from references 11,17,18, and 19. These data are from the most severely affected litters.
[b] ND = not determined.

to reach adulthood is shown in Table 2. Exposure to maternal anti-NGF, either prenatally or postnatally, destroys sympathetic neurons; only prenatal exposure results in destruction of DRG neurons. These data indicate that DRG neurons go through a phase prenatally during which NGF is required for their *survival*, and this dependence is lost postnatally.

Several other catecholamine-synthesizing tissues were also examined. No changes in catecholamine levels and/or TH activity were found in the adrenal gland, vas deferens (innervated by short adrenergic neurons), or in the central nervous system (CNS) (brain stem, spinal cord, forebrain). These results suggest that NGF is not necessary for survival of either short adrenergic neurons or adrenal medullary cells. No conclusion can be reached from this negative data on brain since we have no data on the access of antibody to the developing CNS.

The ability to use this experimental approach to explore the role of NGF in early developmental events is limited by the amount of antibody passively transferred from mother to fetus and the time in gestation when this transfer occurs. There are marked species differences in the time and quantity of antibody transferred during gestation. General patterns in different species are shown in Table 3, which is taken from the monograph by Brambell (20). As shown in the table, in the rat relatively little antibody is transferred prenatally; most antibody is transferred postnatally via the milk. Our results in the rat are consistent with this pattern of transfer. One would expect more dramatic effects in those species in which large amounts of maternal antibody are passively transferred prenatally. Of the common laboratory animals, this occurs in rabbits and guinea pigs. Higher primates and humans also passively transfer large quantities of antibody prenatally.

Because of these properties of passive transfer, we continued our studies in rabbits and guinea pigs. In our experience, outbred rabbits and guinea pigs produce higher titers of anti-NGF than do the Sprague-Dawley rats. Again, although considerable variability occurs, titers of 8000 against mouse NGF are not unusual. At the time of this writing, our analysis of the effects of maternal anti-NGF in rabbits is preliminary. It is clear, however, that the permanent destruction of the rabbit sympathetic nervous system is not as great as might be anticipated, and that the effects of maternal anti-NGF are far less profound than those in the guinea pig (16). Offspring, born to anti-NGF-producing female rabbits, which survive to adulthood show no obvious sensory deficits. A morphometric analysis of the effects of maternal anti-NGF on the DRG of developing rabbits has shown effects similar to those in the rat (16).

Table 3. Time of Transmission of Passive Immunity from Mother to Offspring in Several Species

Species	Transmission of Passive Immunity		
	Prenatal	Postnatal	(duration)
Horse	0	+++	(24 hours)
Pig	0	+++	(24–36 hours)
Ox, goat, sheep	0	+++	(24 hours)
Wallaby	0	+++	(180 days)
Dog, cat	+	++	(1–2 days)
Fowl	++	++	(5 days)
Hedgehog	+	++	(40 days)
Mouse	+	++	(16 days)
Rat	+	++	(20 days)
Guinea pig	+++	0	
Rabbit	+++	0	
Man, monkey	+++	0	

Source: Taken from monograph by Brambell [(20), p. 14].

The most striking effects of maternal anti-NGF can be seen in the guinea pig. In contrast to rats, at birth newborn guinea pigs have titers of anti-NGF comparable to those of the mothers. Because authentic guinea pig NGF is available, it is possible to test directly the cross-reactivity of guinea pig anti-mouse NGF against guinea pig NGF. There is considerable variability in the degree of cross-reactivity in the antibodies made by individual guinea pigs. Immunized female guinea pigs that make antibodies that cross-react poorly with guinea pig NGF produce pups that are essentially normal. The offspring of female guinea pigs that make antibodies that cross-react well with guinea pig NGF show marked abnormalities. These offspring are normal in appearance and size at birth and appear to be as well coordinated as a newborn control guinea pig. By 2 days of age, however, the affected pups are clearly abnormal. They lose rather than gain weight and develop bilateral corneal opacities. A bizarre occurrence noted in some litters is that the sows chew the ears off the pups. Upon closer examination it is apparent that the offspring are unresponsive to pinches, pin pricks, heat, cold, or noxious irritants. A particularly impressive demonstration of their lack of sensation is that a solution of capsaicin, the active principle of hot peppers, can be instilled directly onto the cornea with absolutely no response from the animal. The loss of body weight in these animals appears to be due to an inability to suckle, as animals killed within the first few days after birth have little or no milk in their stomachs. If left unaided, these animals die within a few days. We have prolonged the life of a few animals to about 2 weeks by removing them from their mother, feeding them with a syringe,

Table 4.   Effects of Exposure to Maternal Antibodies to NGF on Neuronal Numbers in Peripheral Ganglia of Newborn Guinea Pigs

Status of Mother	Ganglion[a]		
	Superior Cervical	8th Cervical DRG	Nodose
Control (unim-munized)	57,600 ± 5080 (3)	15,500 ± 180 (3)	15,900 ± 980 (3)
NGF-im-munized			
Litter 1	280 ± 130 (5)	3,120 ± 96 (3)	15,500 ± 1530 (3)
Litter 2		2,280 ± 156 (3)	

Source: Data taken from and methods described in reference 18.
[a] Values are mean ± SEM of number of animals shown in parentheses.

and attending to their other problems, such as the eye ulcers. With this nursing, the animals gain weight for a few days but eventually revert to the downhill course and die. At death, the most obvious gross anomaly is a greatly enlarged bladder, possibly due to lack of sensation necessary to induce micturition. The precise reason(s) for their demise has not yet been determined.

A morphometric analysis of three different ganglia was carried out by Dr. John Pearson (18). Cell counts in the SCG, the eighth cervical DRG, and the nodose ganglia are shown in Table 4. The SCG was reduced to a minute thread that contained less than 1% of the neurons in ganglia from normal neonatal guinea pigs. The number of neurons in eighth cervical DRG was reduced by 80% in one litter and by 85% in a litter from a different immunized guinea pig. In contrast with the DRG, the nodose ganglion showed no change in the number of neurons. The nodose ganglion (Xth nerve) is derived embryologically from the epidermal placodes rather than from neural crest as are the DRG. These data argue that at least 85% of the

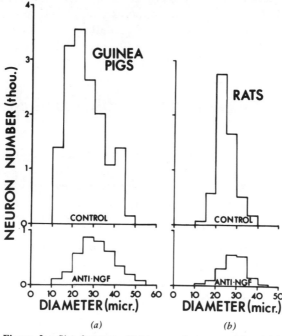

Figure 2. Size-frequency histograms of neurons of the eighth cervical DRG in (a) normal animals and (b) animals exposed *in utero* to maternal antibodies to NGF. Guinea pigs were killed within 2 days of birth. Rats were killed at 16–20 weeks of age. Data taken from and methods described in reference 18.

sensory neurons of neural crest origin go through a phase of NGF dependence, but that sensory neurons of placodal origin do *not* go through a phase of NGF dependence. The latter conclusion is consistent with some (21), but not all (22), of the literature on the effect of NGF *in vitro* on neurons from the nodose ganglia.

Size-frequency histograms of the neurons in the DRG of rats and guinea pigs exposed to maternal anti-NGF *in utero* are shown in Fig. 2. In both species there was a greater loss of neurons of smaller diameters than of neurons of large diameters. This was especially true in the rat. It is clear, however, that in the guinea pig, sensory neurons of large diameters were also decreased in number.

Despite the dramatic effects on DRG neurons and long adrenergic neurons, other cell types that are to some extent responsive to exogenous NGF were not affected. We found little or no effect on norepinephrine levels in vas deferens, thus providing further evidence that short adrenergic neurons do not require NGF for survival. We likewise observed no adverse effects on the developing adrenal medulla of any of the species studied. Examination of adrenals by light microscopy, histofluorescence, or TH activity provided no evidence for degeneration of adrenal medullary cells, such as has been described by Aloe and Levi-Montalcini (10), even in those animals that had suffered massive destruction of sympathetic and sensory ganglia.

5.   UTILITY OF THE AUTOIMMUNE APPROACH TO DEFINE FURTHER THE ROLE OF NGF

The results of our studies to date demonstrate the potential of this experimental autoimmune approach in the study of the biological roles of NGF. The animals produced, particularly the guinea pigs, are unique in terms of anatomical lesions and functional deficits. Many questions regarding the physiological role of NGF remain to be explored in these animals:

1.   Are there detrimental effects on other neural-crest-derived cell types (e.g., enteric nervous system) when a fetus is deprived of NGF?.

2.   What is the basis for the survival of the 15–20% of DRG neurons that do not die? What sensory modalities are impaired and to what degree?

3.   What secondary changes occur in the CNS when the sympathetic and a large part of the sensory nervous system are lost early in development?

4.   At what stage of development do neurons die when deprived of NGF?

5. Are discernible sensory deficits produced in adult animals immunized with NGF?

6. How closely do the lesions in these experimental animals mimic those seen in human diseases such as familial dysautonomia or idiopathic orthostatic hypertension?

6. PROBLEMS AND LIMITATIONS OF THE AUTOIMMUNE APPROACH

An inherent limitation in this experimental approach is the dependence on the properties of passive transfer of antibodies from mother to fetus, specifically how much antibody is transferred and when it is transferred. A summary of properties of passive transfer of different species, taken from the excellent monograph by Brambell (20), is shown in Table 3. Mammals fall into three groups. The young of cattle, sheep, goats, horses, and pigs receive little or no passive immunity prenatally but obtain maternal antibody from the colostrum or milk during the first few hours and days of life. These species for this and other reasons are not likely candidates for study using this experimental approach. Rats, mice, dogs, and cats fall into an intermediate group in which passive immunity is transferred to some extent prenatally and to a larger extent postnatally via the milk. In the rat and the mouse, absorption of maternal antibody from milk occurs for a few weeks postnatally. Our data on the passive transfer of anti-NGF in the rat is consistent with this pattern.

The most likely candidates for the autoimmune approach would be those species in which large quantities of maternal antibody are transferred prenatally. This occurs in rabbit, guinea pig, monkey, and man, in which newborns have antibody titers comparable to those of the mother. Again, our experience with anti-NGF in the rabbit and guinea pig is consistent with this pattern. Thus it is not surprising that we observed greater effects of maternal anti-NGF in guinea pigs than in rats. In fact, it is somewhat surprising, given the low amounts of antibody passively transferred prenatally, that we observed such marked anatomical and biochemical effects in the rat.

Obviously, conclusions regarding the role of NGF in developmental events can be made only at the time when maternal antibody is present in significant concentrations in the fetus. The amount of maternal antibody in the fetus is not constant during gestation but rather is undetectable early and increases toward term. For example, studies in guinea pigs (23,24) indicate that maternal antibody is first detectable in the fetus at about the thirty-fifth day of gestation and then rises sharply to reach concentrations similar to those in maternal serum at about the fiftieth day of gestation. Antibody concentrations then remain constant or increase until parturition (day 65–70). These data indicate that only developmental events occurring after about day 35 of gestation can be examined by the autoimmune approach. We have as yet made no attempt to determine the time course of transfer of maternal anti-NGF in any of the species examined.

A major problem we have encountered using this experimental approach is a high degree of variability. In all species immunized with mouse NGF, we have obtained animals with antibody titers that vary by more than 10-fold. This high variability is not unexpected. Even in rats, rabbits, or guinea pigs with comparable titers of anti-mouse NGF, there was variability in the severity of the effect in the immunized animals and/or in the offspring of these animals. The most likely explanation for this variability is that antibodies vary in the degree of cross-reactivity with the NGF of the species under study. For example, although two rats may both have titers of 1000 against mouse NGF, the antibodies from one animal may cross-react well with rat NGF whereas the antibodies from the other rat may cross-react very poorly with rat NGF (see discussion in reference 25). Predictably, the animal making antibodies that cross-react well with rat NGF would itself be adversely affected and would produce severely affected offspring, whereas animals making poorly cross-reactive antibodies would show minimal effects. We were unable to test this notion directly in rat or rabbit because we do not have authentic NGF from these species. Because of the recent discovery of NGF in guinea pig prostate, we were able to test the cross-reactivity in guinea pigs.

Our results were as expected: those guinea pigs having good titers against guinea pig NGF (>2000) produced severely affected litters; those with low titers against guinea pig NGF did not have severely affected litters. Offspring of animals with modest titers against guinea pig NGF ($>500<1500$) produced animals with clear effects in sympathetic ganglia but modest or no obvious sensory deficits.

We were very fortunate that the first two female guinea pigs we immunized with mouse NGF produced very high titers of antibody that cross-reacted well with guinea pig NGF; these females produced severely affected litters. These are the animals on which we have previously reported (18). Of the subsequent 25 guinea pigs obtained from the same supplier and similarly immunized, we obtained only two more such animals. Hence, as we have previously reported in rats, only a small percentage of immunized animals produce severely affected litters. However, once a female that produces severely affected litters is identified, every litter she generates is similarly affected.

The low percentage of animals that produce high titers of cross-reacting antibody creates logistical problems in conducting systematic experiments such as some of those discussed previously. It has been frustrating to spend so much time and effort immunizing animals and determining titers, since the majority of animals must be discarded. There appear to be two approaches available to resolve the problem.

The first approach depends upon the reasonable assumption that a great deal of the variability in the properties of the immunological response is under genetic control. In previous studies we used outbred rats, rabbits, and guinea pigs. The variability in responses might be greatly reduced if inbred strains of animals were used. We are now systematically examining several inbred strains of rats and guinea pigs in an effort to find a strain that produces high titers of cross-reacting antisera. The second approach involves the use of monoclonal antibodies. One would need to select for clones of anti-NGF that cross-react with homologous NGF (e.g., immunize a rat with mouse NGF and select clones neutralizing rat NGF, thus effectively making rat anti-rat NGF) and are efficiently transferred from mother to fetus. This homologous monoclonal anti-NGF could then be administered to pregnant animals. Thus the titer of antibody in the mother and fetus could be titrated, and one could, to some extent at least, control the time of the exposure. Even with the monoclonal approach, it would be advisable to stay within a given inbred strain of animal in order to prevent an immunological response of the pregnant animal to allotypic differences in the immunoglobins of animals of different strains.

7. APPLICABILITY OF THE AUTOIMMUNE APPROACH TO OTHER "GROWTH FACTORS"

Nerve growth factor is presumably one of many "growth factors" that play a role in development. The physiological role of NGF is probably better understood than that of any other growth factor. This understanding is due to a large extent to the ability to deprive the developing animal of NGF by immunological means, which has allowed the correlation of the effect of NGF deprivation *in vivo* with effects of NGF *in vitro*. Other growth factors are being studied primarily, if not exclusively, *in vitro* in a variety of explants or cell-culture systems. Many of these are discussed extensively in other chapters of this volume.

We propose that the experimental approach we have applied to the study of the physiological roles of NGF may be applicable to other putative growth factors. There are two critical criteria for applying this approach. First, the animal must make antibodies against heterologous growth factor that cross-react well with the homologous growth factor in the animal under study. Our data indicate that in the case of NGF this occurs in a minority of outbred animals. Chemical properties of different factors will significantly alter chances for success. Larger molecules, which have more immunological determinants, are more likely to generate cross-reacting antibodies. In the case of small molecules, such as epidermal growth factor, either derivatization (e.g., with dinitrophenol) or coupling to a larger molecule may increase chances of generating cross-reacting antibodies. The ability to establish the degree of cross-reactivity of antibodies depends on the availability of the factor under study in the species to be examined. Second, this approach can only be used to study developmental events occurring after maternal antibody reaches the fetus.

Satisfying these criteria and using this approach to the study of NGF has been relatively straightforward because of the large literature available on the chemistry and biology of NGF and also because of the availability of sufficient quantities of NGF from mouse and guinea pig with which to work. Application of the approach to less chemically and biologically defined factors will be more difficult. We think, however, that this is a potentially useful experimental approach, and our efforts to resolve some of the problems we have encountered will facilitate the efforts of other workers studying other factors.

8.   POSSIBLE RELATIONSHIP TO BIRTH DEFECTS

Nerve growth factor is undoubtedly one of many chemicals that must be present at appropriate times and in appropriate concentrations for the normal development of the fetus. Many of these chemicals may play no role in the functioning of the *mature* organism. Our data demonstrate that maternal antibody can have devastating effects on the fetus and produce permanent anatomical defects in the offspring, that is, birth defects. It is, to our knowledge, the first such demonstration. Clearly, then, if a pregnant female were making antibodies to one of these "growth factors," this maternal antibody might adversely affect her fetus. The potential for such an effect would be greatest in those species, such as man, in which large amounts of maternal antibody reach the fetus prenatally. If this growth factor played little or no role in the *mature* organism, such antibodies would have no adverse effect on the mother and hence would go undetected. We suggest that whether induced by a failure of immune regulation, by an infection with an agent presenting a cross-reacting antigen, or by some other mechanism, maternal antibody against developmental factors may be a hitherto unrecognized teratogen responsible for some birth defects.

ACKNOWLEDGMENTS

This work was initiated with and much of it carried out by Dr. Pamela Gorin. Collaborations with Dr. John Pearson and Dr. Joan Schwartz have been invaluable, as has the assistance of Patricia Osborne, Russell Rydel, and Leslie Brandeis. The author also thanks Dr. Ralph A. Bradshaw for his generosity and advice over the years.

This work was supported by grants from the March of Dimes Birth Defects Foundation and NIH grant HL20604 to E. Johnson, by NIH training grant 5T32 HL07275, and by the Dysautonomia Foundation and NIH grant HD12260 to John Pearson. E. Johnson is an Established Investigator of the American Heart Association.

REFERENCES

1. Levi-Montalcini, R., and Booker, B., *Proc. Natl. Acad. Sci. USA*, **46**, 324 (1960).

2. Cohen, S., *Proc. Natl. Acad. Sci. USA*, **46**, 302 (1960).

3. Levi-Montalcini, R., and Angeletti, P. U., *Pharmacol. Rev.*, **18**, 619 (1966).

4. Thoenen, H., and Barde, Y.-A., *Physiol. Rev.*, **60**, 1284 (1980).

5. Angeletti, P. U., Levi-Montalcini, R., and Caramia, F., *Brain Res.*, **27**, 343 (1971).

6. Bjerre, B., Wiklund, L., and Edwards, D. C., *Brain Res.*, **92**, 257 (1975).

7. Ennis, M., Pearce, F. L., and Vernon, C. A., *Neuroscience*, **4**, 1391 (1979).

8. Goedert, M., Otten, U., Schafer, Th., and Thoenen, H., *Brain Res.*, **201**, 399 (1980).

9. Kessler, J. A., Cochard, P., and Black, I. B., *Nature*, **280**, 141 (1979).

10. Aloe, L., and Levi-Montalcini, R., *Proc. Natl. Acad. Sci. USA*, **76**, 1246 (1979).

11. Gorin, P. D., and Johnson, E. M., *Proc. Natl. Acad. Sci. USA*, **76**, 5382 (1979).

12. Harper, G. P., Barde, Y.-A., Burnstock, G., Carstairs, J. R., Dennison, M. E., Suda, K., and Vernon, C. A., *Nature*, **279**, 160 (1979).

13. Levi-Montalcini, R., Meyer, H., and Hamburger, V., *Cancer Res.*, **14**, 49 (1954).

14. Fenton, E. L., *Exp. Cell Res.*, **59**, 383 (1970).

15. Gorin, P. D., and Johnson, E. M., *Brain Res.*, **198**, 27 (1980).

16. Johnson, E. M., Gorin, P. D., Osborne, P. A., Rydel, R. E., and Pearson, J., *Brain Res.*, **240**, 131 (1982).

17. Gorin, P. D., and Johnson, E. M., *Dev. Biol.*, **80**, 313 (1980).

18. Johnson, E. M., Gorin, P. D., Brandeis, L. D., and Pearson, J., *Science*, **210**, 916 (1980).

19. Ross, M., Lofstrandh, S., Gorin, P. D., Johnson, E. M., and Schwartz, J., *J. Neurosci.*, **1**, 1304 (1981).

20. Brambell, B. W. R., *Frontiers in Biology*, Elsevier, New York, **18** (1970).

21. Lindsay, R. M., *Nature*, **282**, 80 (1979).

22. Hedlund, K.-O., and Ebendal, T., *J. Neurocytol.*, **9**, 665 (1980).

23. Barnes, J. M., *J. Path. Bact.*, **77**, 371 (1959).

24. Leissring, J. C., and Anderson, J. W., *Am. J. Anat.*, **109**, 149 (1961).

25. Harper, G. P., and Thoenen, H., *J. Neurochem.*, **34**, 893 (1980).

4

BIOCHEMISTRY AND BIOLOGY OF PLATELET-DERIVED GROWTH FACTOR

Bengt Westermark
Carl-Henrik Heldin
Bo Ek
Ann Johnsson
Karin Mellström
Monica Nistér
Åke Wasteson

CONTENTS

Abbreviations

ASV	Avian sarcoma virus
CTAP III	Connective tissue activating peptide III
DMEM	Dulbecco's modified Eagle's medium
DNase I	Deoxyribonuclease I
ECM	Extracellular matrix
EGF	Epidermal growth factor
FGF	Fibroblast growth factor
FITC	Fluorescein isothiocyanate
FSH	Follicle-stimulating hormone
HPLC	High-performance liquid chromatography
HSA	Human serum albumin
LH	Lutropin
ODGF	Osteosarcoma-derived growth factor
PAGE	Polyacrylamide gel electrophoresis
PBP	Platelet basic protein
PDGF	Platelet-derived growth factor
PF-4	Platelet factor 4
LA-PF-4	Low affinity platelet factor 4
PGI$_2$	Prostacyclin
PLase	Phospholipase
RIA	Radioimmunoassay
SDS	Sodium dodecyl sulfate
SV 40	Simian sarcoma virus 40

β-TG   β-Thromboglobulin
TdR   Thymidine

1. INTRODUCTION

The original discovery of a growth factor in platelets was made by Balk in 1971. In a comparative study on the growth behavior of normal and transformed chick fibroblasts in calcium-depleted medium, Balk observed that whereas both cell types prolifcrated in serum-containing medium, only the transformed cells were capable of growth in plasma-containing medium (1). Balk's conclusion was that serum contains a growth factor required by normal cells when grown at low calcium concentration, and that this growth factor is liberated from plasma precursors or released from the platelets during blood coagulation. It was speculated that such a factor might act as a wound hormone that could initiate or promote cell division in an injured tissue (2). Balk's findings were independently confirmed and extended in other laboratories. Kohler and Lipton (3) reported that rat or human serum stimulates mouse 3T3 cells more than the corresponding plasma, and that human platelets can be used as an enriched source of growth-promoting activity. Ross et al. (4) showed that serum derived from platelet-poor plasma is much less efficient in sustaining growth of monkey arterial smooth muscle cells than is serum prepared from whole blood. Furthermore, the growth-promoting activity of the platelet-poor plasma is restored by the addition of platelets, and a growth-promoting activity is released from fresh platelets when they are exposed to thrombin. The latter experiment thus demonstrated that the growth-promoting activity is a normal platelet-release product. Busch et al. (5) confirmed this finding by using a variety of platelet-releasing agents. Further proof of the growth-promoting activity in platelets appeared when Westermark and Wasteson (6,7) demonstrated that a lysate prepared from human outdated platelets contained large amounts of mitogenic activity for human glial cells. In these studies the cationic character of the factor became evident. When the lysate was run on a cation exchanger at neutral pH, all activity became absorbed to the column (7). The lack of growth-promoting activity in the breakthrough fraction was later shown to be an artifact due to the presence of a thymidine-degrading enzyme, thymidine phosphorylase (8). However, most of the studies to date on the growth-promoting activity of platelets have been done on the cationic factor, and it is also this factor that has been given the name *platelet-derived growth factor* (PDGF). For previous reviews on PDGF, see references 9 and 10.

Independent of the studies on platelets, Antoniades and collaborators isolated a factor from human serum with growth-promoting activity on mouse 3T3 cells (11). They claimed that this factor was a 13,000-dalton cationic polypeptide, and using a radioimmunological method later showed that the factor was derived from platelets and identical to the cationic PDGF (12).

2.   ORIGIN AND LOCALIZATION OF PDGF

In order to understand the function of PDGF, it is important to consider that it is stored in particulate form within the platelet and therefore is not normally generally available to other cells. *In vitro*, PDGF may be liberated from its storage site in the platelet release reaction (5); inhibitors of the platelet release reaction also prevent the liberation of PDGF (13). Under conditions of selective release, PDGF is accompanied by platelet factor 4 (PF-4) and β-thromboglobulin (β-TG), two polypeptides of the platelet α-granule, but remains separate from the dense-granule constituents or the acid hydrolases (14,15). These findings indicate that PDGF is stored in the platelet α-granules. Separation of platelet homogenates on sucrose gradients supports this notion in that the highest levels of PDGF are found in the same fraction as those enriched in PF-4 and β-TG (14,16). However, in both the release experiments and the subcellular-fractionation studies, PDGF was identified by an assay for growth-promoting activity; therefore, other platelet growth factors (8) may have contributed to the observed activities. A different line of evidence derives from observations on patients with storage-pool deficiencies, a heterogeneous group of platelet abnormalities in which either dense granules or dense granules and α-granules are missing or diminished. Cases showing partial or pronounced granule deficiency had correspondingly reduced levels of PF-4, β-TG, and PDGF, but were normal in their acid hydrolases (17). In the gray platelet syndrome, sometimes classified as a subgroup of the storage-pool deficiencies (17), there is an isolated deficiency in the α-granules; in two such cases there was a marked reduction in both PF-4, β-TG, and PDGF (18). Taken together these observations support the view that PDGF is an α-granule constituent.

   The site of biosynthesis of PDGF has not been determined; however, the low rate of protein synthesis in circulating platelets raises the possibility that PDGF is not produced in the platelet proper. A more likely alternative is that PDGF is synthesized by the platelet precursor cells, for example, megakaryocytes. Indirect support for this derives from experiments in which growth factor activity was demonstrated in megakaryocyte-enriched fractions of guinea pig (19) as well as human (20) bone marrow. However, neither the identity of PDGF nor the biosynthesis of the factor was established in these studies. Similarly, the conditioned medium of rat promegakaryoblasts in culture has been found to contain a growth-promoting activity (21). Whether this activity is related to PDGF remains, however, to be examined. A third possibility is that PDGF is produced in a different tissue in the body and secondarily stored in megakaryocytes/platelets. However, no experimental support for this alternative is available; attempts to demonstrate uptake of [^{125}I]PDGF by platelets *in vitro* have been unsuccessful (Heldin et al., unpublished).

3. GROWTH FACTORS IN PLATELETS

Several laboratories have reported that, in addition to PDGF, platelets contain a number of other growth-promoting activities. In this chapter these platelet-derived factors are reviewed and compared with PDGF, which is by far the most well characterized platelet mitogen and the major topic of this review. The characteristics of the known growth factor activities from platelets are summarized in Table 1.

Paul et al. (27) have reported the purification of a platelet protein with mitogenic activity for Swiss 3T3 cells. This peptide had a high isoelectric point (10.0–11.0) and was therefore denoted platelet basic protein (PBP). It had an apparent molecular weight on gel electrophoresis in sodium dodecyl sulfate (SDS-PAGE) of 11,000–15,000 compared with cationic standard proteins (histones) and 14,000–17,000 compared with conventional standards. Optimal mitogenic activity was found with 10–40 ng of PBP per milliliter in the cell-culture medium. The PBP had immunological determinants in common with low affinity PF-4 (LA-PF-4) and β-TG. However, PDGF did not compete with PBP for binding to anti-PBP antibodies (27), and antibodies against PDGF did not recognize ^{125}I-labeled PBP (Heldin et al., unpublished observations). Thus PBP differs from PDGF with regard to both its mobility in SDS-PAGE and its immunological properties. Further, the activity of PBP on 3T3 cells could be neutralized by heparin (34), whereas the biological activity of PDGF on glial cells was unaffected by the presence of heparin up to 10 μg/ml (Heldin et al., unpublished observations).

Castor and collaborators (28,29) described a cationic platelet peptide, denoted connective tissue activating peptide III (CTAP III), that stimulated DNA synthesis in cultures of human synovial cells and dermal fibroblasts. CTAP III had a molecular weight of 9300 as determined from the mobility of a stained component in SDS-PAGE. The amino acid sequence was identical to that of β-TG, except for the presence of an extra N-terminal tetrapeptide (35). It was suggested that CTAP III is identical to LA-PF-4 (35,36). However, other investigators found no biological activity of LA-PF-4 (29,36). Further,

Table 1. Growth Factors in Platelets

Designation	Reference	Molecular Weight	Isoelectric Point	Concentration Used[a] (ng/ml)	Responsiveness Demonstrated in
PDGF	4, 22–26	29,000–33,000	10	2	3T3 cells, fibroblasts, glial cells, smooth muscle cells
PBP	27	14,000–17,000	10–11	10–40	3T3 cells
CTAP III	28, 29	9,300	8.5	13,000	Synovial cells, fibroblasts
—	8	About 40,000 and <10,000	5	100,000	Glial cells
—	30, 31	30,000–50,000 and <10,000	?	200,000	Mammary tumor cells and 24 other cell lines
—	32	?	?	200,000	Neuroblastoma cells, renal adenocarcinoma cells, Leydig testicular cells, mammary tumor cells
—	33	72,000	7.8–8.3	5,000	SV 40 transformed cells

[a] Note that the figures give only a rough estimate of the specific activity of the preparations used. The figures cannot be compared directly with each other since different degrees of activity were obtained in different experiments.

rather large concentrations of CTAP III [several μg/ml (28)] were needed to achieve any biological effects, which makes it possible that the observed activity was due to a minor contamination by PDGF in the preparation; less than 1% would be sufficient. Further studies are required to establish the exact relation between PDGF, PBP, and CTAP III.

Chromatography of a platelet lysate on CM-Sephadex led to the recovery of mitogenic activity for normal human glial cells both in the adsorbed fraction (PDGF) and in the unadsorbed fraction (8). The growth factor activity that passed unadsorbed through CM-Sephadex appeared in the unadsorbed fraction also when rechromatographed on the same column. This indicates that the growth factor activity is truly anionic and not, for example, carrier-associated PDGF in equilibrium with free PDGF. Further, the anionic growth factor activity was not recognized by antibodies against PDGF (37). Thus platelet lysate contains anionic growth factors distinct from the cationic growth factor activities described above. Initial characterization by gel chromatography revealed at least two active components (8), one of apparent molecular weight 40,000 and one of lower molecular weight, less than 10,000. These factors stimulate glial cells (8), but their target-cell specificity has not been further characterized. In addition, crude platelet lysate has been shown to contain growth factor activity for other cell types (30–33).

Eastman and Sirbasku (30) identified a platelet protein with growth-promoting activity on a rat mammary tumor cell line. It is labile to heat treatment at 70°C and had an apparent molecular weight of 30,000–50,000 on Sephadex G-100 chromatography. In a subsequent study (31), human platelet lysate was found to be mitogenic for 24 cell lines out of 29 tested. The responsive ones included cells from man, rat, mouse, Syrian hamster, Chinese hamster, and monkey. Similarly, Hara et al. (32) reported the presence in platelet lysate of growth factor activity for four established tumor cell lines: mouse neuroblastoma cells, mouse renal adenocarcinoma cells, rat Leydig testicular cells, and mouse mammary tumor cells. They concluded that the active molecule may be a glycoprotein, since the activity is completely destroyed by periodate oxidation. In addition, Kepner and Lipton (33) demonstrated that platelet lysate contains a growth factor activity for simian sarcoma virus 40 (SV 40)-transformed 3T3 cells, distinct from the 3T3-cell-stimulating activity (i.e., PDGF). The growth factor for SV-40 transformed-3T3 cells had an apparent molecular weight of about 72,000 daltons on a Sephadex G-100 column and was heat labile and labile to oxidation with periodate.

Thus the platelet-derived growth factor activities described by Eastman and Sirbasku (30,31), Hara et al. (32), and Kepner and Lipton (33), and the anionic growth factor activity described by Heldin et al. (8) have features in common, such as susceptibility to heat and periodate oxidation and have, by and large, similar estimated molecular weights. However, none of the proteins have been purified and too little is known about their physico-chemical characteristics to permit a careful comparison.

4.   PURIFICATION AND STRUCTURE OF PDGF

Progress in the purification of PDGF has been hampered by the limited availability of platelets and the fact that PDGF occurs in platelets in only minute amounts. In retrospect it is also possible to ascribe some of the difficulties in purifying PDGF to the chemical properties of the factor (Table 2). The basic character (pI 10) and some hydrophobicity probably contribute

Table 2.   Chemical and Physical-Chemical Properties of PDGF

Property	Method	Reference
Resistant to		
4 M Guanidine-HCl	Determination of biological activity	8
6 M Urea	Determination of biological activity	38
1% SDS	Determination of biological activity	8
1 M Acetic acid	Determination of biological activity	22, 23, 39
Heat (80°C, 100°C)	Determination of biological activity	7, 22
Susceptible to		
Trypsin	Determination of biological activity	7
Reduction	Determination of biological activity	22
Affinity for		
Pentyl-Sepharose	Column chromatography	23
Cibacron blue F3GA	Column chromatography	23
Phenyl-Sepharose	Column chromatography	40
Lichrosorb RP-8	Column chromatography	41
Molecular weight		
Unreduced		
33,000	Ultracentrifugation	24
25,000–35,000	Gel chromatography	8, 23
26,000–33,000	Gel electrophoresis in SDS	8
Reduced		
Chain A 14,000–18,000	Gel electrophoresis in SDS	41
Chain B 16,000	Gel electrophoresis in SDS	41
Isoelectric point 9.5–10.4	Isoelectric focusing	8, 22, 25

to the strong tendency of PDGF to adsorb to a variety of materials. This makes PDGF activity elusive unless the appropriate precautions are taken. Most important is probably the use of a suitable solvent, strong enough to keep PDGF in solution. Fortunately, PDGF is resistant toward a number of denaturing agents, including 4 M guanidine hydrochloride, 6 M urea, 1 M acetic acid, and 1% SDS, the latter two solvents being particularly important. The demonstration that PDGF is stable to SDS enabled direct analysis of PDGF activity in electrophoretic gels run in the presence of SDS (8). Later the same principle was utilized as a final preparative step for PDGF (22,23). Acetic acid, being a volatile solvent, has found universal use in both handling and storage of PDGF (22,23,38,39). The most important parameters utilized in the purification of PDGF are charge [e.g., cation-exchange chromatography (8,22,23,25,40) or preparative isoelectric focusing (8,22,25], hydrophobicity [e.g., chromatography on Blue Sepharose (23); phenyl-Sepharose (40); or high-performance liquid chromatography (HPLC) on RP-8, an octyl sub-stituted matrix (41)], hydrodynamic size [e.g., gel chromatography on BioGel P-150 in 1 M acetic acid (22,23)], or molecular weight [migration in elec-trophoretic gels in the presence of SDS (22,23)]. The preparation of small amounts of PDGF in near-homogeneous form was described independently in 1979 by Antoniades et al. (22) and by Heldin et al. (23). Modified procedures have since been published that avoid the use of SDS in the preparation and produce larger amounts of PDGF at higher yields (24, 25,41,42). Analysis of the isolated product by gel electrophoresis in SDS showed the absence of stainable components other than PDGF (Fig. 1). The high specific biological activity of the preparation, as demonstrated by its stimulatory effect on DNA synthesis in cultured glial cells, also indicated high purity (>95%). Gel electrophoresis in SDS further showed that the stainable material appeared in a region of the gel rather than in one distinct band. This is in accordance with the previous suggestion that PDGF is heterogeneous with respect to molecular weight (8,23). The migration rate in SDS-containing gels indicates a molecular weight range of 28,000–33,000 daltons; analysis for biological activity indicates equal potency of the different molecular-weight classes in this region. Under reducing conditions the entire material was converted to faster-moving species with protein-stainable bands corresponding to molecular weights of 14,000–18,000 daltons (23). Since the molecular-weight data were important for our conception of the molecular model for PDGF, and since a markedly different view of the molecular weight of PDGF was maintained by others (22), an independent molecular-weight analysis was carried out by sedimentation-equilibrium studies in the ultracentrifuge. The resulting figure [molecular weight 33,000 daltons for unreduced PDGF (24)]was in close agreement with that obtained by gel electrophoresis in SDS or gel chromatography in various solvents (8,23),

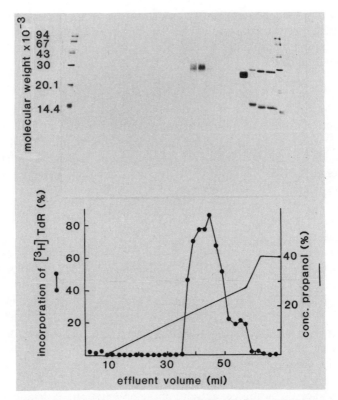

Figure 1. Purification of PDGF by HPLC. Semipure PDGF (approximately 30% pure), obtained from the BioGel P-150 step described in reference 24, was chromatographed on a Lichosorb RP-8 column essentially as described (41). Aliquots of effluent fractions were pooled and analysed by gel electrophoresis in SDS (*top*) or by an assay for stimulation of DNA synthesis (8) (*bottom*). The distribution of protein-stainable material demonstrates: (1) heterogeneity in the PDGF material, (2) absence of other components in the PDGF-containing fractions, (3) powerful resolution of PDGF from contaminants, and (4) appearance of biological activity exclusively in the PDGF-containing region.

thus confirming our previous molecular-weight data and lending support to the notion that PDGF is a 30,000-dalton protein, consisting of two disulfide-linked polypeptide chains. In addition to the molecular-weight heterogeneity of PDGF, which has now been verified by other groups (25,42), there is also a charge heterogeneity, demonstrable, for example, in isoelectric-focusing experiments (8,22,25).

Amino acid analysis of different preparations of highly purified PDGF gives essentially similar results (24,25); a conspicuous feature is the high proportion of basic amino acids and the high content of half-cystine residues. In addition, Deuel et al. identified mannose, galactose, *N*-acetylglucosamine, *N*-acetylgalactosamine, and fucose and suggest that PDGF is a glycoprotein, containing up to 7% of carbohydrate (25).

High-performance liquid chromatography of reduced and alkylated PDGF on a hydrophobic matrix (RP-8) led to resolution of the two polypeptide chains constituting the native molecule (41). Gel electrophoresis in SDS indicated that the highest-molecular-weight component of these, designated A, consists of four molecular-weight species, with molecular weights 18,000, 15,000, 14,000, and 11,000. The other one, designated B, is essentially made up of a single 16,000-dalton species. The structural model for PDGF that can be deduced from these observations is outlined in Fig. 2. According to this model PDGF is a two-chain protein with a molecular weight of about 30,000; the molecular weight is somewhat variable in the range 28,000–33,000 as determined by gel electrophoresis in SDS under nonreducing conditions. PDGF consists of two different polypeptide chains, designated A and B in the figure. The A chain is heterogeneous in size, showing one major 18,000-dalton form and in addition distinct fragments of somewhat shorter length. The B chain is more homogeneous, consisting only of one major 16,000-dalton form. Disulfide bonds link the two polypeptides; the high number of half-cystine residues in PDGF (24,25) allows for several (6–9) disulfide bridges in the molecule. These structures probably have a stabilizing effect on the PDGF molecule, since native PDGF is remarkably resistant to denaturation by heat or dissociative solvents, but irreversibly inactivated by reducing agents (Table 2). The molecular-weight variability in the A chain may explain the heterogeneity in intact PDGF observed previously. This feature of the A chain is remarkable, considering the ho-

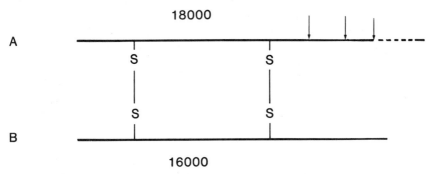

Figure 2. Tentative molecular model of PDGF. The two polypeptide chains, A and B, are linked by an unknown number of disulfide bridges. The arrows indicate possible sites of proteolytic attack, leading to A chains of varying lengths. The dotted line indicates a region of the A chain that may vary without change in biological activity of the PDGF molecule.

mogeneous appearance of peak A in HPLC. The most likely interpretation is a proteolytic degradation of the A chain, producing fragments of different lengths, but with a common hydrophobic determinant. It remains to be clarified whether this process is a specific event, for example, related to the maturation of the molecule, or an unspecific but limited attack by proteases in the course of preparation. It is noteworthy, however, that partial modification, for example, as indicated by the dashed line in the figure, is compatible with a retained biological activity of the molecule.

5.   USE OF ANTIBODIES AGAINST PDGF

In order to facilitate further characterization and purification of PDGF, attempts have been made to produce antibodies against the molecule. Rabbit antibodies capable of inhibiting the mitogenic effect of PDGF when added together with the growth factor in the cell-culture medium have been obtained (37,43).

Heldin et al. (37) showed that the anti-PDGF immune serum selectively recognized [^{125}I]PDGF when exposed to iodinated proteins from a semipure preparation of PDGF. Thus when exposed to likely contaminants in the preparation used to immunize the rabbit, the antiserum seemed specific for PDGF. The antiserum was used to investigate the immunological relationship between PDGF and other growth factors or other platelet proteins. Mouse epidermal growth factor (EGF), bovine fibroblast growth factor (FGF), or the anionic growth factors in human platelets (8) were not recognized by the antibodies. In contrast, osteosarcoma-derived growth factor (ODGF), a growth factor produced by a human osteosarcoma cell line (44, and Section 8), cross-reacted immunologically with PDGF (37). But PF-4 and β-TG, both peptides stored together with PDGF in the platelet α-granules, did not show any immunological cross-reactivity with PDGF (37).

The possible use of these antibodies in the preparation of pure PDGF was also demonstrated. When a platelet lysate was passed over a column of immobilized anti-PDGF immunoglobulin, PDGF was retained on the column and could be recovered after elution of the column with acid.

A radioimmunoassay (RIA) was developed using [^{125}I]PDGF in conjunction with anti-PDGF antibodies immobilized on Sephadex (37). The sensitivity of the assay permits the detection of 5 ng of PDGF per milliter. The concentration of PDGF in human serum was about 100 ng/ml as measured by the RIA. Good correlation was found between the concentration of PDGF and the concentration of PF-4 in different sera (Fig. 3). In platelet-poor plasma, 30–40 ng of PDGF per milliliter was found. The explanation of

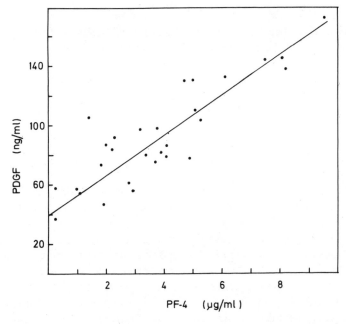

Figure 3. Levels of PDGF in human sera having varying concentrations of PF-4. Serum samples were assayed for PF-4 and PDGF content by RIAs (37).

this finding is not clear. It may be due to unspecific interactions between serum proteins and the antibody/antigen used in the RIA or, alternatively, it may suggest that PDGF is derived from sources other than the platelets.

6. CELLULAR BINDING AND PROCESSING OF [125I]PDGF

The availability of pure radiolabeled PDGF made it possible to demonstrate a specific high-affinity receptor for PDGF on the fibroblast cell surface (45). Scatchard analysis of binding data indicates a single class of receptors with a dissociation constant of $1 \times 10^{-9}M$. The number of receptors is about 3×10^5 per cell. Thus, human foreskin fibroblasts have 3–5 times more PDGF receptors than EGF receptors. The receptor was specific for PDGF in the sense that other growth factors like EGF, FGF, or insulin did not compete with [125I]PDGF for binding (45). However, a semipure preparation of ODGF did (Heldin et al., unpublished observations), indicating that ODGF is not only immunologically (see Section 4), but also functionally related to PDGF.

In our studies PDGF receptors were found on skin fibroblasts, normal and malignant glial cells, smooth muscle cells, 3T3 cells, and osteosarcoma cells (see Table 3). In contrast, epithelial-derived cells, endothelial cells, neuroblastoma cells, and peripheral blood lymphocytes showed no significant specific binding. Apparently, only connective-tissue-derived cells and glial cells have receptors for PDGF. Thus the target-cell specificity of PDGF is narrower than that of EGF, which also stimulates epithelial-derived cells (see Table 3). Our results on the PDGF receptor on various types of cells have recently been confirmed by Bowen-Pope and Ross (46). However these authors found a markedly lower value for the dissociation constant for the interaction between PDGF and its receptor.

In our studies of [^{125}I]PDGF binding to human fibroblasts at 37°C, the cellular binding first increased to reach a maximum after about 30 minutes and then decreased. This decrease in binding was due both to degradation of [^{125}I]PDGF by the cells and to down-regulation of the PDGF receptor, that is, exposure of the cells to PDGF caused a decreased subsequent cellular PDGF-binding capacity (47). The degradation was complete rather than partial in the sense that intermediary-size fragments could not be found in the cell-culture medium. It was blocked by low concentrations of lysosomotropic agents like chloroquine, ammonium chloride, or methylamine. This suggests that PDGF is internalized after binding and degraded in the lysosomes. Down-regulation of the PDGF receptor was optimal after a 60-minute incubation with PDGF at 37°C. It was dose dependent; half maximal down-regulation occurred at a concentration of 0.5 nM. When the PDGF-containing medium was changed to medium without PDGF, the binding capacity increased again; after down-regulation to 40% of initial binding capacity, the binding increased to 80% after 4 hours of incubation at 37°C. This reappearance of PDGF receptors on the cell surface was dependent on protein synthesis; it was totally blocked by cycloheximide. Thus either the receptor has to be synthesized *de novo* after internalization or some step in the recycling of "used" receptors is dependent on protein synthesis (47).

Some initial structural characterization of the PDGF receptor has been performed by affinity labeling it with [^{125}I]PDGF and stabilizing the binding with covalent cross-linkers. Homobifunctional succinimidyl esters (Glenn et al., personal communication, and Heldin et al., unpublished observations) or heterobifunctional photoreactive cross-linkers (Heldin et al., unpublished observations) have been used. Analysis on SDS gel electrophoresis revealed a molecular weight of the [^{125}I]PDGF–receptor complex of about 180,000 on 3T3 cells (Glenn et al., personal communication) and 180,000–230,000 on human fibroblasts (Heldin et al., unpublished observations). The estimated molecular weight of the complex was about the same under reducing conditions as under nonreducing conditions, indicating that the PDGF receptor is a single-chain protein.

Table 3.   Distribution of PDGF and EGF Receptors on Various Cell Types

CELL TYPE	PDGF RECEPTOR	EGF RECEPTOR
Human fibroblasts	+	+
Human glial cells	+	+
Human glioma cells	+/−	+
Porcine smooth muscle cells (renal artery)	+	+
Human osteosarcoma cells	+/−[a]	+
Porcine thyroid cells	−	+
Human thyroid cancer cells	−	+
Human squamous carcinoma of the lung	−	+
Human epidermal carcinoma (A-431 cells)	−	+
Human neuroblastoma cells	−	−
Human umbilical vein endothelial cells	−	−
Mouse 3T3 cells	+	+
Human blood lymphocytes	−	−

Source: Data taken from reference 44 and Heldin et al., unpublished observations.
[a] PDGF receptors were found on one osteosarcoma cell line (393 OS), but not on another (2 OS; this cell line produces ODGF).

7.   EFFECTS OF PDGF ON CULTURED CELLS

A summary of the various effects of PDGF on cultured cells is given in Table 4. Some of the effects are discussed in the following sections.

7.1.   Stimulation of Tyrosine-Specific Phosphorylation by PDGF

A new aspect of the mechanism of action of polypeptide growth factors has emerged with the recent finding that EGF causes a rapid phosphorylation of membrane-associated proteins (90). The protein kinase activity seems to be an intrinsic property of the EGF receptor itself, since it has not been possible to dissociate the EGF-binding capacity physically from the kinase activity of detergent-solubilized receptor (91). Moreover, the receptor functions as a phosphoacceptor in the kinase reaction (91).

It has recently been observed that PDGF also causes a rapid stimulation of the phosphorylation of membrane-associated proteins (80). The PDGF-induced stimulation of protein kinase activity was demonstrated by incubating the growth factor and [^{32}P]ATP together with plasma membranes isolated from human foreskin fibroblasts and glial cells. A marked stimulation of

Table 4. Effects of PDGF on Cultured Cells

Effect	Cell Type	Reference
Stimulation of cell replication	Balb/c 3T3 cells	3, 11, 12, 22,[a] 48–50
	Swiss 3T3 cells	39, 42,[a] 46,[a] 51–53
	Human glial cells	6, 7, 8, 23,[a] 24,[a] 54[a]
	Human dermal fibroblasts	55–58
	Monkey dermal fibroblasts	26
	Chicken fibroblasts	1, 2, 59, 60
	Monkey vascular smooth muscle cells	4, 26, 51, 61
	Human vascular smooth muscle cells	15
	Rat vascular smooth muscle cells	62, 63
	Rat cardiac fibroblasts	64
	Rat calvaria cells	65
Induction of anchorage-independent growth	BHK 21 C113 cells	66
Stimulation of fluid endocytosis	Monkey aortic smooth muscle cells	67–69
	Swiss 3T3 cells	67
Stimulation of cell migration	Human venous smooth muscle cells	70
	Human umbilical vein endothelial cells	71
Stimulation of chemotaxis	Sheep aortic smooth muscle cells	72

Induction of actin reorganization	Human glial cells	[b]
	Human foreskin fibroblasts	[b]
Increase in low-density-lipoprotein-binding capacity	Monkey aortic smooth muscle cells	73
	Human skin fibroblasts	74
Decrease in EGF-binding capacity	3T3 cells	75
	Human skin fibroblasts	47[a]
Increase in somatomedin-C-binding capacity	Balb/c 3T3 cells	76
Stimulation of PLase activity and release of prostaglandins	3T3 cells	77[a]
	Bovine arterial endothelial cells	78[a]
	Bovine adrenal capillary endothelial cells	78[a]
	Bovine aortic smooth muscle cells	78,[a], 79[a]
Stimulation of phosphorylation	Human fibroblast and glial cell membranes	80[a]
Expression of specific genes	Balb/c 3T3	81,[a] 82[a]
Increase in LH-binding capacity and steroid synthesis	Rat ovarian granulosa cells	83, 84
Increase in production of somatomedin C	Human fibroblasts	85
Increase in cholesterol synthesis	Arterial smooth muscle cells	86
Increase in acetate incorporation	Human skin fibroblasts	87
Stimulation of collagen synthesis	Monkey smooth muscle cells	88
Inhibition of adipose conversion of preadipocytes	3T3-F442A Strain	89

[a] Indicates that pure PDGF was used in the investigation.
[b] Mellstrom et al., submitted.

the phosphorylation of components of molecular weights 175,000* and 130,000 was seen in both membrane preparations (80). PDGF also stimulated the phosphorylation of some other components, albeit to a lesser extent. A comparison of the phosphoprotein patterns obtained by treating the cells with EGF with those obtained from PDGF-treated cells clearly demonstrated that the two factors stimulated the phosphorylation of different components, with one exception; the phosphorylation of a 35,000-dalton protein was increased both by EGF and PDGF and might therefore be a common substrate for the two growth-factor-induced kinase reactions. Whether this protein is identical to one of the early proteins with the same apparent molecular weight (81), synthesized by 3T3 cells during competence formation, is not known but is an interesting possibility. This implies that cells respond to PDGF by both a posttranslational modification and an increased synthesis of the same protein, the latter reaction yielding more substrate for the former.

Both PDGF (80) and EGF (92) stimulate phosphorylation of tyrosine residues; this type of phosphorylation is rare in normal, untransformed cells, but not in certain virus-transformed cells. It has recently been shown that the transforming proteins of several tumor viruses are tyrosine-specific protein kinases. Perhaps the best-studied example is the avian sarcoma virus (ASV) system, in which the transforming *onc* gene product is a phosphoprotein with tyrosine-specific kinase activity, denoted pp60^{src} (93, 94). Untransformed cells carry a homologous gene (*c-src*) and synthesize a homologous kinase, pp60^{c-src}, which has an unknown function in normal cells (95,96). It has been an enigma in tumor biology that the expression of one single gene of a transforming virus such as ASV can give rise to all the properties of the transformed phenotype. The finding that several of the *onc*-gene products are tyrosine-specific protein kinases must be regarded as a major breakthrough in this field of research. It is not difficult to envisage that such enzymes may modify the function of several substrate proteins and thus give rise to a plethora of phenotypic changes. Whether this is the result of an increase in the degree of phosphorylation of the substrates for the normal pp60^{c-src} or involves the phosphorylation of aberrant substrates is not known (reviewed in reference 97).

It follows from the discussion above that transformation induced by ASV and stimulation of cell replication by polypeptide growth factors such as EGF and PDGF have a common feature in the stimulation of tyrosine-specific phosphorylation. Moreover, a transformed cell and a cell stimulated by EGF or PDGF also have several phenotypical properties in common, for

---

* Mellström, K., Höglund, A. -S., Nistér, M., Heldin, C. -H., Westermark, B., and Lindberg, U., submitted for publication.

example, morphology, growth pattern, surface motility, and calcium dependence (see below). The *in vitro* transformed property that is believed to be the best correlate to *in vivo* malignancy is growth in semisolid media (98). Neither EGF nor PDGF seem to induce such anchorage independency of normal, diploid cell lines. However, PDGF has been reported to induce growth of the pseudonormal BHK-C113 cells in methocel (66). Some other properties of the transformed cell, such as the loss of pericellular fibronectin, are not mimicked by growth factors; EGF has even been reported to increase the production of fibronectin in 3T3 cells (99). A graphic representation of the similarities and differences between the phenotype of the EGF- and the PDGF-stimulated cell and the ASV-transformed cell is given in Fig. 4. The overlapping areas, representing common features, include properties that are attributable to common substrates for tyrosine-specific phosphorylation. This oversimplified, highly schematic model can serve as a testable working hypothesis for virus transformation and growth stimulation. Several other authors have also pointed out the similarities between transformation and growth stimulation by EGF (100–102). Now that it has also been shown that there are similarities in the behavior of the PDGF-stimulated cell and the transformed cell on one hand and with the EGF-stimulated cell on the other hand, it will be of particular importance to identify the cellular substrates for the three different tyrosine-specific kinases in order to elucidate their mode of involvement in the reactions common to virus transformation and growth stimulation.

Erikson's group has recently shown that in A-431 cells exposed to EGF, a 34-kilodalton protein is phosphorylated on tyrosine residues (103) and that this phosphoprotein is homologous to, and has the same molecular weight as, one of the substrates for pp60^{src} in ASV-transformed cells. The

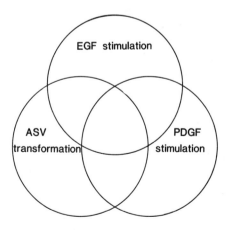

Figure 4. Schematic representation of the phenotypic characteristics of cells transformed by ASV and cells exposed to growth factors (EGF or PDGF). Overlapping areas represent similarities, e.g., growth pattern, membrane mobility, and calcium dependence. These properties are proposed to result from tyrosine phosphorylation of regulatory proteins, which are common to the respective kinase activities. Excluded areas represent properties unique for each situation.

function of this pp60^{src} substrate is not known; it has been shown to be physically associated with the detergent-resistant cytoskeleton (104). An interesting possibility, which we are currently probing, is that this 34-kilodalton protein is homologous to the 35-kilodalton phosphoprotein found in membranes after exposure to EGF or PDGF (80).

7.2.   Effects of PDGF on Cell Morphology, Cell Locomotion, Membrane Motility, and Actin Organization

Platelet-derived growth factor has both acute and long-term effects on the morphology and growth pattern of responsive cells. Thus human glial cells maintained in serum-free medium supplemented with PDGF differ markedly in morphology from unexposed control cells (54), with an irregular growth pattern and long cytoplasmic projections as the most prominent features. Human skin fibroblasts grown under the same conditions become extremely elongated, with long, slender projections, most probably retraction fibrils resulting from an increased locomotory activity. Even more notable is the effect of PDGF on cell morphology when the growth factor is added to confluent, stationary monolayers of 3T3 cells (Fig. 5). In a regular growth medium, such as Dulbecco's modified Eagle's medium (DMEM) with 5% calf serum, these cells show a regular "cobblestone" growth pattern. When exposed to PDGF for 24–48 hours, the cells round up, become spindle-shaped, and grow in an irregular crisscross pattern. Large membrane ruffles, often associated with macropinocytotic vesicles, can be seen on most of the cells. Morphologically, the PDGF-treated cells look "transformed" since a reduced cell-substratum adhesion, growth in crisscross pattern, and a vivid membrane ruffling are features typical of transformation. The similarity in phenotype of transformed and PDGF-treated cells is consistent with the hypothesis that transformation and PDGF might at least partially have a common metabolic pathway (see also Section 7.1).

Comparison of the locomotor activity of arterial smooth muscle cells in media supplemented with whole-blood serum and plasma-derived serum, respectively, has given circumstantial evidence that PDGF is a stimulator of cell locomotion, that is, a chemokinetic factor. As to the migration properties of arterial endothelial cells, conflicting data have been published. Wall et al. (71), using a platelet-release material, found a positive effect on endothelial cell migration, whereas Thorgeirsson et al. (70) found no difference in activity in plasma-derived serum and whole-blood serum, respectively. This discrepancy clearly demonstrates the hazard of using crude PDGF instead of pure factor to establish genuine effects of PDGF.

A true chemotactic effect of PDGF on arterial smooth muscle cells has been demonstrated by Grotendorst et al. using a modified Boyden chamber

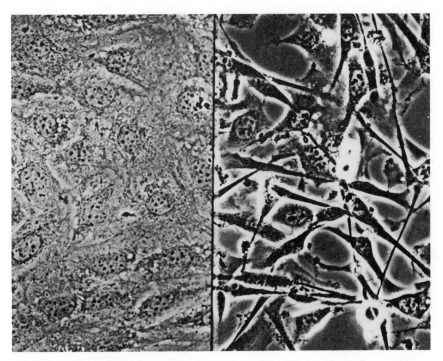

Figure 5. Effect of PDGF on cell morphology and growth pattern. (*Left*) Confluent stationary culture of Balb/c 3T3 cells grown for 5 days in DMEM, 5% fetal bovine serum. Note the regular, cobblestonelike growth pattern. (*Right*) Sister culture, exposed for 24 hours to 20 ng of PDGF per milliliter. Note the crisscross growth pattern, spindle-shaped morphology, and vivid ruffling activity. Two mitoses are seen (*arrows*).

(72). Both crude and pure PDGF were shown to act as chemotactic agents, that is, to induce a directed migration of cells toward a high concentration of PDGF. This may be an important finding in view of the supposed role of PDGF in the pathogenesis of atherosclerosis. According to the model proposed by Ross and co-workers, migration of smooth muscle cells from the arterial media to the intimal layer and increased mitotic activity are the key events in the formation of the early atherosclerotic lesion (105,106). Thus PDGF released from aggregated platelets and diffusing into the arterial wall may be a stimulant of both these events.

Using cultures of human glial cells in a serum-free medium, the early effects of PDGF on membrane motility and actin organization can be studied without interferences of other serum or plasma factors. A dramatic effect of PDGF can then be revealed by phase contrast microscopy. A few minutes after addition of PDGF, large, often circular ruffles can be seen on the dorsal cell surface (not shown). In some cases the ruffles are associated with macropinocytotic vesicles. This peculiar ruffling activity is transitory, and after 2–3 hours only remnants can be seen.

The inner structure of ruffles is formed by a lattice of actin filaments, and polymerization of actin may constitute the molecular basis of ruffle formation (107). The early effect of PDGF on ruffling activity would thus imply that the growth factor can cause rapid changes in the dynamic structure of the actin cytoskeleton. Indeed, by using an indirect immunofluorescence technique, based on the sequential addition of deoxyribonuclease I (DNase I), rabbit anti-DNase I, and fluorescein isothiocyanate (FITC)-conjugated goat anti-rabbit immunoglobulin, it has been demonstrated that PDGF causes profound, acute changes in the distribution of actin* (cf. Fig. 6). Within 1 minute, a patchy fluorescence appears on the upper surface, probably corresponding to small ruffles observed in the scanning electron microscope (Nistér et al., unpublished). After 5–15 minutes a lattice of rather coarse filaments is seen, and in many cells an intensive circular actin staining is visible, corresponding to the circular ruffles observed by phase contrast microscopy.

Similar effects on actin staining as those induced by PDGF can also be seen in EGF-treated cells, albeit less pronounced. In A 431 cells, EGF has a more profound acute influence on ruffling activity (100), and in these cells, EGF causes a reorganization of actin (102) very similar to that seen in PDGF-treated glial cells. Thus although EGF and PDGF bind to separate receptors, they induce a similar or even identical change in the dynamic organization of the actin filaments. Since the activated EGF receptor (91) and possibly also the PDGF receptor (80) are tyrosine-specific protein kinases, it is tempting to speculate that the effect of the growth factors on the structure of actin is caused by a tyrosine phosphorylation of proteins involved in the regulation of actin polymerization and/or actin-filament bundling. Identi-

---

* Mellström, K., Höglund, A. -S., Nistér, M., Heldin, C. -H., Westermark, B., and Lindberg, U., submitted for publication.

Figure 6. Rapid effect of PDGF on actin organization. Human glial cells were trypsinized, plated on coverslips, and grown for 2 days in serum-free MCDB 105 medium as described (54). The cultures were then given 40 ng of PDGF per milliliter, fixed at intervals in paraformaldehyde, and postfixed in acetone. Actin was visualized by a double-sandwich technique, by sequentially adding DNase I, rabbit anti-DNase I, and FITC-conjugated goat anti-rabbit immunoglobulin. Pictures were taken in a Leitz epifluorescence microscope. 1(a). Control showing actin in stress fibers and in diffusely stained perinuclear area. 2(b). One minute after the addition of PDGF. Note the increased ruffling activity and the patchy actin staining, probably representing small ruffles or microvilli. 3(c). Five minutes after the addition of PDGF. Actin is now redistributed in a coarse, weblike pattern. 4(d). Fifteen minutes after the addition of PDGF. Note the enormous, flowerlike ruffle on the dorsal surface.

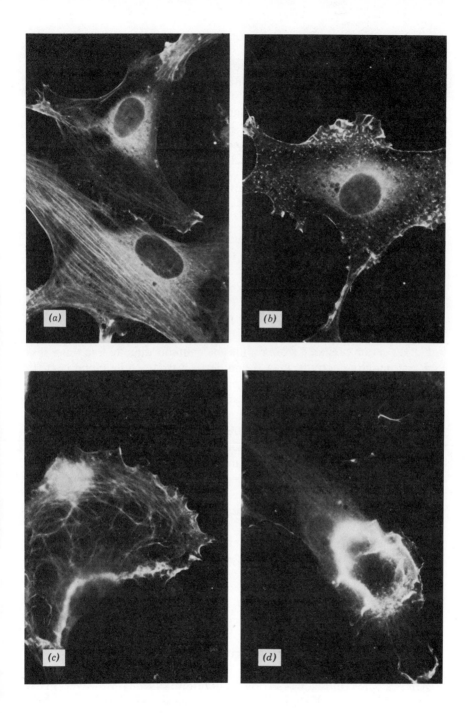

fication of such proteins in combination with studies on the EGF- and PDGF-mediated protein phosphorylation may prove or disprove the validity of such a hypothesis.

The possible relation between the mitogenic effect of PDGF and the effects on membrane motility, cell morphology, and locomotor activity has not been clarified. In several other instances, however, intense ruffling activity is positively correlated with cell proliferation (108). This relationship points to a coupling between membrane motility and the initiation of DNA synthesis.

7.3. Stimulation of Phospholipase A₂ Activity and Prostaglandin Synthesis by PDGF

The initial step in the synthesis of prostaglandins is the release of arachidonic acid from membrane phospholipids (109), brought about by the enzyme phospholipase A_2 (PLase). Increased PLase activity is an early response to serum treatment of quiescent 3T3 cells (110) that can mainly be ascribed to PDGF; serum prepared from rat plasma contains three to five times less PLase-stimulating activity than serum derived from whole blood (77). In addition, purified PDGF added at 1 ng/ml has a considerable PLase-stimulating activity. Prostaglandin release has been shown to be induced by PDGF both in endothelial cells and in arterial smooth muscle cells (77–79). The finding that PDGF has an effect on endothelial cells is surprising, since such cells do not bind [125I]PDGF (45). However, we cannot exclude the possibility that endothelial cells carry a small number of PDGF receptors that are not detectable by the radioreceptor assay. The alternate explanation, that is, that the effect of PDGF on prostaglandin release and PLase activity is not mediated by the PDGF receptor seems less likely. Coughlin et al. demonstrated that PDGF and serotonin act synergistically as stimulators of prostacyclin (PGI_2) release by vascular smooth muscle cells in culture (79). Prostacyclin is a vasodilator and a very potent inhibitor of platelet aggregation, and the authors speculate on the possibility that PDGF, released from aggregated platelets *in vivo*, stimulates smooth muscle cells to produce PGI_2, which protects against excessive platelet aggregation and thrombus formation.

7.4. Expression of PDGF Mitogenicity in Culture

PDGF is a potent mitogen in various cell-culture systems. However, PDGF seems to have a relatively narrow range of tissue specificity, since so far only mesenchymal cells and human glial cells have been shown to be responsive. No effect has been observed on the replication of endothelial cells, epithelial cells, or hematopoietic cells. These findings correlate well with the distribution of PDGF receptors (see Table 3). The concentration dependence of the mitogenic activity of pure PDGF has been studied in detail on Balb/c 3T3 cells (22), Swiss 3T3 cells (46), and human glial cells (23,24). A maximal growth response has been obtained with 1–4 ng of PDGF per milliliter. Comparison between the concentration dependence of receptor occupancy and of cell replication in one study on human fibroblasts indicated that about one order of magnitude higher concentration of PDGF was needed for half-maximal binding than for half-maximal growth stimulation (45). This would indicate the presence of "spare receptors." However, other investigators found about the same concentration dependency of receptor occupancy and growth stimulation on Swiss 3T3 cells, suggesting the absence of "spare receptors" (46). Obviously, further studies are required to clarify this point. One should bear in mind that the half-maximal doses for binding and mitogenicity, respectively, are determined under entirely different experimental conditions. Mitogenicity is measured by a long-term assay at 37°C, that is, under conditions where the concentration of PDGF is continuously decreasing because of cell binding, internalization, and degradation (46,47), whereas the binding assay is performed in the cold.

During the last one or two decades, numerous attempts have been made to design nutrient media that will sustain long-term growth in a serum-free environment (see Chapter 9). A number of laboratories have devoted their work to the purification of serum growth factors, which has turned out to be a formidable task, mainly due to the minute concentrations in serum of the essential factors.

Ham and colleagues have focused their interest on the synthetic part of the medium and been able to design media that sustain growth of even diploid cells at a very low serum concentration. These so-called MCDB media are derived from the nutrient medium F-12 and differ from this in that they contain several trace metals and that the concentration of each ingredient is individually optimized for a specific cell type (111). The hope that PDGF would turn out to be the universal growth factor of serum has not been fulfilled, because of the lack of responses of epithelial cells, hematopoietic cells, and endothelial cells. In the case of human glia-like cells, arterial smooth muscle cells, and human fibroblasts, however, PDGF has been shown to be a useful growth factor for serum-free culture.

In regular serum-free media, such as DMEM or F-10, PDGF had a very low mitogenic activity, which, however, could be potentiated by the addition of human serum albumin (HSA)(6). When one of Ham's media, MCDB 105, originally designed for human diploid lung fibroblasts, was used, the requirement for albumin was abolished, that is, pure PDGF could sustain

the multiplication of human diploid glia-like cells in serum-free culture
(54). A miniclonal analysis showed that a fraction of the cells underwent
several cell-cycle rounds in this defined medium. However, the cells did
not survive a prolonged incubation and attempts to grow the cells serially
in such medium have failed. Although PDGF can substitute for the mitogenic
activity of serum, additional factors are required for long-term cell survival.
Indeed, Ham and collaborators recently succeeded in designing a medium
(MCDB 110) that sustains clonal growth of human diploid fibroblasts after
supplementation with EGF (112). The authors also mention that PDGF can
substitute for EGF. It thus seems as if growth factors such as EGF or PDGF
will find a role as essential components in defined media for serial passage
of normal diploid cells.

The study of growth factor requirement of arterial smooth muscle cells
derives its main interest from the modern "endocrine" atherosclerosis model
(see also Section 9). Weinstein et al. (63) demonstrated that smooth muscle
cells can be serially propagated in selenite-supplemented DMEM fortified
with a mixture of hormones (EGF, insulin, hydrocortisone, and PDGF),
transferrin, and fibronectin. Based on this multiple-hormone dependency,
Weinstein et al. constructed an elaborate model for atherosclerosis in which
all the mentioned factors are involved. Mounting evidence supports the
notion that calcium plays an important role in the regulation of cell proliferation. A deep penetration into this matter is beyond the scope of this
chapter, but some findings directly related to PDGF should be discussed.
Several investigators have recorded a lack of PDGF responsiveness in cells
grown at physiological calcium concentrations. Thus Balk's initial observation (1) with chicken pectoral fibroblasts was that only at an unphysio-
logically low calcium concentration is the proliferation rate faster in serum-
containing medium than in medium supplemented with plasma. This observation was confirmed by Balk and his collaborators in more recent investigations (59,60). Scher and collaborators (56) reported that human diploid
fibroblasts are rather unresponsive to PDGF at a physiological calcium
concentration, and our group recently confirmed this finding using cultures
of human foreskin fibroblasts in serum-free MCDB 105 medium. In such a
medium, even if no growth factor is added, there is a clear concentration-
dependent stimulation of cell proliferation by calcium ions. A mitogenic
effect of PDGF and EGF is demonstrable at 1 mM Ca^{2+}, but considerably
more pronounced at low calcium concentrations. This finding is in agreement
with results obtained on EGF and human lung fibroblasts by McKeehan and
McKeehan (113) and on prostate epithelial cells by Kaighn and Lechner
(114). The latter groups have approached the problem by applying enzyme
kinetics to determine quantitatively the effect of ions and growth factors

on proliferation rate and have found that EGF reduces the requirement for extracellular calcium. Using a similar kinetic approach, Ohno and Kaneko (57) showed that PDGF and calcium are competitive stimulators of cell proliferation in fibroblast cultures. The simplest explanation of these findings is that calcium is a regulator in postreceptor messsenger systems, transmitting PDGF or EGF effects. Direct experimental support of this hypothesis is, however, lacking.

Differentiation and cellular growth properties are influenced not only by soluble factors, but also by interactions between neighboring cells and between cells and extracellular matrix (ECM). The importance of the ECM for cell proliferation is demonstrated by the behavior of smooth muscle cells in culture; when cultured on a regular plastic surface, these cells require serum growth factors (i.e., PDGF) and consequently do not grow in plasma. On an ECM, such as detergent-treated endothelial cells, these cells grow equally well in serum and plasma (61). It has been speculated that the ECM makes the cells respond to growth factors in plasma; such factors may thus be of physiological importance *in vivo*, but without any effect in a regular tissue-culture system. These findings demonstrate the complexity of the regulation of cell proliferation and stress the need of defined culture systems by which the interaction of cells, ECM, and growth factors can be critically studied.

Fibronectin is a major glycoprotein of many cells *in vitro* and *in vivo* (115). One of the effects of fibronectin in cell culture is to mediate cell adhesion and spreading. Many cell types synthesize fibronectin in culture, but fibronectin is also a constituent of plasma and serum and is identical to cold-insoluble globulin. Various nonproducing cell lines require exogenously added fibronectin for growth in serum-free medium (116). The role of fibronectin in such culture systems is probably to mediate or facilitate cell adhesion. Immunofluorescence using antibodies directed against fibronectin shows that both human glial cells and foreskin fibroblasts grown in MCDB 105 without serum secrete fibronectin, which becomes adsorbed to the solid substratum and trapped in ECM (Mellström et al., unpublished observations). It is therefore possible that these cells do require fibronectin but are able to furnish this substance themselves.

7.5. PDGF and the Cell Cycle

The cell cycle of proliferating normal anchorage-dependent cells can operationally be divided into two parts, one deterministic (serum independent) portion (beginning and end of G1 plus S, G2, and M), which the cells can run through even in serum-free medium of simple composition, and one serum-dependent part formed by the remaining portion of G1 (117). Serum growth factors are thus required for the completion of the G1 phase; in the absence of such factors, the cells become blocked in G0/G1. Density-arrested cells are also blocked in G0/G1, and upon reinitiation of the cell cycle, for example, by the addition of fresh serum, there is a lag exceeding the length of the G1 of cycling cells before the cells start synthesizing DNA. Such is the case in confluent, stationary Balb/c 3T3 cells. After the addition of serum, there is a 12-hour lag before DNA synthesis starts, whereas the mean of the G1 length of cycling cells is 6 hours (48,118).

Considering the fact that serum contains several hormonal growth factors, at least two possibilities may be envisaged for serum-induced stimulation of cell replication in stationary cultures, and maintenance of G1 traverse in cycling cells.

1. One growth factor is sufficient to induce DNA synthesis, and all cell-cycle events can thus be triggered by a single factor, the various hormonal growth factors in serum acting more or less in the same way by eliciting a "pleiotrophic response" (119).

2. The cells require several complementary growth factors for the completion of the cell cycle. The growth factors act in concert and affect individual metabolic events, which may be localized to different stages in the prereplicative phase. The addition of only one growth factor therefore does not lead to initiation of DNA synthesis. It also follows that several growth factors can act synergistically.

By sequentially adding PDGF and plasma to confluent stationary cultures of Balb/c 3T3 cells and by measuring the rate of entrance into the S phase, Pledger and collaborators obtained data that favor the second hypothesis. The major observation was that PDGF alone does not stimulate DNA synthesis; only in combination with plasma, that in itself is nonstimulatory, is PDGF mitogenic (48). This finding was later confirmed in Swiss 3T3 cultures (39). A brief exposure to plasma followed by incubation with PDGF does not lead to initiation of DNA synthesis, whereas a brief exposure to PDGF followed by a continuous incubation in plasma-containing medium induces DNA synthesis (48,49). On the basis of these observations, Pledger and co-workers have proposed that PDGF renders the cells competent for DNA replication and cell division. Competence alone does not lead to the completion of the cell-cycle traverse. For this to occur, the cells also need progression factors that are constituents of plasma. Using this terminology, PDGF is a competence factor and has no progression activity. This property is not unique for PDGF; competence can also be induced by FGF, calcium phosphate precipitates, low cell density (50), or a short alkaline pulse (120).

The competent state is stable and persists for many hours after the removal of PDGF (48). Competence is also dependent upon PDGF concentration and time of exposure. However, the rate and extent of competence formation has not been investigated in terms of PDGF binding. No data are therefore available on competence formation in relation to number of PDGF receptors occupied per unit of time.

The observation that a brief exposure to PDGF is sufficient to render the cells competent has not been unequivocally substantiated. In all experiments based on the complete removal of PDGF from the cultures, one has to consider seriously the difficulty of removing nonspecifically bound PDGF. Platelet-derived growth factor is a basic and hydrophobic protein that readily adsorbs to most solid surfaces, including plastic, glass, and extracellular matrix. After removal of all free PDGF, the nonspecifically bound PDGF may be recruited and may specifically bind to cellular receptors. In some of the experiments on competence formation, mercaptoethanol has been used to inactivate remaining PDGF (48); whether this treatment really abolished all PDGF activity has not been clearly demonstrated. A strong argument, however, is that competence formation is temperature dependent. Exposure to PDGF at a high concentration at 4°C, a wash with mercaptoethanol, and then shift to 37°C do not lead to competence formation (48). However, since biologically active, radioactively labeled PDGF is now available, it should be possible to reinvestigate competence formation in experiments in which all parameters are controlled: specific binding, internalization, and degradation of PDGF, as well as the recruitment from the pool of nonspecifically bound PDGF.

Challenging cells with PDGF in the absence of plasma proteins makes it possible to study metabolic events related to competence formation *per se* in the absence of processes involved in progression and growth. After exposure to PDGF for 1.5–4.5 hours under such conditions, stationary 3T3 cells start to synthesize a family of five cytoplasmic proteins denoted PI to PV (81). One of these, PI, a 29-kilodalton protein, is detected by [^{35}S] methionine labeling as early as 40 minutes after addition of PDGF. The exact relation between the synthesis of these proteins and competence formation has not been elucidated. However, only competence factors cause a major increase in the synthesis of these proteins, and other growth factors such as insulin or EGF are reported to affect their synthesis but little. Plasma has no detectable effect.

The finding that competence formation after a short exposure to PDGF is linked to initiation of *de novo* protein synthesis implies that PDGF, in addition to having a posttranslational effect (i.e., protein phosphorylation) has an effect at the transcriptional or translational level. Using an elegant experimental approach, Smith and Stiles demonstrated that the competent state can be transferred from a competent donor cell to a noncompetent recipient by Sendai-virus-induced cell fusion (82). Competence formation in the recipient cell could not be abolished by inhibitors of protein synthesis, but was abrogated when inhibitors of RNA synthesis were added to the donor cell. There is thus experimental evidence that exposure to PDGF leads to the formation of new, stable RNA species, which may be messengers for all or some of the proteins detected by [^{35}S]methionine labeling early after exposure to PDGF. Cell-fusion technique and perhaps also microinjection of cell sap from competent donor cells into noncompetent recipients will probably prove to be valuable tools in further experiments on early metabolic events after PDGF stimulation.

Mapping of the progression phase of 3T3 cells has been done by analyzing the rate of DNA-synthesis initiation in competent cell lines after subliminal exposure to plasma, reinforced either by adding suboptimal concentrations of plasma or by exposing the cells to plasma for a short period of time, insufficient to elicit a maximal response. By such an experimental approach, several growth-arrest points have been identified (49). One such point, the V point, is localized in mid-G1 of stimulated, density-arrested Balb/c 3T3 cells. Arrest in the V point can be induced by amino acid starvation, suboptimal concentrations of plasma, and high concentrations of cyclic AMP. Another arrest point, termed W, is localized just prior to the start of DNA synthesis.

The progression activity of plasma can be ascribed partially to its content of somatomedins. These are growth-hormone-dependent polypeptide hormones that in many studies have been shown to possess a weak mitogenic activity on mesenchymal cells (121). That the somatomedins may be required for progression of 3T3 cells was demonstrated by the inability of plasma from hypophysectomized rats to induce progression (50). The progression activity of such plasma can be restored by supplementation with somatomedin C. In the absence of plasma, somatomedin C can release cells blocked in the V point and can also bring them through the W point. Furthermore, EGF can replace plasma in the early progression phase (122). Thus in the stimulation of DNA replication in density-arrested Balb/c 3T3 cells, serum can be replaced by a hormonal cocktail consisting of PDGF, EGF, and somatomedin C (123).

It should be emphasized that the need for individual growth factors that seem to trigger an ordered sequence of events in the prereplicative phase has only been demonstrated for stationary Balb/c 3T3 cells, clone A 31. This cell line is, like all types of 3T3 cells, aneuploid and selected for high serum dependence, growth in monolayer, and low terminal cell density. If not repeatedly recloned, the cells lose these properties and obtain the phenotype of transformed cells. Whether the controlled growth of 3T3 cells in all features resembles that of normal diploid cells has not been elucidated. One could, for instance, envisage that these cells have been selected for "low endogenous progression activity" and therefore require the addition of exogenous factors. In contrast, density-arrested human diploid fibroblasts exposed to PDGF enter S phase even in somatomedin-free plasma from hypophysectomized rats (58). This is probably attributable to an endogenous production of somatomedin C (85), since repeated medium changes in PDGF-stimulated cultures prevent DNA replication in control medium, but not in medium to which somatomedin C has been added (58). Furthermore, high levels of somatomedin C antigen have been found in conditioned media of fibroblast cultures (85). An interesting observation is that the somatomedin C production is stimulated both by PDGF and by human growth hormone. Future studies will show if somatomedin C production is a general feature of mesenchymal cells in culture; if so, the 3T3 cells might represent "somatomedin C̄ mutants," which would explain their need for exogenous somatomedins.

Opposing the view held by Pledger and collaborators, we have proposed that PDGF alone can induce DNA synthesis in stationary cells, provided the cells are given a perfectly balanced defined medium containing all essential low-molecular-weight nutrients (54). One such medium is the MCDB 105 medium, originally designed for human diploid fibroblasts (124). Human diploid fibroblasts and glial cells can be trypsinized and plated in serum-free MCDB 105 medium and stay viable in a stationary phase. After the addition of either PDGF or EGF, DNA synthesis and cell replication are induced; PDGF thus induces both competence and progression in these cells (54). Progression in the fibroblast cultures may be related to an endogenous production of somatomedins. This event is probably less likely to be limiting in the glial cultures, since these cells have previously been shown to be unresponsive to this group of growth factors (125).

Our finding that both human glial and fibroblast cultures are responsive to PDGF and EGF in sparse cultures is also hard to reconcile in terms of the competence/progression cell-cycle model as based on findings with 3T3 cells. Since sparsity alone is a competence factor (50), PDGF should be without function. The model also clearly proposes a difference in action in the cell cycle between PDGF and EGF, the first being a competence factor and the second a progression factor (50). Whether this is true for cells other than 3T3 remains to be elucidated. It would be surprising, though, since the two growth factors when added to other cells that carry receptors for both, are very similar in action; both stimulate tyrosine-specific phosphorylation, both induce the same kind of rapid surface motility and actin reorganization, and both reduce the requirement for calcium (see Sections 7.1, 7.2 and 7.4).

Progression is dependent on low-molecular-weight nutrients. The responsiveness to PDGF and similar "competence" factors then depends on the extracellular concentration of these nutrients and on the presence of hormones, which regulate the transmembranous transport and intracellular availability of these components. Furthermore, hormonal (nonnutritional) growth factors also regulate the requirement for some of the nutritional growth factors such as calcium, magnesium, and pyruvate. Progression is then dependent on several parameters, all or some of which may be cell-type specific: availability of low-molecular-weight nutrients extracellularly (i.e., composition of the nutrient medium), requirement for low-molecular-weight nutrients, exogenously added hormonal growth factors, endogenously produced hormonal growth factors, and the sparing effect of these growth factors on the requirement for low-molecular-weight nutrients. Some of these parameters may be interrelated and mutually exchangeable, and it is possible that a deficient nutrient medium might be matched by the addition of growth factors such as the somatomedins. In addition to analyzing the effects of hormonal growth factors, it therefore seems important to put some effort into designing an optimal nutrient medium.

For example, we have found that glial cells grown in F-10 or F-12 medium are unresponsive to EGF or PDGF unless the medium is supplemented with HSA. Under these circumstances, HSA clearly acts as a progression factor. When the cells are grown in MCDB 105, however, they no longer require HSA (54). The need for HSA as a progression factor can therefore entirely be ascribed to the use of an inadequate nutrient medium.

It will certainly be a challenge in future experimental work to test whether the competence/progression concept for the prereplicative phase is true and generally applicable or rather if the 3T3 cells form an exception since they have been positively selected for growth control.

7.6. Effects of PDGF on Binding and Synthesis of Other Hormones

The effect of PDGF on the expression of other hormone receptors has been investigated in a few cell-culture systems. Platelet-derived growth factor modulates the number of EGF receptors on 3T3 cells (126) and human fibroblasts (47) in a dose-dependent manner. Exposure of the cells to PDGF causes a rapid decrease in EGF binding capacity; the phenomenon can be observed after 2 minutes of incubation at 37°C and is maximal after 10 minutes. However, EGF does not modulate the number of PDGF receptors (47), thus lending no support to the idea (126) that the receptors for EGF and PDGF are processed in a common pathway.

In cultures of Balb/c 3T3 cells, the addition of PDGF leads to an increase in the number of somatomedin C receptors (76). This finding is of particular interest in view of the somatomedin requirement for the completion of the G1 traverse of 3T3 cells rendered competent by PDGF (see also Section 7.5). An increase in binding capacity may thus increase the responsiveness to somatomedins. In human fibroblast cultures, exposure to PDGF leads to an increased synthesis and release of somatomedin C (see also Section 7.5).

Virtually all studies of PDGF on cultured cells have been related to cell proliferation, whereas considerably less is known about its possible effects on differentiated functions. One interesting exception concerns the effect of PDGF on cultured ovarian granulosa cells (83,84). Under the influence of follicle-stimulating hormone (FSH) these cells acquire *in vivo* (127) and *in vitro* (128) receptors for lutropin (LH), which is a prerequisite for ovulation and development of the corpus luteum. It was reported that PDGF potentiates the FSH-dependent LH-receptor induction both in serum-free and in serum-containing medium (84), whereas both EGF and FGF have the opposite effect. In addition, PDGF increases the steroidogenic response to human choriogonadotropin; EGF inhibits steroidogenesis in granulosa cell cultures (129).

These findings are intriguing in several ways. First, the reported effects of PDGF on granulosa cells can only be regarded as preliminary findings, since an impure commercial preparation of PDGF was used. If pure PDGF can be shown to affect hormonally active epithelial cells, this would be remarkable in light of the restricted distribution of PDGF receptors (Table 3). Such studies in conjunction with [^{125}I]PDGF binding experiments are therefore highly warranted. Second, PDGF is normally stored in platelet α-granules and therefore is not apparently accessible to granulosa cells *in vivo*. It is thus difficult to understand how platelet-bound PDGF would act as a physiological regulator of LH-receptor expression. In this context it may be worthwhile to consider the interesting possibility of an extraplatelet pool of PDGF with functions other than those related to cell regeneration (see also Section 5 and Fig. 3). Third, the finding of opposed effects of PDGF and EGF is surprising because of the similarities in their action on fibroblasts (see Section 7.1, 7.2, and 7.4).

8.   ODGF—A SARCOMA-DERIVED EQUIVALENT OF PDGF

Temin et al. originally suggested that the production of endogenous growth factors by certain tumor cells *in vitro* may help the cells maintain their own growth under serum-free conditions (130). Several different cell lines have since been found to secrete growth-promoting activity into the cell-culture medium. Among these is an established osteosarcoma cell line, derived from a human osteogenic sarcoma (6,131). The conditioned medium from this cell line was found to contain growth-promoting activity (osteosarcoma-derived growth factor, ODGF) for glial cells and fibroblasts. The accumulation of this activity occurred at a constant rate over a period of 25 days, suggesting *de novo* synthesis rather than passive release of stored material. Application of purification principles similar to those utilized for PDGF indicated similar behavior of ODGF and PDGF and resulted in a preparation of ODGF with an estimated purity of 50%. Analysis of the susceptibility of ODGF to denaturing solvents, heat, trypsin, or reducing agents yielded results similar to those previously obtained with PDGF. The macromolecular properties of the two factors, including their apparent molecular weights in the non-reduced (about 30,000) and the reduced (14,000–18,000) state were also similar and suggest that both proteins are made up of two different polypeptide chains linked via disulfide bonds. These findings, in conjunction with the observation that ^{125}I-labeled ODGF was recognized by an antibody to PDGF and competed with PDGF for binding to glial cells, led to the conclusion that PDGF and ODGF are closely related or identical (44). It is interesting to note that other examples of sarcoma-derived growth factors have been described (see Chapter 7). The major group consists of EGF-like substances produced by sarcoma-virus-transformed cells, chemically-induced tumor cells, or spontaneously occurring sarcomas (132). These factors are denoted transforming growth factors because of their ability to induce a transformed phenotype in a variety of test cells. Analogously, multiplication-stimulating-activity-like substances are produced by other tumor cells (133) (see Chapter 11). It is tempting to speculate that these different groups of sarcoma-derived growth factors may be of importance for the biology of sarcomas *in vivo*, perhaps maintaining the growth of the tumor cells themselves and/or that of the surrounding normal cells.

9.   ROLE OF PDGF IN NORMAL AND PATHOLOGICAL CELL PROLIFERATION *IN VIVO*

The fact that PDGF is a stimulatory factor for connective-tissue-derived cells *in vitro* has led to the idea that PDGF may be involved in repair processes *in vivo*. The exposure of subendothelial structures following various kinds of tissue damage is bound to cause local adherence and possibly also aggregation of platelets, with subsequent release of the granule contents. Since PDGF is stored in the α-granules, there is a potential for liberation of PDGF whenever the integrity of the vascular lining is disturbed. Mobilization of a proliferation- and chemotaxis-stimulating factor like PDGF could thus be a purposeful event in repair processes. In other situations the reparative response may lead to pathological reactions. One such process is the development of atherosclerotic lesions, long held to be an inflammatory or proliferative response to injuries inflicted by various agents upon the vascular intima. Ross and co-workers have formulated a hypothesis according to which PDGF specifically participates in this reaction by stimulating the proliferation of exposed subintimal smooth muscle cells (105, 106, 134). This attractive model has stimulated much interest and research in the PDGF field. Although still unproved it is supported by a number of observations.

Mechanical injury to the arterial wall, causing local deendothelialization, leads to thickening of the intima with proliferation of smooth muscle cells and formation of connective-tissue matrix. Although basically reversible in nature, this fibromusculoelastic lesion tends to become irreversible and progressive if hypercholesterolemia is maintained in the experimental animal. This phenomenon was, however, not demonstrable in animals made severely thrombocytopenic by administration of anti-platelet antiserum (135, 136). This indicates that platelet-derived components are important for the atherosclerotic lesion to develop. Similarly, the proliferative lesions induced by homocysteine infusion into baboons were dependent on platelet function. Thus, the incidence of lesions was markedly reduced by dipyridamole treatment, which interferes with the ability of platelets to aggregate (137). A third line of evidence comes from studies on swine with von Willebrand's disease, a bleeding disorder involving defective platelet adherence. When subjected to experimental hypercholesterolemia, the affected animals were much less prone to develop atherosclerotic lesions than were the control animals, again suggesting a central role for the platelet in the origin of such lesions (138). However, direct proof for the involvement of PDGF is still lacking. The use of antibodies specifically directed against PDGF in conjunction with atherosclerotic model systems may help clarify this problem. Another approach may be the identification and clinical assessment of putative conditions in which PDGF function is selectively impaired. The gray platelet syndrome, although known to involve α-granule constituents in general, may be an interesting object for such studies.

ACKNOWLEDGMENTS

This work was supported by the Swedish Medical Research Council (4486), the Swedish Cancer Society (56, 689, 786, and 1794), Konung Gustaf V:s 80-årsfond, and Centrala Försöksdjursnämnden, Department of Agriculture (80–120).

REFERENCES

1. Balk, S. D., *Proc. Natl. Acad. Sci. USA*, **68**, 271 (1971).
2. Balk, S. D., Whitfield, J. F., Youdale, T., and Braun, A. C., *Proc. Natl. Acad. Sci. USA*, **70**, 675 (1973).

3. Kohler, N., and Lipton, A., *Exp. Cell Res.*, **87**, 297 (1974).

4. Ross, R., Glomset, J., Kariya, B., and Harker, L., *Proc. Natl. Acad. Sci. USA*, **71**, 1207 (1974).

5. Busch, C., Wasteson, Å., and Westermark, B., *Thromb. Res.*, **8**, 493 (1976).

6. Westermark, B., and Wasteson, Å., in R. Luft and K. Hall, Eds., *Advances in Metabolic Disorders*, Academic, New York, 1975, Vol. 8., p. 85.

7. Westermark, B., and Wasteson, Å., *Exp. Cell Res.*, **98**, 170 (1976).

8. Heldin, C.-H., Wasteson, Å., and Westermark, B., *Exp. Cell Res.*, **109**, 429 (1977).

9. Ross, R., and Vogel, A., *Cell*, **14**, 203 (1978).

10. Scher, C. D., Shepard, R.C., Antoniades, H. N., and Stiles, C. D., *Biochim. Biophys. Acta*, **560**, 217 (1979).

11. Antoniades, H. N., Stathakos, D., and Scher, C. D., *Proc. Natl. Acad. Sci. USA*, **72**, 2635 (1975).

12. Antoniades, H. N., and Scher, C. D., *Proc. Natl. Acad. Sci. USA*, **74**, 1973 (1977).

13. Ihnatowycz, I. O., Cazenave, J.-P., Mustard, J.-F., and Moore, S., *Thromb. Res.*, **14**, 311 (1979).

14. Kaplan, K. L., Broekman, M. J., Chernoff, A., Lesznik, G. R., and Drillings, M., *Blood*, **53**, 604 (1979).

15. Witte, L. D., Kaplan, K. L., Nossel, H. L., Lages, B. A., Weiss, H. J., and Goodman, D. S., *Circ. Res.*, **42**, 402 (1978).

16. Kaplan, D. R., Chao, F. C., Stiles, C. D., Antoniades, H. N., and Scher, C. D., *Blood*, **53**, 1043 (1979).

17. Weiss, H. J., Witte, L. D., Kaplan, K. L., Lages, B. A., Chernoff, A., Nossel, H. L., Goodman, D. S., and Baumgartner, H. R., *Blood*, **54**, 1296 (1979).

18. Gerrard, J. M., Phillips, D. R., Rao, G. H. R., Plow, E. F., Walz, D. A., Ross, R., Harker, L. A., and White, J. G., *J. Clin. Invest.*, **66**, 102 (1980).

19. Chernoff, A., Levine, R. F., and Goodman, D. S., *J. Clin. Invest.*, **65**, 926 (1980).

20. Castro-Malaspina, H., Rabellino, E. M., Yen, A., Nachman, R. L., and Moore, M. A. S., *Blood*, **57**, 781 (1981).

21. Weinstein, R., Stemerman, M. B., MacIntyre, D. E., Steinberg, H. N., and Maciag, T., *Blood*, **58**, 110 (1981).

22. Antoniades, H. N., Scher, C. D., and Stiles, C. D., *Proc. Natl. Acad. Sci. USA*, **76**, 1809 (1979).

23. Heldin, C.-H., Westermark, B., and Wasteson, Å., *Proc. Natl. Acad. Sci. USA*, **76**, 3722 (1979).

24. Heldin, C.-H., Westermark, B., and Wasteson, Å., *Biochem J.*, **193**, 907 (1981).

25. Deuel, T. F., Huang, J. S., Proffitt, R. T., Baenziger, J. U., Chang, D., and Kennedy, B. B., *J. Biol. Chem.*, **256**, 8896 (1981).

26. Rutherford, R. B., and Ross, R., *J. Cell Biol.*, **69**, 196 (1976).

27. Paul, D., Niewiarowski, S., Varma, K. G., Rucinski, B., Rucker, S., and Lange, E., *Proc. Natl. Acad. Sci. USA*, **77**, 5914 (1980).

28. Castor, C. W., Ritchie, J. C., Scott, M. E., and Whitney, S. L., *Arthrit. Rheum.*, **20**, 859 (1977).

29. Castor, C. W., Ritchie, J. C., Williams, J. C., Scott, M. E., Whitney, S. L., Myers, S. L., Sloan, T. B., and Anderson, B. *Arthrit. Rheum.*, **22**, 260 (1979).

30. Eastman, C. T., and Sirbasku, D. A., *J. Cell. Physiol.*, **97**, 17 (1978).

31. Eastman, C. T., and Sirbasku, D. A., *In Vitro*, **16**, 694 (1980).

32. Hara, Y., Steiner, M., and Baldini, M. G., *Cancer Res.*, **40**, 1212 (1980).

33. Kepner, N., and Lipton, A., *Cancer Res.*, **41**, 430 (1981).

34. Paul, D., Niewiarowski, S., Varma, K. G., and Rucker, S., *Thromb. Res.*, **18**, 883 (1980).

35. Walz, D. A., and Castor, C. W., *Clin. Res.*, **27**, 649 A (1979).

36. Niewiarowski, S., Walz, D. A., James, P., Rucinski, B., and Kueppers, F., *Blood*, **55**, 453 (1980).

37. Heldin, C.-H., Westermark, B., and Wasteson, Å., *Exp. Cell Res.*, **136**, 255 (1981).

38. Heldin, C.-H., Westermark, B., and Wasteson, Å., in G. Sato and R. Ross, Eds., *Hormones and Cell Culture*, Cold Spring Harbor Laboratory, Cold Spring Harbor, N.Y., 1979, p. 17.

39. Vogel, A., Raines, E., Kariya, B., Rivest, M.-J., and Ross, R., *Proc. Natl. Acad. Sci. USA*, **75**, 2810 (1978).

40. Ross, R., Vogel, A., Davies, P., Raines, E., Kariya, B., Rivest, M.-J., Gustafson, C., and Glomset, J., in G. Sato and R. Ross, Eds., *Hormones and Cell Culture*, Cold Spring Harbor Laboratory, Cold Spring Harbor, N.Y., 1979, p. 3.

41. Johnsson, A., Heldin, C.-H., Westermark, B., and Wasteson, Å., *Biochem. Biophys. Res. Commun.*, **104**, 66 (1982).

42. Raines, E., and Ross, R., *J. Biol. Chem.*, **257**, 5154 (1982).

43. Owen, A. J., Geyer, R. P., and Antoniades, H. N., *Fed. Proc.*, **40**, 773 A (1981).

44. Heldin, C.-H., Westermark, B., and Wasteson, Å., *J. Cell. Physiol.*, **105**, 235 (1980).

45. Heldin, C.-H., Westermark, B., and Wasteson, Å., *Proc. Natl. Acad. Sci. USA*, **78**, 3664 (1981).

46. Bowen-Pope, D. F., and Ross, R., *J. Biol. Chem.*, **257**, 5161 (1982).

47. Heldin, C.-H., Wasteson, Å., and Westermark, B., *J. Biol. Chem.*, **257**, 4216 (1982).

48. Pledger, W. J., Stiles, C. D., Antoniades, H. N., and Scher, C. D., *Proc. Natl. Acad. Sci. USA*, **74**, 4481 (1977).

49. Pledger, W. J., Stiles, C. D., Antoniades, H. N., and Scher, C. D., *Proc. Natl. Acad. Sci. USA*, **75**, 2839 (1978).

50. Stiles, C. D., Capone, G. T., Scher, C. D., Antoniades, H. N., Van Wyk, J. J., and Pledger, W. J., *Proc. Natl. Acad. Sci. USA*, **76**, 1279 (1979).

51. Ross, R., Nist, C., Kariya, B., Rivest, M.-J., Raines, E., and Callis, J., *J. Cell. Physiol.*, **97**, 497 (1978).

52. Yen, A., and Riddle, V. G. H., *Exp. Cell Res.*, **120**, 349 (1979).

53. Vogel, A., Ross, R., and Raines, E., *J. Cell Biol.*, **85**, 377 (1980).

54. Heldin, C.-H., Wasteson, Å., and Westermark, B., *Proc. Natl. Acad. Sci. USA*, **77**, 6611 (1980).

55. Slayback, J. R. B., Cheung, L. W. Y., and Geyer, R. P., *Exp. Cell Res.*, **110**, 462 (1977).

56. Scher, C. D., Pledger, W. J., Martin, P., Antoniades, H. N., and Stiles, C. D., *J. Cell. Physiol.*, **97**, 371 (1978).

57. Ohno, T., and Kaneko, I., *Cell Struct. Funct.*, **6**, 83 (1981).

58. Clemmons, D. R., and Van Wyk, J. J., *J. Cell. Physiol.*, **106**, 361 (1981).

59. Balk, S. D., *Proc. Natl. Acad. Sci. USA*, **77**, 6606 (1980).

60. Balk, S. D., Levine, S. P., Young, L. L., LaFleur, M. M., and Raymond, N. M., *Proc. Natl. Acad. Sci. USA*, **78**, 5656 (1981).

61. Gospodarowicz, D., and Ill, C. R., *Proc. Natl. Acad. Sci. USA*, **77**, 2726 (1980).

62. Taggart, H., and Stout, R. W., *Atherosclerosis*, **37**, 549 (1980).

63. Weinstein, R., Stemerman, M. B., and Maciag, T., *Science*, **212**, 818 (1981).

64. Frelin, C., *J. Mol. Cell. Cardiol.*, **12**, 1329 (1980).

65. Canalis, E., *Metabolism*, **30**, 970 (1981).

66. Currie, G. A., *Br. J. Cancer*, **43**, 335 (1981).

67. Davies, P. F., and Ross, R., *J. Cell Biol.*, **79**, 663 (1978).

68. Davies, P. F., and Ross, R., *Exp. Cell Res.*, **129**, 329 (1980).

69. Habenicht, A. J. R., Glomset, J. A., Ross, R., and Gronwald, R., *Biochim. Biophys. Acta*, **631**, 495 (1980).

70. Thorgeirsson, G., Robertson, A. L., Jr., and Cowan, D. H., *Lab. Invest.*, **41**, 51 (1979).

71. Wall, R. T., Harker, L. A., and Striker, G. E., *Lab. Invest.*, **39**, 523 (1978).

72. Grotendorst, G. R., Seppä, H. E. J., Kleinman, H. K., and Martin, G. R., *Proc. Natl. Acad. Sci. USA*, **78**, 3669 (1981).

73. Chait, A., Ross, R., Albers, J. J., and Bierman, E. L., *Proc. Natl. Acad. Sci. USA*, **77**, 4084 (1980).

74. Witte, L. D., and Cornicelli, J. A., *Proc. Natl. Acad. Sci. USA*, **77**, 5962 (1980).

75. Wrann, M., Fox, C. F., and Ross, R., *Science*, **210**, 1363 (1980).

76. Clemmons, D. R., Van Wyk, J. J., and Pledger, W. J., *Proc. Natl. Acad. Sci. USA*, **77**, 6644 (1980).

77. Schier, W. T., *Proc. Natl. Acad. Sci. USA*, **77**, 137 (1980).

78. Coughlin, S. R., Moskowitz, M. A., Zetter, B. R., Antoniades, H. N., and Levine, L., *Nature*, **288**, 600 (1980).

79. Coughlin, S. R., Moskowitz, M. A., Antoniades, H. N., and Levine, L., *Proc. Natl. Acad. Sci. USA*, **78**, 7134 (1981).

80. Ek, B., Westermark, B., Wasteson, Å., and Heldin, C.-H., *Nature*, **295**, 419 (1982).

81. Pledger, W. J., Hart, C. A., Locatell, K. L., and Scher, C. D., *Proc. Natl. Acad. Sci. USA*, **78**, 4358 (1981).

82. Smith, J. C., and Stiles, C. D., *Proc. Natl. Acad. Sci. USA*, **78**, 4363 (1981).

83. Mondschein, J. S., and Schomberg, D. W., *Science*, **211**, 1179 (1981).

84. Mondschein, J. S., and Schomberg, D. W., *Endocrinology*, **109**, 325 (1981).

85. Clemmons, D. R., Underwood, L. E., and Van Wyk, J. J., *J. Clin. Invest.*, **67**, 10 (1981).

86. Habenicht, A. J. R., Glomset, J. A., and Ross, R., *J. Biol. Chem.*, **255**, 5134 (1980).

87. Cheung, L. W. Y., Slayback, J. R. B., and Geyer, R. P., *Proc. Soc. Exp. Biol. Med.*, **158**, 292 (1978).

88. Burke, J. M., and Ross, R., *Exp. Cell Res.*, **107**, 387 (1977).

89. Hayashi, I., Nixon, T., Morikawa, M., and Green, H., *Proc. Natl. Acad. Sci. USA*, **78**, 3969 (1981).

90. Carpenter, G., King, L., Jr., and Cohen, S., *Nature*, **276**, 409 (1978).

91. Cohen, S., Carpenter, G., and King, L., Jr., *J. Biol. Chem.*, **255**, 4834 (1980).

92. Ushiro, H., and Cohen, S., *J. Biol. Chem.*, **255**, 8363 (1980).

93. Brugge, J. S., and Erikson, R. L., *Nature*, **269**, 346 (1977).

94. Hunter, T., and Sefton, B. M., *Proc. Natl. Acad. Sci. USA*, **77**, 1311 (1980).

95. Stehelin, D., Varmus, H. E., Bishop, J. M., and Vogt, P. K., *Nature*, **260**, 170 (1976).

96. Collett, M. S., Brugge, J. S., and Erikson, R. L., *Cell*, **15**, 1363 (1978).

97. Erikson, R. L., Purchio, A. F., Erikson, E., Collett, M. S., and Brugge, J. S., *J. Cell Biol.*, **87**, 319 (1980).

98. Shin, S.-I., Freedman, V. H., Risser, R., and Pollack, R., *Proc. Natl. Acad. Sci. USA*, **72**, 4435 (1975).

99. Chen, L. B., Gudor, R. C., Sun, T. T., Chen, A. B., and Mosesson, M. W., *Science*, **197**, 776 (1977).

100. Chinkers, M., McKanna, J. A., and Cohen, S., *J. Cell Biol.*, **83**, 260 (1979).

101. Hunter, T., and Cooper, J. A., *Cell*, **24**, 741 (1981).

102. Schlessinger, J., and Geiger, B., *Exp. Cell Res.*, **134**, 273 (1981).

103. Erikson, E., Shealy, D. J., and Erikson, R. L., *J. Biol. Chem.*, **256**, 11381 (1981).

104. Cheng, Y.-S. E., and Chen, L. B., *Proc. Natl. Acad. Sci. USA*, **78**, 2388 (1981).

105. Ross, R., and Glomset, J. A., *N. Engl. J. Med.*, **295**, 369 (1976).

106. Ross, R., and Glomset, J. A., *N. Engl. J. Med.*, **295**, 420 (1976).

107. Höglund, A.-S., Karlsson, R., Arro, E., Fredriksson, B.-A., and Lindberg, U., *J. Muscle Res. Cell Motil.*, **1**, 127 (1980).

108. Brunk, U., Schellens, J., and Westermark, B., *Exp. Cell Res.*, **103**, 295 (1976).

109. Samuelsson, B., Goldyne, M., Granström, E., Hamberg, M., and Hammarström, S., *Annu. Rev. Biochem.*, **47**, 997 (1978).

110. Hong, S-C. L., and Levine, L., *Proc. Natl. Acad. Sci. USA*, **73**, 1730 (1976).

111. Ham, R. G., and McKeehan, W. L., in W. B. Jakoby and I. H. Pastan, Eds., *Methods in Enzymology*, Academic, New York, 1979, Vol. 58, p. 44.

112. Bettger, W. J., Boyce, S. T., Walthall, B. J., and Ham, R. G., *Proc. Natl. Acad. Sci. USA*, **78**, 5588 (1981).

113. McKeehan, W. L., and McKeehan, K. A., *Exp. Cell Res.*, **123**, 397 (1979).

114. Lechner, J. F., and Kaighn, M. E., *Exp. Cell Res.*, **121**, 432 (1979).

115. Vaheri, A., and Mosher, D. F., *Biochim. Biophys. Acta*, **516**, 1 (1978).

116. Barnes, D., and Sato, G., *Cell*, **22**, 649 (1980).

117. Smith, J. A., and Martin, L., *Proc. Natl. Acad. Sci. USA*, **70**, 1263 (1973).

118. Yen, A., and Pardee, A. B., *Exp. Cell Res.*, **116**, 103 (1978).

119. Herschko, A., Mamout, P., Schield, R., and Tomkins, G., *Nature New Biol.*, **232**, 206 (1971).

120. Zetterberg, A., and Engström, W., *Proc. Natl. Acad. Sci. USA*, **78**, 4334 (1981).

121. Van Wyk, J. J., and Underwood, L. E., in G. Litwack, Ed., *Biochemical Actions of Hormones*, Academic, New York, 1978, Vol. 5, p. 101.

122. Leof, E. B., Wharton, W. R., Van Wyk, J. J., and Pledger, W. J., *J. Cell Biol.*, **87**, 5A (1980).

123. Van Wyk, J. J., Underwood, L. E., D'Ercole, A. J., Clemmons, D. R., Pledger, W. J., Wharton, W. R., and Leof, E. B., in M. Ritzén, A. Aperia, K. Hall, A. Larsson, A. Zetterberg, and R. Zetterström, Eds., *The Biology of Normal Human Growth*, Raven Press, New York, 1981, p. 223.

124. McKeehan, W. L., Genereux, D. P., and Ham, R. G., *Biochem. Biophys. Res. Commun.*, **80**, 1013 (1978).

125. Wasteson, Å., Westermark, B., and Uthne, K., in R. Luft and K. Hall, Eds., *Advances in Metabolic Disorders*, Academic, New York, 1975, Vol. 8, p. 101.

126. Wrann, M., Fox, C. F., and Ross, R., *Science*, **210**, 1363 (1980).

127. Zeleznik, A. J., Midgley, A. R., Jr., and Reichert, L. E., Jr., *Endocrinology*, **95**, 818 (1974).

128. Eriksson, G. F., Wang, C., and Hsueh, A. J. W., *Nature*, **279**, 336 (1979).

129. Hsueh, A. J. W., Welsh, T. H., and Jones, P. B. C., *Endocrinology*, **108**, 2002 (1981).

130. Temin, H. M., Pierson, R. W., Jr., and Dulak, N. C., in G. H. Rothblat and J. Cristofalo, Eds., *Growth, Nutrition and Metabolism of Cells in Culture*, Academic, New York, 1972, Vol. 1, p. 49.

131. Pontén, J., and Saksela, E., *Int. J. Cancer*, **2**, 434 (1967).

132. Todaro, G. J., De Larco, J. E., Fryling, C., Johnson, P. A., and Sporn, M. B., *J. Supramol. Struct. Cell. Biochem.*, **15**, 287 (1981).

133. Marquardt, H., Wilson, G. L., and Todaro, G. J., *J. Biol. Chem.*, **255**, 9177 (1980).

134. Harker, L. A., and Ross, R., in *Seminars in Thrombosis and Hemostasis*, 1979, Vol. 5, p. 274.

135. Moore, S., Friedman, R. J., Singal, D. P., Gauldie, J., Blajchman, M., and Roberts, R. S., *Thromb. Hemostas.* **35**, 70 (1976).

136. Friedman, R. J., Stemerman, M. B., Wenz, B., Moore, S., Gauldie, J., Gent, M., Tiell, M. L., and Spaet, T. H., *J. Clin. Invest.*, **60**, 1191 (1977).

137. Harker, L. A., Ross, R., Slichter, S. J., and Scott, C. R., *J. Clin. Invest.*, **58**, 731 (1976).

138. Fuster, V., Bowie, W. E. J., Lewis, J. C., Fass, D. N., Owen, C. A., Jr., and Brown, A. L., *J. Clin. Invest.*, **61**, 722 (1978).

NOTE ADDED IN PROOF

For previous reviews on PDGF see also ref. 1.

Bjornson Childs et al. have described another growth factor of probable platelet origin. This factor has transforming properties, i.e., induces colony formation in soft agar by anchorage-dependent mouse or rat cells (2).

Antoniades et al. have isolated two forms of PDGF with different molecular weights, illustrating the molecular weight heterogeneity of the factor (3).

Further development of the RIA for PDGF has lowered the background and increased the sensitivity, the present lower detection level being about 1 ng/ml. Application of the improved method to whole serum results in PDGF readings of about 20 ng/ml; estimates of PDGF in plasma-derived serum yields about 2.5 ng/ml (Heldin et al., unpublished).

Huang et al. have demonstrated specific high-affinity binding of PDGF to 3T3 cells (4). Protamine sulfate displaced bound PDGF from the 3T3 cells indicating that the binding was reversible. Williams et al. have described a similar high-affinity binding of PDGF to vascular smooth muscle cells (5). Crosslinking experiments by Glenn et al. indicate a molecular weight of 164,000 for the PDGF receptor (6). Smith et al. have demonstrated that PDGF bound to an extracellular substrate may be mitogenically active, indicating that the PDGF receptor may recognize and utilize not only soluble PDGF, but also PDGF sequestered in an insoluble form (7).

Witte et al. have extended their studies of the effects of PDGF on the low-density lipoprotein receptor pathway in cultured human fibroblasts, exploring in detail the relationships between the effects of PDGF on low-density lipoprotein metabolism, cholesterol metabolism, and DNA synthesis (8).

Nishimura and Deuel have shown that PDGF stimulates the phosphorylation of the serine residues of an M_r 33,000 protein in 3T3 cells (9). More recently they have also demonstrated a tyrosine-specific phosphorylation of 3T3 cell membrane proteins, M_r 180,000 and 160,000, respectively (10). These cells thus seem to contain a kinase activity similar to that present on human fibroblast membranes. Extended characterization of the latter enzyme indicated that it phosphorylated an M_r 185,000 and an M_r 130,000 protein and was clearly distinct from the EGF-stimulated kinase present in the same preparation (11). Further, the components participating in the PDGF-dependent phosphorylation reaction could be solubilized from the membranes by treatment with Triton X-100, without loss of activity.

PDGF has been shown to be chemotactic for fibroblasts (12) and for monocytes and neutrophils (13). These observations are in agreement with the idea that PDGF has a function in inflammatory and repair processes following tissue damage.

Shupnik et al. (14) and Tashjian et al. (15) have presented further evidence for an enhancing effect of PDGF on prostaglandin E_2 formation; the stimulating effect of PDGF on bone resorption was thought to be mediated via this pathway. Shier et al. have suggested that the stimulation by PDGF of prostaglandin formation is due to the release of arachidonic acid and propose that this effect, rather than increased prostaglandin formation, is essential for the expression of the proliferative response to PDGF (16). Whereas previous investigators have ascribed the effect of PDGF on arachidonic acid release to an increase in PLase A_2 activity, Habenicht et al. suggest that, rather, PDGF regulates the activity of PLase C (17).

Weinstein et al. have used a serum-free defined medium for the growth of human foreskin fibroblasts (18). In their experimental system, which included the addition of several macromolecular components and the use of fibronectin-coated culture dishes, PDGF was not a limiting factor for cellular growth.

Wharton et al. have reported that the formation of the state of competence in Balb/c-3T3 cells is potentiated by increases in cyclic AMP, brought about, e.g., by the addition of cholera toxin or isobutylmethylxanthine (19,20). Since this effect was accompanied by both a decrease in the number of EGF receptors and a lowered requirement for EGF in the progression phase, the authors speculate that the internalization of EGF receptors is somehow part of an overall growth response by the cell (19).

Dicker et al. have pointed out that fibroblast-derived growth factor, a product of SV-40 transformed baby hamster kidney cells, has properties in common with PDGF (21). Although the comparison was not taken into any detail, it is possible that fibroblast-derived growth factor, like ODGF belongs to the same family of growth factors as PDGF.

Braunstein et al. have observed a fibroblast-stimulating effect of platelets injected subcutaneously into rats (22). However, the response was delayed and apparently linked to an inflammatory reaction; therefore it was considered to be secondary to neutrophil activation. Inglot and Inglot (23) and Witkoski et al. (24) have demonstrated an enhancing effect on tumor growth in vivo of (a) factor(s) present in human platelets; the nature of the active component is, however, unknown.

References to the Addendum

1. Ross, R., in Baserga, R., Ed., Handbook of Experimental Pharmacology, Springer, Berlin, 1981, Vol. 57, p. 133.
2. Bjornson Childs, C., Proper, J. A., Tucker, R. F., and Moses, H. F., *Proc. Natl. Acad. Sci. USA*, **79**, 5312 (1982).
3. Antoniades, H. N., *Proc. Natl. Acad. Sci. USA*, **78**, 7314 (1981).
4. Huang, J. S., Huang, S. S., Kennedy, B., and Deuel, T. F., *J. Biol. Chem.*, **257**, 8130 (1982).
5. Williams, L. T., Tremble, P., and Antoniades, H. N., *Proc. Natl. Acad. Sci. USA*, **79**, 5867 (1982).
6. Glenn, K., Bowen-Pope, D. F., and Ross, R., *J. Biol. Chem.*, **257**, 5172 (1982).
7. Smith, J. C., Singh, J. P., Lillquist, J. S., Goon, D. S., and Stiles, C. D., *Nature*, **296**, 154 (1982).
8. Witte, L. D., Cornicelli, J. A., Miller, R. W., and Goodman, D. S., *J. Biol. Chem.*, **257**, 5392 (1982).
9. Nishimura, J., and Deuel, T. F., *Biochem. Biophys. Res. Commun.*, **103**, 355 (1981).
10. Nishimura, J., Huang, J. S., and Deuel, T. F., *Proc. Natl. Acad. Sci. USA*, **79**, 4303 (1982).
11. Ek, B., and Heldin, C.-H., *J. Biol. Chem.*, **257**, 10486 (1982).
12. Seppä, H., Grotendorst, G., Seppä, S., Schiffmann, E., and Martin, G. R., *J. Cell Biol.*, **92**, 584 (1982).

13. Deuel, T. F., Senior, R. M., Huang, J. S., and Griffin, G. L., *J. Clin. Invest.*, **69**, 1046 (1982).

14. Shupnik, M. A., Antoniades, H. N., and Tashjian, A. H., Jr., *Life Sci.*, **30**, 347 (1982).

15. Tashjian, A. H., Jr., Hohmann, E. L., Antoniades, H. N., and Levine, L., *Endocrinology*, **111**, 118 (1982).

16. Shier, W. T., and Durkin, J. P., *J. Cell. Physiol.*, **112**, 171 (1982).

17. Habenicht, A. J. R., Glomset, J. A., King, W. C., Nist, C., Mitchell, C. D., and Ross, R., *J. Biol. Chem.*, **256**, 12329 (1981).

18. Weinstein, R., Hoover, G. A., Majure, J., van der Spek, J., Stemerman, M. B., and Maciag, T., *J. Cell. Physiol.*, **110**, 23 (1982).

19. Wharton, W., Leof, E., Pledger, W. J., and O'Keefe, E. J., *Proc. Natl. Acad. Sci. USA*, **79**, 5567 (1982).

20. Wharton, W., Leof, E. B., Olashaw, N., Earp, H. S., and Pledger, W. J., *J. Cell. Physiol.*, **111**, 201 (1982).

21. Dicker, P., Pohjanpelto, P., Pettican, P., and Rozengurt, E., *Exp. Cell Res.*, **135**, 221 (1981).

22. Braunstein, P. W., Jr., Cuénod, H. F., Joris, I., and Majno, G., *Am. J. Pathol.*, **99**, 53 (1980).

23. Inglot, A. D., and Inglot, O., *Arch. Immunol. Ther. Exp.*, **29**, 431 (1981).

24. Witkoski, E., Kepner, N., Leitzel, K., Rogers, C., Jefferson, L. S., and Lipton, A., *Cancer Res.*, **42**, 2350 (1982).

5

EPIDERMAL GROWTH FACTOR: CELLULAR BINDING AND CONSEQUENCES

Harry T. Haigler

CONTENTS

Abbreviations

EGF	Epidermal growth factor
SDS	Sodium dodecyl sulfate
Fl-EGF	Fluorescein isothiocyanate derivative of epidermal growth factor (fluorescent)
F-EGF	Ferritin conjugate of epidermal growth factor
EM	Electron microscope
LDL	Low-density lipoprotein
α_2-**M**	α_2-macroglobulin
Fl-α_2-M	Fluorescein-labeled α_2-macroglobulin
R-EGF	Rhodamine conjugate of epidermal growth factor
NRK	Normal rat kidney
TCA	Trichloroacetic acid

Epidermal growth factor (EGF) is a small, very stable polypeptide hormone that was first isolated and described by Stanley Cohen. It is a potent mitogen for a wide variety of cells *in vivo* and in tissue culture. Specific cellular receptors for EGF have been demonstrated in vertebrates ranging from the dogfish shark to humans, and it appears that both the hormone and its receptor have been conserved during the process of evolution. Although this suggests that EGF plays an important role in the metabolism and/or development of the intact organism, the exact role has not yet been determined.

Most recent studies of EGF have been performed on cultured cells. The interactions of EGF with cultures of target cells provide useful systems for studying growth control and the biochemistry and cell biology of polypeptide-hormone–receptor interactions. It has been shown that cell-bound EGF rapidly clusters in the plane of the plasma membrane in clathrin-coated pits and is internalized into endocytic vesicles that eventually fuse with lysosomes, where the hormone is degraded. This area of research, and a comparison with the internalization of other polypeptide ligands, is covered in detail. Another focus of this article concerns experiments showing that a tyrosine-specific protein kinase activity is associated with the EGF receptor. This highly unusual activity is shared with certain tumor viruses, and this raises the possibility that EGF and these viruses stimulate cell growth by similar mechanisms. Before covering these topics, the existing knowledge concerning the biochemistry and biology of EGF are discussed. Since several excellent reviews of research involving EGF are available (1–5), this chapter does not present a general comprehensive coverage, but focuses on recent studies and studies relevant to the cellular internalization and receptor-associated protein kinase problems.

1.   ISOLATION AND PHYSIOCHEMICAL PROPERTIES

During the isolation of nerve growth factor from mouse submaxillary glands, Stanley Cohen (6) observed that injection of extracts of these glands into newborn mice resulted in precocious opening of eyelids and eruption of incisors. These morphological alterations were the consequence of enhanced epidermal growth. The factor responsible for these effects was isolated and designated EGF (7). A rapid two-step procedure was devised that permits the isolation of milligram quantities of EGF from the submaxillary gland of mice (8). Since mouse EGF can be isolated in relatively large quantities, it has been possible to characterize its physical and chemical properties in detail. It is a single-chain polypeptide with a molecular weight of 6045; the complete amino acid sequence and location of the three disulfide bonds have been reported (9). The hormone contains no alanine, phenylalanine, or lysine and is extremely stable (10).

Under appropriate extraction conditions, EGF can be isolated from the mouse submaxillary gland as a high-molecular-weight complex in which EGF is associated with a specific arginine esteropeptidase (11,12). It has been demonstrated that a pro-EGF of approximately 9000 daltons is synthesized that is then specifically cleaved at an arginine residue by the binding protein to form EGF (13). Nerve growth factor can also be isolated from the submaxillary gland as a high-molecular-weight complex with an arginine esteropeptidase that has sequence homology with, but is not identical to, the EGF binding protein (14,15).

A polypeptide, designated human EGF, has been isolated from human urine (16). It possesses all of the biological activities of mouse EGF *in vivo* and *in vitro* and cross-reacts to some extent with antibodies prepared against mouse EGF. An unexpected aspect of the biology of EGF emerged with the publication of the amino acid sequence of human urogastrone (17).

Urogastrone had been studied for over 20 years as a urinary substance that inhibits gastric HCl secretion (3,18). The sequence and subsequent biological studies suggest that human EGF and urogastrone are identical molecules. The sequence of urogastrone is 70% identical to that of mouse EGF. This and other evidence (19) strongly suggest that human EGF (urogastrone) and mouse EGF are homologous proteins that arose from a common ancestral gene.

Moore (20) has isolated an EGF from rat submaxillary glands that has a similar, but not identical, amino acid composition to EGF from either mouse or human sources.

2. BIOLOGICAL EFFECTS OF EGF

2.1. Effects *in Vivo*

Epidermal growth factor stimulates cell replication in a number of tissues *in vivo* including skin (21,22), liver (23), cornea (24,25), lung (26), and trachea (26). In addition to its mitogenic effects, EGF also affects several differentiated cellular functions. For example, intravenous injection of EGF inhibits histamine-induced gastric acid secretion in rats and dogs (27), and these effects are correlated with morphological changes in the surface of parietal cells (28). Epidermal growth factor has been reported to promote the healing of stomach ulcers (18). And EGF also appears to stimulate the synthesis and secretion of alveolar surface-active material in fetal rabbit lungs (29).

Although it has long been known that the placenta contains a high concentration of EGF-binding activity (30), the possible role played by EGF in fetal development only recently has attracted much research effort. Nexo et al. (31) showed that EGF and its cellular receptors are present in mouse embryos as early as day 13 of gestation. Especially high concentrations of receptors were found in the secondary palate, and this suggests that EGF may have a role in palate closure. High concentrations of EGF receptors have also been found in the mouse amnion at 13 days of gestation (32).

Mouse EGF is synthesized in the submaxillary gland, and quite high concentrations are stored in the tubular duct cells (see references 1 and 33 for reviews). The amount stored in the gland is dependent on the androgen status of the animal, and the release of EGF into the saliva and the circulatory system is under α-adrenergic control. Although the synthesis and storage of EGF in the mouse submaxillary gland is under physiological control, the gland does not seem to be crucial in the regulation of plasma levels of EGF; the plasma concentration of EGF has been observed to remain at normal levels 2 weeks after removal of the submaxillary glands (33). Therefore, other sites of synthesis of EGF must exist. In humans, EGF (urogastrone) has been localized to the submaxillary gland and to the Brunner's gland of the duodenum (34,35).

The exact role EGF plays in development and metabolism remains to be established. Historically, endocrinologists have investigated the physiological role of a particular hormone by removing the gland where it is synthesized and observing the ensuing effects. However, this route of investigation of EGF is not available because it appears that there is not a single discrete site of synthesis. Although new approaches may be required, studies of the biology of EGF in the intact animal should attract more research effort in the future since its growth-promoting activity makes it a potentially useful agent for the clinical treatment of severe burns, corneal wounds, and ulcers.

2.2. Effects in Organ and Tissue Culture

The mitogenic effects of EGF seen *in vivo* can also be demonstrated in organ culture. In cultures of skin tissue from chick embryos and fetal humans, EGF stimulated ornithine decarboxylase activity, RNA, protein, and DNA synthesis, and ultimately cell division in the epidermis (36,37). A mitogenic effect on cultures of human and bovine corneal epithelium has also been reported (38,39).

EGF is a potent mitogen for certain cultured cells and has been used extensively as a model for studying growth control (see references 1,2, and 40 for reviews). In the intact animal and in organ culture, EGF seems only to stimulate the growth of epidermal and epithelial cells. However, in tissue culture EGF is mitogenic for a wide variety of cells including murine and human fibroblasts (41–43), human glial cells (44), human keratinocytes (45), rabbit chondrocytes (46), bovine smooth muscle cells (47), bovine and human granulosa cells (48,49), rat hepatocytes (50), human vascular endothelial cells (51), human mesenchymal cells (52), rabbit endometrial cells (53), and monkey kidney epithelial cells (54).

Diploid human cells plated in the presence of 0.1 nM EGF and optimal concentrations of serum reach a fourfold higher saturation density, and EGF can support the growth of cells at low concentrations of serum (55). In this and other respects, normal cells stimulated with EGF are similar to cultured tumor cells. However, EGF does not support the growth of normal cells in soft agar.

The addition of EGF to confluent quiescent monolayers of human fibroblasts stimulates DNA synthesis, with the maximal stimulation occurring approximately 24 hours after addition (55). If EGF is removed 4 hours after addition, the amount of thymidine incorporated is reduced by over 90%, indicating that the initial interaction (binding) of the mitogen with the cell-surface receptors is not sufficient to stimulate DNA synthesis; that is, the cell-surface receptors have to be occupied over an extended period to exert their mitogenic effect. Since EGF–receptor complexes are rapidly removed from the plasma membrane by endocytosis (see below), these results can be explained by one of the following hypotheses: (1) a small fraction of the occupied EGF receptors escape internalization and remain on the cell surface, or (2) all occupied receptors are rapidly internalized, and the continued presence of occupied receptors on the surface is due to the binding of EGF to newly inserted receptors. Haigler and Carpenter used an antibody against the EGF receptor to obtain evidence in support of the second hypothesis (56), however, Schechter et al. (57) have presented data that they interpret to be in support of the first hypothesis.

In addition to the "long-term" effects of EGF (i.e., DNA synthesis and mitosis), several "short-term" effects that occur with 4 hours of treatment have been reported in cultured cells. The following short-term effects of EGF may be a general preprogrammed response to prepare a cell for replication rather than a specific response to EGF: increased uptake of $^{86}Rb^+$ (58), deoxyglucose (59), and aminoisobutyrate (60); increased incorporation of glucosamine into extracellular matrix glycoproteins (61); increased glycolytic rate (62); and an increase in the specific activity of phosphofructokinase (63). The biochemical basis of these early events has been reviewed by Rozengurt (64).

A number of reports have described specific effects of EGF on differentiated cell function that apparently are not directly related to the mitogenic response. Physiological concentrations of EGF promote the secretion of fibronectin in 3T3 cells (65). In cultured rat pituitary cells, EGF increases the synthesis of prolactin and inhibits the synthesis of growth hormone (66), and in cultured human choriocarcinoma cells, EGF stimulates chorionic gonado-tropin secretion (67). Epidermal growth factor regulates the number of gonadotropin receptors in cultured Leydig tumor cells (68) and granulosa cells (69). Sun and Green have shown that EGF influences the differentiated state of cultured keratinocytes (70).

3.   EGF RECEPTORS

3.1.   Characterization of Cellular Binding of EGF

Cells that are responsive to EGF contain specific saturable cell-surface receptors for the hormone that can be studied using ^{125}I-labeled EGF. Most cultured cells that are responsive to EGF contain approximately 25,000–150,000 binding sites per cell with apparent dissociation constants of approximately 0.5 nM (see references 1,2, and 5 for reviews). Cultures of the epithelioid carcinoma cells A-431 (71,72) and KB (73) have approximately 2 million and 400,000, respectively, receptors per cell and are thus useful for certain types of experiments.

In a series of studies concerning the fate of cell-bound [^{125}I]EGF in cultured human fibroblasts, Carpenter and Cohen (74) made the following observations: (1) cell-bound [^{125}I]EGF is rapidly degraded to [^{125}I]monoiodotyrosine at 37°C, (2) the degradation, but not the binding, requires metabolic energy, and (3) the degradation is inhibited by drugs that inhibit lysosomal function, such as chloroquine and ammonium chloride. Based on these and other indirect observations, they postulated that after the initial binding of [^{125}I]EGF to specific plasma-membrane receptors, the EGF–receptor complex is internalized, and the hormone, probably along with its receptor, eventually is degraded by lysosomes. Additional experimental support for this hypothesis was provided by Das and Fox (75). They labeled a putative EGF receptor with a photoreactive derivative of [^{125}I]EGF and located degradation products of the receptor in the "lysosomal" fraction of the cell. Internalization and degradation of [^{125}I]EGF has been observed in a number of other cell lines (43,76–80, 84). The direct visualization of the binding and internalization has been achieved by several morphological methods and is discussed in detail below.

Cytogenetic analysis of somatic-cell hybrids have shown that in humans the gene coding for the EGF receptor is located in chromosome 7 (81,82).

3.2. Modulation of Binding Activity

[^{125}I]EGF binding activity on cultured cells can be modulated in a number of ways. Cohen and co-workers (74,83) showed that in the presence of EGF, the amount of EGF-binding activity rapidly decreases. They suggested (74) that the loss of receptor activity is due to the internalization of EGF–receptor complexes, with a slower rate of insertion of new receptors.

The cellular binding of [^{125}I]EGF can be reduced by incubating the cells with phorbol ester tumor promoters and by transformation with certain tumor viruses. These topics are reviewed by Horowitz and Weinstein and by DeLarco, respectively, in this volume. The cellular binding of [^{125}I]EGF to pheochromocytoma and 3T3 cells is reduced by nerve growth factor and platelet-derived growth factor, respectively (85,86). Glucocorticoids (87,88) and retinoids (89) increase the number of EGF receptors.

3.3. Chemical Nature of the Receptor

Carpenter and Cohen suggested (90), based on the ability of various lectins to inhibit EGF binding reversibly, that the EGF receptor is a glycoprotein. Experiments by Pratt and Pastan (91) showing that a cell mutant defective in glycoprotein synthesis has a marked reduction in EGF-binding capacity support the glycoprotein nature of the EGF receptor. The ability of the carbohydrate moities of the EGF receptor to interact with immobilized lectins has been used by Hollenberg and co-workers (92,93) to purify the detergent-solubilized EGF receptor from human placenta. The main component of the purified receptor preparation had a molecular weight of approximately 160 kilodaltons on sodium dodecyl sulfate (SDS) polyacrylamide gel electrophoresis.

Cohen et al. (94) purified a putative EGF receptor to near homogeneity from Triton-solubilized A-431 membranes on an EGF affinity column. The purified protein ran as a doublet of 150 and 170 kilodaltons on SDS polyacrylamide gel electrophoresis.

Several groups have attempted to identify the EGF receptor by covalently cross-linking the receptor to [^{125}I]EGF. Using a photoaffinity derivative of [^{125}I]EGF, Das et al. (95) labeled a protein with an apparent molecular weight of 190 kilodaltons in 3T3 cells. Two placental proteins of apparent molecular weights 180 and 160 kilodaltons were labeled by similar methods (96). Very low yields were obtained by both methods (95,96).

It was later found that [^{125}I]EGF that was not coupled to a heterobifunctional cross-linking agent could also be covalently coupled to its putative receptors in human fibroblasts (97), 3T3 cells (98), epidermoid carcinoma cells A-431 (99), and placenta (100) that had apparent molecular weights ranging from 170 to 190 kilodaltons. But it has recently been shown by Comens, Simmer, and Baker (101) that the "spontaneous" cross-linking of [^{125}I]EGF to its cellular receptor is a function of chloramine T treatment during the iodination procedure and does not reflect a physiological process. They found that the amount of spontaneous cross-linking was increased with increasing amounts of chloramine T used in the iodination procedure; very little cross-linking was seen using the iodination conditions originally used by Carpenter and Cohen (74). The EGF that was iodinated by a lactoperoxidase procedure (102) did not become covalently linked to its receptor unless it was subsequently exposed to chloramine T (101). Comens et al. (101) also showed that under appropriate conditions, chloramine T-treated [^{125}I]EGF is a useful reagent for radiolabeling EGF receptors.

4. INTERNALIZATION OF EGF

It is generally agreed that small hydrophobic hormones such as steroids passively diffuse through the plasma membrane and exert their biological effects by interacting with intracellular receptors. In contrast, polypeptide hormones are unable to passively cross the plasma membrane and until recently were thought to exert their biological effects by a transmembrane signal generated while the hormones were bound to their receptors located on the cell surface (103). However, there is not an absolute barrier between extracellular proteins and the cytosol, because it has long been known that certain proteins such as diphtheria toxin can gain access to the cell's interior (104).

In an innovative set of experiments, Carpenter and Cohen presented the first evidence that [^{125}I]EGF is internalized in cultured fibroblasts (74). It is now clear that many, if not most, polypeptide hormones can enter cells by the process of receptor-mediated endocytosis. It appears that these polypeptide hormones share the same basic cellular pathway for internalization with a number of other ligands including vitellogenin (105), low-density lipoproteins (106), α_2-macroglobulin (107–109), lysosomal hydrolases (110,111), transcobalamin II (112), asialoglycoproteins (113–115), and certain viruses (116,117). Common features of the pathway include a clustering of the ligand–receptor complexes in clathrin-coated pits, internalization into endocytic vesicles, and eventual sequestration in lysosomal structures. This pathway has been extensively studied using radioactive, fluorescent, and ferritin conjugates of EGF. A coherent story has emerged from these different methods that forms a framework for future attempts to understand the physiological role that internalization and degradation of cell-bound EGF plays in the cellular action of EGF.

4.1. Fluorescent EGF

The direct visualization of EGF binding to target cells first was accomplished using fluorescent derivatives of the hormone. The N-terminal amino group of EGF was modified by reacting with fluorescein isothiocyanate, and the resulting conjugate (Fl-EGF) was purified by ion-exchange chromatography (71). The Fl-EGF retained 45% of the binding activity of the native hormone and was approximately as mitogenic for cultured fibroblasts as the unmodified hormone. Visualization of cellular binding of Fl-EGF was greatly facilitated by using the A-431 cell line isolated by Fabricant et al. (72) that contained an extraordinarly high binding capacity—approximately 2.5×10^6 receptors per cell (71).

To determine the initial distribution of EGF in the plane of the plasma membrane, A-431 cells were incubated with Fl-EGF at 6°C; at this temperature, the EGF receptor cannot diffuse laterally in the plane of the membrane. The fluorescence (Fig. 1a) and Nomarski (Fig. 1b) photomicrographs show that under these conditions, the cellular borders were prominently stained, and the fluorescence on the remainder of the membrane was uniform.

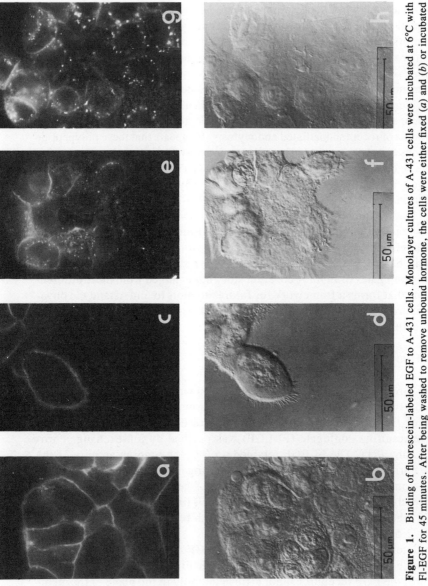

Figure 1. Binding of fluorescein-labeled EGF to A-431 cells. Monolayer cultures of A-431 cells were incubated at 6°C with Fl-EGF for 45 minutes. After being washed to remove unbound hormone, the cells were either fixed (a) and (b) or incubated at 37°C for 2 minutes (c) and (d), 10 minutes (e) and (f), or 20 minutes (g) and (h) prior to fixation. (a), (c), (e), and (g): Fluorescence micrographs under epi-illumination. (b), (d), (f), and (h): Photographs by Nomarski optics of the same cells and in the same focal plane. Bar = 50 μm. Reprinted with permission from reference 71.

An identical pattern was seen when the cells were fixed prior to staining with Fl-EGF.

To determine the distribution of Fl-EGF at physiological temperatures, cells were pretreated with Fl-EGF at 6°C and then were incubated at 37°C for varying lengths of time and examined for the pattern of fluorescence. No detectable alterations were noted after 2 minutes at 37°C (Figs. 1c,1d); however, at 10 minutes randomly distributed spheres of fluorescence could be detected (Figs. 1e,1f). From the plane of focus and immunofluorescent studies (not shown), these spheres clearly were inside the cell and were interpreted to be endocytic vesicles. After 20 minutes at 37°C (Figs. 1g,1h), these endocytic vesicles had redistributed to form a perinuclear ring. At 2 hours (not shown), the fluorescence at the cell borders and membrane was markedly decreased, but that in the perinuclear vesicles was still detectable.

Fluorescent derivatives of EGF have also been studied in cultured cells containing approximately 100,000 receptors per cell (e.g., 3T3 cells) by observing the cell-bound derivatives with a silicon-intensifier-target television camera system developed by Willingham and Pastan (118). This system allows detection of very low levels of emitted light. By using low amounts of excitation light, the cellular damage caused by illumination can be reduced to the point that it is possible to visualize fluorescent probes in living cells for extended periods of time. Using this system, Schlessinger et al. (119,120) also found that EGF initially bound to the cell surface in a diffuse manner and after 10–30 minutes was located in endocytic vesicles. Videotapes showed that the fluorescent endocytic vesicles moved about the cytoplasm in a saltatory manner. Schlessinger et al. (119) used a fluorescence-photobleaching recovery method to determine that at 23°C the fluorescent EGF–receptor complex was mobile in the plane of the membrane and had a diffusion coefficient of approximately 4×10^{-10} cm^2/second. This rate of diffusion is consistent with the distance and time course involved in redistribution of cell-surface-bound ferritin-labeled EGF (see below).

4.2. [^{125}I]EGF

Gordon et al. (121) used a quantitative electron microscope (EM) autoradiographic approach to visualize the events involved in the binding process. When human fibroblasts were exposed to [^{125}I]EGF for 2 hours at 4°C or 2 minutes at 37°C, the grains primarily localized to the plasma membrane. With increasing time at 37°C, the amount of labeled EGF on the cell surface decreased with a corresponding increase in the number of grains localized to lysosomes. At steady state (2 hours at 37°C), greater than ⅔ of the label was intracellular. Because of radiation scatter, this method was not able to determine the nature of the structures involved in the shuttling of the cell-surface EGF to the lysosomes. However, the resolution was sufficient to determine that the cell-surface binding showed some preference for coated pits.

4.3. Ferritin-Conjugated EGF

In order to visualize and quantitatively study the events that occur prior to and during the internalization of the hormone–receptor complex, Haigler, McKanna, and Cohen (122) prepared a conjugate of ferritin and EGF. By exploiting the fact that EGF contains only one free amino group, it was possible to design a synthetic procedure that yielded a conjugate containing EGF and ferritin in a 1:1 molar ratio. After purification by gel filtration and affinity chromatography, a biologically active ferritin-EGF (F-EGF) conjugate was isolated. Monolayers of A-431 cells were incubated with F-EGF at 4°C and processed for the EM. Electron micrographs of sections show that the F-EGF was located exclusively on the extracellular face of the plasma membrane (Fig. 2A). Most of the ferritin cores were randomly distributed, although a few were found in small groups. The average density of ferritin cores over the entire cells surface was 200 particles/μm^2. This corresponds to approximately 6×10^5 particles per cell and is in good agreement with the amount of binding of [^{125}I]EGF obtained under these conditions (approximately 1×10^6 molecules per cell). Binding of F-EGF was very specific; when an excess of unlabeled EGF was added simultaneously with the conjugate, fewer than 2 particles/μm^2 were observed.

The fate of cell-bound F-EGF was investigated by binding the conjugate to monolayers at 4°C, removing unbound F-EGF, and then warming the cultures to 37°C. The F-EGF rapidly redistributed on the cell surface such that within 30 seconds 47% was located in small clusters. At peripheral regions the cells were thin enough to permit penetration of the electron beam through an *en face* presentation of the intact cell (123). In such electron micrographs, the tightly packed clusters of F-EGF can be seen in discrete locations (Fig. 2B). These clusters are fairly uniform in size and in the number of ferritin particles (approximately 10–15 per cluster) and are presumably the sites of endocytosis of the hormone. In such clusters, the ferritin cores are separated by center-to-center distances of approximately 12 nm (123). This corresponds to a hexagonal close-packing pattern for the ferritin particles (123,124) and defines an upper limit of 12 nm for the diameter of the. F-EGF–receptor complex. This corresponds to an EGF-receptor density of 8000 receptors/μm^2. The 250-kilodalton acetylcholine receptor has an average diameter of 8 nm and appears to assume the conformation of randomly close packed discs in the postsynaptic membrane (125). This corresponds to approximately 10,000 acetylcholine receptor

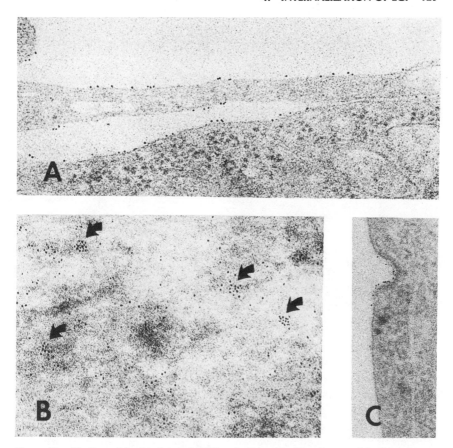

Figure 2. Binding of ferritin-labeled EGF to A-431 cells. Monolayers of A-431 cells were incubated with F-EGF for 40 minutes at 4°C, then washed to remove unbound hormone. The cells were either fixed (*A*) or warmed to 37°C for 2.5 minutes and (*B*) and (*C*) prior to fixation. Cells were fixed with glutaraldehyde, postfixed with osmium tetroxide, and were examined unstained. Both (*A*) and (*C*) are 60-nm thick sections; (*B*) is an *en face* view of a thin peripheral region of an intact cell. Arrows indicate a location of clustered F-EGF. [Magnification: (*A*) and (*B*) × 80,000, (*C*) × 65,000.]

monomers/μm^2. Thus it seems possible that the 170-kilodalton EGF–receptor complex may assume a density greater than 8000 receptors/μm^2 if the EGF is not coupled to the relatively large ferritin molecule.

Since the initial density of the receptor is 200 receptors/μm^2, the clustered distribution of the ferritin cores represents a 40-fold increase in density of the hormone–receptor complex. It is shown below that most of the cell-surface-bound hormone is rapidly endocytosed. Therefore, the process of

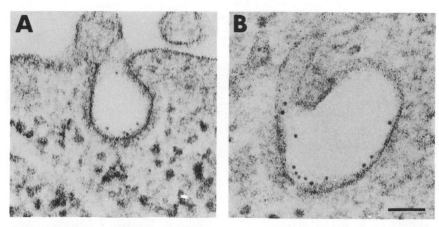

Figure 3.   Binding of ferritin-labeled EGF to Swiss 3T3 cells. Monolayers of Swiss 3T3 cells were incubated with F-EGF at 4°C, then warmed to 37°C for either 2 minutes (*A*) or 8 minutes (*B*) prior to fixation and processing for electron microscopy. The ferritin particles are shown in a coated pit (*A*) and in a receptosome (*B*). (Bar = 100nm.)

concentrating the hormone in discrete locations that are specifically internalized provides a mechanism by which all of the hormone–receptor complex can be removed from the cell surface while only a small fraction of the cell-surface membrane and other cell-surface proteins are internalized. The molecular mechanism of clustering is not known. It does not require metabolic energy because the process occurs in the presence of azide and 2-deoxyglucose in glucose-free media (122).

Certain ligands such as low-density lipoproteins that are internalized by receptor-mediated endocytosis cluster in specialized regions of the plasma membrane known as coated pits. These indentations are coated on their cytoplasmic face with the protein clathrin. Although in the experiments described above, some of the ferritin-EGF clusters in A-431 cells were located in coated pits, the majority were located on areas of the membrane with no distinguishing features. However, in the relatively rare instances in which a cell-surface cluster was seen in the process of invaginating to form endocytic vesicles, the cytoplasmic face of the indented membrane was usually coated (Fig. 2C). This raises the possibility that a clathrin coat may have formed under all hormone clusters prior to invagination and endocytosis. The involvement of coated pits was more clear when the fate of F-EGF was studied in cells (Swiss 3T3, Balb, and NRK) that have fewer EGF receptors and are mitogenically responsive to EGF. In these cells, the hormone also was initially diffusely distributed on the cell surface and in a time- and temperature-dependent manner redistributes to form clusters

(Haigler, Willingham, and Pastan, in preparation). When Swiss 3T3 cells were labeled with F-EGF at 4°C, then warmed to 37°C for 45 seconds, approximately 90% of the cell bound ferritin was located in coated pits (Fig. 3A).

When A-431 cells that were prelabeled at 4°C with F-EGF were warmed to 37°C for 2.5 minutes, 32% of the ferritin was located in endocytic vesicles with a diameter of approximately 120 nm. Clathrin coats were not observed on these vesicles. The number of ferritin cores per vesicle was very similar to the number of particles per cell-surface cluster. After 2.5 minutes, there was a decrease in the amount of conjugate within small vesicles and a concomitant accumulation of F-EGF in multivesicular bodies and secondary lysosomes as a result of fusion between these structures. Figure 4 shows a multivesicular body and several endocytic vesicles in a cell that had been incubated at 37°C for 30 minutes. The F-EGF was not observed to associate with any other cellular organelles. Close examination of Fig. 4 shows that the ferritin was not free in the lumen of the structures, but was associated with the luminal face of the membrane. This is interpreted as evidence that

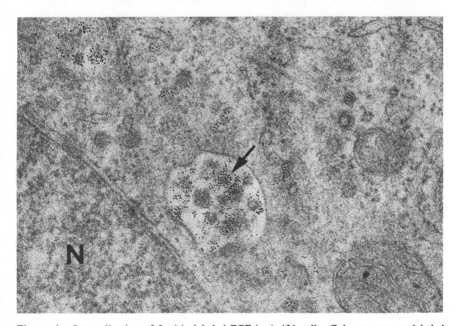

Figure 4.   Internalization of ferritin-labeled EGF in A-431 cells. Cultures were prelabeled with F-EGF at 4°C as in Fig. 2 and warmed to 37°C for 30 minutes. Ferritin cores were observed inside multivesicular bodies located primarily on the convex surface of internal vesicles (*arrow*) and also in cytoplasmic vesicles. Note the absence of F-EGF in the nucleus (*N*). (Magnification: × 65,000.)

the EGF receptor is internalized along with the ligand, and the F-EGF remains associated with the receptor. At later times (45–60 minutes), the ferritin was frequently observed in pools free in the lumen. This is interpreted as evidence of disruption of the F-EGF–receptor complex due to digestion of one or several components. This interpretation is supported by parallel biochemical experiments that showed that the onset of release of [^{125}I]tyrosine from cells labeled with [^{125}I]EGF corresponded to the time of appearance of free ferritin in the lysosomes in F-EGF-labeled cells. Furthermore, the addition of drugs such as chloroquine, ammonium chloride, and methylamine that are known to inhibit lysosomal function, resulted in the maintenance of the characteristic relationship between F-EGF and the lysosomal membrane and blocked the appearance of free ferritin in the lumen (123).

Figure 5 shows the temporal relationship between the binding of F-EGF to the plasma membrane, clustering within the plane of the plasmalemma, internalization into endocytic vesicles, and accumulation of the hormone in lysosomes in A-431 cells. Figure 6 illustrates the probable sequence of events by which these processes occur. As illustrated in the drawing, the cytoplasmic vesicles appear to fuse with and enter the multivesicular bodies by a mechanism that results in an inversion of the sidedness of the vesicles.

The internalization of F-EGF has also been studied in Swiss 3T3, KB, Balb, and NRK cells (Haigler, Willingham, and Pastan, in preparation).

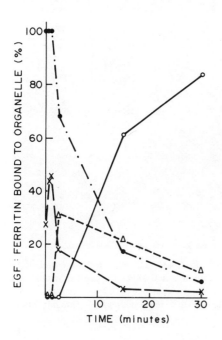

Figure 5. Fate of ferritin-labeled EGF in A-431 cells. Monolayers were incubated with F-EGF for 40 minutes at 4°C, unbound conjugate was removed, and the cells were warmed to 37°C for the indicated times and processed for EM observation. The amount of F-EGF associated with the indicated organelle was quantitated, and the results are expressed as percentage of total cell-bound conjugate. For the purpose of this tabulation, all multivesicular bodies were scored as lysosomes. The curves show percentage of conjugate that was associated with the plasma membrane (●), cell-surface groups containing five or more ferritin particles (x), cytoplasmic vesicles (Δ) or lysosomes (o). Reprinted by permission from reference 122.

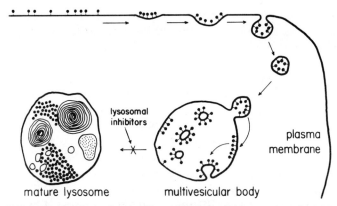

Figure 6. Composite drawing illustrating the probable sequence of events by which EGF is internalized and degraded in A-431 cell. Clathrin-coated pits are involved in endocytosis of some of the hormone, but the extent of involvement has not been evaluated quantitatively. Reprinted by permission from reference 123.

The time course of internalization and degradation of the hormone in these cells and in A-431 cells is very similar. The only significant difference between these cells and the A-431 cells is in the endocytic vesicle that the hormone enters when being endocytosed from the coated pits. The endocytic vesicles in A-431 cells are approximately 120 nm in diameter and roughly spherical. In the other cell lines, the endocytic vesicles are larger (150–350 nm in diameter). They frequently contain intravesicular membrane structures and eccentrically located vesicular protrusions into the cytoplasm. Figure 3B shows an example of an F-EGF-labeled endocytic vesicle from a Swiss 3T3 cell that protrudes into the cell cytoplasm. Endocytic vesicles with these morphological characteristics that participate in receptor-mediated endocytosis have been named *receptosomes* by Willingham and Pastan (126). They proposed that they are specialized structures that deliver receptor-associated ligands from coated pits to the cell interior and showed that different receptor-bound ligands are endocytosed in the same receptosome (127). Unlike phase-dense lysosomes and phase-lucent macropinosomes, receptosomes cannot be distinguished from the cytoplasm by phase-contrast microscopy.

It is worth noting that in our studies of F-EGF in a variety of cultured cell types, we have not observed F-EGF in endocytic vesicles that could unambiguously be identified as clathrin coated. Evaluation of the possible role of coated vesicles presents a number of technical difficulties including the following: (1) the plane of section of a cell can be such that a deeply invaginated coated pit appears not to be in communication with the cell surface and, (2) coated vesicles could be very transient structures that are not readily preserved within the time course of conventional fixation procedures. It has been proposed (128) that the clathrin coat remains associated with the plasma membrane, and the uncoated receptosome is the initial endocytic vesicle. This is in contrast to experiments in numerous other laboratories that present evidence for a coated pit→coated vesicle pathway of receptor-mediated endocytosis (see 129 for review). Certain subcellular fractionation studies also suggest a role for coated vesicles. Fine et al. (130) labeled 3T3 cells with [^{125}I]EGF and observed a time-and temperature-dependent accumulation of label in a subcellular fraction on sucrose gradients that corresponded to the density of coated vesicles from brain. Furthermore, the vesicles labeled with the [^{125}I]EGF could be precipitated by antiserum specific for coated vesicles. Although this evidence clearly places EGF in coated vesicles, it does not prove that the coated vesicles exist in the cytoplasm. Homogenization of the cells could cause the formation of closed clathrin-coated structures from EGF-containing coated pits located on the plasma membrane.

Clathrin-coated vesicles clearly exist in cells and appear to be involved in the intracellular transport of newly synthesized proteins (131–133), and evidence has been presented that they are involved in receptor-mediated endocytosis of several ligands (129). However, there is no morphological evidence that they are involved in the internalization of EGF that is clustered in coated pits. These negative results must be considered with caution in light of the technical limitations of the EM methods and conflicting subcellular-fractionation studies.

4.4.   Other Mechanisms of Endocytosis

In addition to the coated-pit pathway described above, other cellular mechanisms for receptor-mediated endocytosis have been described. Huet, Ash, and Singer (134) showed that divalent antibodies directed against β_2-microglobulin caused cross-linking of HLA antigens into cell-surface patches. These patches were found in uncoated surface invaginations that were endocytosed into uncoated vesicles. Bretscher et al. (135) showed that endocytosis of θ and H63 antigens did not involve clustering in coated pits. The multivalent-ligand concanavalin A was also internalized by the non-coated-pit pathway (136). Anti-IgM antibodies induced endocytosis of cell surface IgM molecule via coated and noncoated pits in cultured lymphoblastoid cells (137).

The types of pinocytosis for the internalization of EGF via coated pits and for the ligands discussed above at uncoated regions are known as adsorptive endocytosis or receptor-mediated endocytosis. Receptor-mediated endocytosis is a selective, saturable process that involves the binding of a ligand to a cell-surface receptor before internalization. Most eukaryotic cells can also internalize soluble material by engulfing droplets of solution in a process known as fluid-phase pinocytosis (see reference 138 for a review). Fluid-phase pinocytosis can occur via the small endocytic vesicles (less than 150 nm) that form at coated and noncoated regions of the membrane, and by macropinocytosis. Macropinocytosis occurs when a cellular ruffle falls back onto, and fuses with, the cell surface, trapping medium in a relatively large (0.5–3.0μm) vesicle. Since binding is not involved, the uptake of solute is directly related to its concentration in the extracellular fluid. By biochemical and histochemical methods, Haigler, McKanna, and Cohen showed that EGF induced a 10-fold increase in the initial rate of fluid-phase pinocytosis in A-431 cells (139). The effect was rapid (within 30 seconds) but transient; the rate of fluid uptake returned to control levels within 15 minutes. Scanning electron microscopy showed that the increased macropinocytosis correlated with a striking increase in cell-surface ruffling and extension of filopods (140). The physiological purpose of the EGF-stimulated ruffling and macropinocytosis is not known. A small percentage of cell-surface-bound F-EGF was internalized into the large macropinosomes. The density of the F-EGF bound to the limiting membrane of these vesicles was the same as the density of the F-EGF on the cell surface. This is in contrast to the clustering and selective internalization of F-EGF that occurred when entering the smaller vesicles as described above.

Comparison of the uptake of EGF by the coated-pit pathway with solute uptake by macropinocytosis clearly illustrates the efficiency of the former process. An average 120 nm vesicle contains approximately 10 molecules of F-EGF. When the thickness of the membrane and glycocalyx is considered, it is calculated that 120 nm (outer diameter of vesicle) contains 1.1×10^{-16} ml of fluid. This corresponds to an EGF concentration inside the vesicle of 1.5×10^5 nM, and this is 15,000-fold more concentrated than an extracellular EGF concentration of 10 nM. This increase in concentration occurs in a two-step process: (1) binding to high-affinity cell-surface receptors (approximately 375-fold increase), and (2) clustering in the plane of the plasma membrane (approximately 40-fold increase). In contrast, solutes taken up by fluid-phase pinocytosis are at the same concentration in the vesicle as in the extracellular fluid.

4.5. Degradation of Internalized EGF

The initial studies by Carpenter and Cohen showed that cell-bound [^{125}I]-EGF is rapidly degraded to [^{125}I]monoiodotyrosine at 37°C and that the appearance of labeled tyrosine is blocked by agents that inhibit lysosomal function (74). Essentially all cell-associated radioactivity is intact EGF; very little, if any, low-molecular-weight radioactive degradation products accumulate in the cell. These studies provide strong evidence that EGF is being degraded by lysosomal hydrolases. In an attempt to determine the point in the EGF internalization pathway at which EGF begins to be degraded, Haigler, Willingham, and Pastan studied the fate of cell-bound EGF in a human epithelioid carcinoma cell line (KB) and a mutant line of KB cells (KB-R$_2$A) that was isolated by Moehring and Moehring (141). The mutant line is resistant to killing by diphtheria toxin and to infection by certain RNA viruses (142,143). Since both diphtheria toxin and viruses enter cells by receptor-mediated endocytosis, a possible explanation of the mutant's resistance to these two agents would be a defect in the internalization and/ or degradation pathway. Such a defect might prove useful in investigating the metabolic fate of EGF. Haigler, Willingham, Moehring, and Pastan (manuscript in preparation) found that both KB and KB-R$_2$A cells bound similar amounts of [^{125}I]EGF and internalized the hormone at nearly identical rates. However, there was a striking difference in the rate of cellular degradation of [^{125}I]EGF. As seen in Fig. 7, TCA-soluble radioactivity was released by KB cells beginning between 10 and 20 minutes and by 60 minutes, 45% of the initial cell-bound hormone had been degraded. In contrast, only 5% was degraded by 60 minutes in the KB-R$_2$A cells. At later times, KB-R$_2$A cells began to degrade the hormone, but at a slower rate. These biochemical results were correlated with the fate of ferritin-labeled EGF under the same conditions. In both cell lines, F-EGF clustered in coated pits and was internalized into receptosomes at a similar rate. In

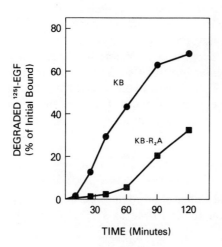

Figure 7. Degradation of cell-associated [^{125}I]EGF. Monolayer cultures of KB (●) and KB-R$_2$A (■) cells were labeled with [^{125}I]EGF at 4°C, unbound hormone was removed, and then the cells were warmed to 37°C. At the indicated time, the medium was removed and analyzed for radioactivity that was soluble in 10% trichloroacetic acid (TCA). To verify the validity of using the TCA-precipitation method as a measure of [^{125}I]EGF degradation, certain samples were also analyzed by gel filtration on BioGel P-10 (74). The two methods gave essentially identical results. In addition to re-leasing degraded hormone into the medium, both cell lines released approximately 15% of the initial cell-bound hormone into the me-dium as intact [^{125}I]EGF. Essentially all of the release of intact hormone occurred within the first 10 minutes at 37°C.

KB cells, F-EGF passed through the receptosome compartment and accumulated in lysosomal structures at a rate comparable to the rate observed in other cell lines we have studied. However, in KB-R$_2$A cells, F-EGF was retained in the receptosome compartment for an extended period of time. Therefore, the lesion that prevents normal degradation of EGF appears either to be distal to the receptosome or to be a defect in the receptosome that prevents it from fusing with the next vesicular compartment. Elucidation of the molecular and cellular nature of this lesion should shed light on the metabolism of EGF and on possible overlapping mechanisms in the processing of diphtheria toxin, viruses, and polypeptide hormones.

It has been reported that colchicine causes a small reduction in the rate of cellular degradation of [^{125}I]EGF in 3T3 cells. This suggests that microtubules may have a role in the cellular processing of the hormone (144).

4.6. Physiological Role of EGF Clustering and Internalization

Two distinctly different possibilities exist for the role EGF internalization plays in EGF-stimulated cell growth. The first possibility is that EGF exerts its biological effect while bound to its receptor on the cell surface, and the hormone–receptor complex is internalized solely for delivery to the lysosomes for catabolism. This scheme predicts that the internalization and degradation would serve the function of an "off" switch. Since the EGF–receptor complex would only generate its mitogenic signal while on the cell surface, internalization would serve as a negative regulator. The second possible role of internalization is to deliver the EGF–receptor complex (or a proteolytic fragment thereof) to an intracellular site of action. In this scheme, internalization would serve an obligatory positive function. Although data has been presented in support of each of the alternatives (145–147), the site at which the mitogenic signal is generated has not been clearly established. However, time-course studies (139) clearly show that EGF stimulation of macropinocytosis can occur while the hormone is located on the cell surface. At least in the case of this rapid effect, a transmembrane signal must be involved.

It has been reported that EGF accumulates in the nucleus of cultured rat pituitary cells, GH$_3$ (148). When these cells were incubated at 37°C for 18 hours with [^{125}I]EGF plus chloroquine (to block lysosomal degradation), labeled EGF was found in the nuclear pellet following detergent lysis. Only trace amounts of radioactivity were found in the nucleus in the absence of chloroquine. In previous studies on other cell lines, ferritin-labeled EGF was not observed in the nucleus even in the presence of lysosomotropic agents (122). However, in the EM studies, the time course of incubation with F-EGF was shorter, so the possibility that nuclear accumulation would have occurred at later times must be considered. Nuclear accumulation of polypeptide hormones is not without precedents; nerve growth factor (149) and insulin (150) have been reported to bind to the nucleus.

It should be noted that the coated-pit pathway of EGF internalization does not offer a complete mechanism by which EGF could enter the nucleus or bind to the nuclear membrane. All observed intracellular F-EGF has been located inside membrane-limited vesicular and lysosomal structures, that is, the hormone is still separated from the cytoplasm. Since the hormone does not enter the cytoplasm, some type of fusion between these vesicles and the nucleus must be proposed.

Theoretical calculations (151) and experimental evidence suggest that clustering of hormone–receptor complexes in the plane of the plasma membrane may be necessary for the hormone to exert its biological effect. This interesting hypothesis is supported by the following innovative experiments by Kahn et al. (152), using antibodies to the insulin receptor. The bivalent antireceptor antibodies bound to the insulin receptor and mimicked insulin action, whereas the monovalent F_{ab} fragment of the antibodies bound to the receptor but did not have insulin-like activity. The interpretation was that the divalent antibodies induced clustering, but the monovalent antibodies did not. This was supported by the fact that cross-linking of the receptor-bound F_{ab} fragments with bivalent anti-F_{ab} antibodies resulted in a restoration of insulin-like activity. In a conceptually similar set of experiments, Schechter et al. (153) showed that the biological activity of a nonmitogenic, non-clustering analogue of EGF could be restored by cross-linking with bivalent anti-EGF antibodies.

The laboratories of Herschman (154) and Shimizu (155) independently have begun a novel approach that promises to provide useful information concerning the role internalization plays in EGF's biological activity. They have covalently coupled EGF to agents that are cytotoxic if they gain entry into the cytoplasm. Since the toxic agents cannot passively enter the cell, they must rely on EGF-receptor-mediated endocytosis of the toxin-EGF complex for entry. These toxin-EGF conjugates are being used to select for mutant cultured cells that are defective in EGF binding and/or internalization properties. The site of the defect in clustering, internalization, and degradation of EGF then can be determined and correlated with the cells' physiological response to EGF.

5.   QUANTITATION OF EGF INTERNALIZATION AND DEGRADATION

When studying the binding of polypeptide hormones to their target cells, investigators usually are interested in the affinity of the binding and the number of binding sites. These values are frequently obtained by measuring the amount of radioactive hormone bound as a function of free hormone concentration and plotting the results according to the method of Scatchard (156,157). However, two conditions must be met for such a treatment to be meaningful: the binding must be reversible, and the system must be at equilibrium. As was seen above, receptor-bound EGF is rapidly removed from the cell surface by endocytosis; thus the internalized EGF is not in equilibrium with the extracellular ligand. Under physiological conditions, the binding of EGF to living cells cannot be viewed solely as the interaction of EGF with its receptor; the cellular processes involved must be considered. A significant advance toward this end recently was made by Wiley and Cunningham (158,159). They reasoned that the interaction of polypeptide ligands with cells, like life in general, can more accurately be modeled on steady-state assumptions than on equilibrium assumptions. They derived steady-state equations for analyzing the binding, internalization, and degradation of ligands. The equations include four new rate constants that correspond to the rate of (1) insertion of new receptors into the cell surface, (2) endocytosis of occupied receptors, (3) turnover of unoccupied receptors, and (4) hydrolysis of internalized ligands. Using the interaction of [125I]EGF with human fibroblasts as a model system, they developed procedures for the experimental determination of these rate constants. These measurements were facilitated by a biochemical method (79) for determining [125I]EGF binding that permits a clear discrimination between cell-surface-bound and internalized [125I]EGF. Computer simulations based on the derived steady-state equations showed a close correspondence to experimental data and indicated that the equations provide an accurate model of the cellular processes involved in the interaction of EGF and cells under physiological conditions. Using these methods, they determined that occupied receptors are internalized greater than 14 times faster than unoccupied receptors, thereby explaining the phenomenon of "down-regulation" (74). Based on the steady-state equations, a technique was developed that permits a rapid and sensitive method for determining the lag time between [125I]EGF internalization and the initiation of degradation. They found this time to be 15 minutes in human fibroblasts (159), and this is in good agreement with the initiation of degradation found in KB cells (Fig. 7). The approach developed by Wiley and Cunningham should be applicable to the study of a wide variety of polypeptide ligands.

6. INTERNALIZATION OF OTHER POLYPEPTIDE LIGANDS

Receptor-mediated endocytosis is involved in the internalization of a number of polypeptide hormones, transport proteins, plant toxins, and viruses.

Since a detailed review is beyond the scope of this chapter, only certain general characteristics are discussed, except in specific instances when information concerning EGF is directly involved. The interaction of polypeptide ligands with intracellular structures has been reviewed by Goldfine (150), and the entry of viruses into cells has recently been reviewed (160). The proceedings of a conference on receptor-mediated binding and internalization of toxins and hormones (161) is a good source of information on this rapidly growing field.

In order to understand the endocytosis of a ligand, it is useful to consider the probable physiological role of internalization. In the case of diphtheria toxin, it is clear that the enzymatically active A fragment must gain entry to the cytosol in order to inactivate the ribosome (see reference 104 for a review). Similarly, the transport protein low-density lipoprotein (LDL) delivers cholesterol esters to lysosomes, where hydrolysis results in the release of cholesterol into the cytoplasm (162). In both these cases, it is clear that the ligand *must* enter the cell in order to exert its effect. In contrast, the function of hormones is to deliver information to the cell. In certain cases, the information is transduced across the plasma membrane by a second messenger; for example, human chorionic gonadotropin stimulates steroidogenesis by activating adenylate cyclase, which forms cyclic AMP (163). Although the polypeptide hormone may be internalized and degraded in the lysosomes, endocytosis is *not necessarily* required for the hormone to exert its biological effect.

By viewing ligands in terms of their physiological role, Kaplan has divided the receptors for polypeptide ligands into two classes (164). Class I receptors regulate cell metabolism and are typified by receptors for hormones. Internalization may or may not be required for biological activity. Class II receptors are involved in delivery of a ligand to the cell's interior and are typified by the receptor for LDL. Internalization of class II ligands is absolutely required for function. Certain characteristics are unique to each class. Divalent cations are required for the binding of ligands to class II receptors, but not to class I receptors. Perhaps the most interesting difference concerns the regulation of receptor number by its ligand, a phenomenon sometimes called down-regulation. Class I receptors are down-regulated by their ligand and in some cases [e.g., EGF (75,123), insulin (165), growth hormone (166)] there is evidence that the loss of binding activity is due to the receptor being internalized and degraded along with the bound hormone. In contrast, class II receptors, in general, are not down-regulated by their ligand, and for some ligands [e.g., α_2-macroglobulin (167,168) and lysosomal hydrolases (169,170)] there is evidence that the receptors are internalized and then recycled to the cell surface. Since it appears that both class I and class II receptors are internalized by the coated-pit pathway (see below), there must be a characteristic molecular difference between the receptors that allows an unknown cellular mechanism to determine which receptors are to be catabolized and which are to be recycled.

It is also possible that the postendocytic compartmentation of a ligand–receptor complex can be influenced by the nature of the ligand. It has been proposed that in the endocytic vesicle, the vitellogenin–receptor complex generates a transmembrane signal that determines the cellular fate of the vesicle (105).

α_2-Macroglobulin (α_2-M) is a large serum protein that is internalized by cultured fibroblasts (108,109) and macrophages (107) by receptor-mediated endocytosis through coated pits. By simultaneously incubating cultured fibroblasts with fluorescein-labeled α_2-M (Fl-α_2-M) and EGF conjugated to rhodamine-labeled lactalbumin, Maxfield et al. (127) found that the two ligands were endocytosed into the same endocytic vesicle. Figure 8 shows the cointernalization of Fl-α_2-M and a direct conjugate of rhodamine and EGF (R-EGF) in NRK-V B_4 cells that were incubated with the two ligands for 20 minutes at 37°C. Note that most, but not all, of the fluorescein and rhodamine localizes to the same cellular location. From parallel EM studies,

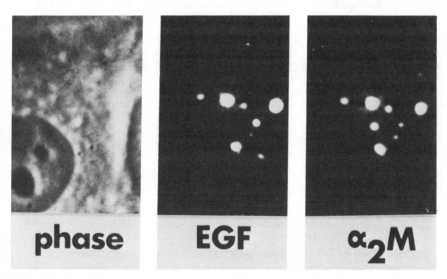

Figure 8. Simultaneous uptake of Fl-α_2-M and R-EGF. Cultures of NRK-V B_4 cells were incubated with Fl-α_2-M and R-EGF for 20 minutes at 37°C. The cells were washed, fixed, and observed using a silicon-intensifier-target television camera. The photographs are from the video monitor and are of the same cell using phase-contrast optics or fluorescent epi-illumination using filters appropriate for either rhodamine (*center*) or fluorescein (*right*). Magnification is approximately × 900.

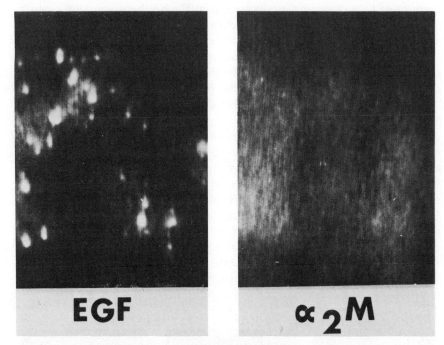

Figure 9.   Effect of bacitracin on uptake Fl-α_2M and R-EGF. Cultures of NRK-V B$_4$ cells were preincubated with bacitracin (1 mg/ml) for 5 minutes then, in the continued presence of bacitracin, were incubated with Fl-α_2M and R-EGF for 20 minutes at 37°C as described in Fig. 8. The gain control on the video monitor was at a higher setting than in Fig. 8 in order to visualize the diffusely distributed Fl-α_2M. Magnification is approximately ×900.

it is known that the ligands are in endocytic vesicles at this time. The location of the vesicles does not correspond to any recognizable images in the phase-contrast micrograph, probably because the vesicles are of approximately the same density as the cytoplasm. The cointernalization of EGF and α_2-M has been confirmed at the ultrastructural level using F-EGF and α_2-M coupled to colloidal gold (171). The two ligands cocluster in the same coated pits and then occupy the same receptosomes.

Davies et al. (172) found that several compounds (e.g., methylamine, bacitracin, dansylcadaverine) that inhibit the cellular enzyme transglutaminase, inhibited the internalization of Fl-α_2-M. They speculated that transglutaminase catalyzes the cross-linking of certain membrane proteins involved in clustering of ligand–receptor complexes and is a necessary step in ligand internalization. The exact role of transglutaminase in this process remains to be determined.

Figure 9 shows that transglutaminase does not play a role in the internalization of EGF. Cultured NRK-V B_4 cells were incubated with R-EGF and Fl-α_2-M as in Fig. 8, but in the presence of the transglutaminase inhibitor bacitracin. As previously reported (172), Fl-α_2-M remained diffusely distributed in the presence of bacitracin; however, the fate of R-EGF was not influenced by the inhibitor (compare Figs. 8 and 9). A similar result was obtained when bacitracin was replaced with methylamine (40 mM). The internalization of R-EGF was inhibited by dansylcadaverine. However, the minimum dose required was approximately 10-fold higher than the dose required to block internalization of Fl-α_2-M and inhibit transglutaminase. The inhibition of internalization by dansylcadaverine was probably due to an effect on some cellular component other than transglutaminase. These results have been confirmed using [125I]EGF by Haigler, Willingham, and Pastan (80) and others (146,121,173,174) and at the ultrastructural level using F-EGF (123). It seems clear that transglutaminase is not involved in EGF clustering or internalization. Thus although EGF (a class I receptor) and α_2-M (a class II receptor) are sequestered in the same endocytic vesicles, the molecular mechanisms of clustering and internalization appear to be different. It was originally reported by Maxfield, Willingham, Davies, and Pastan (175) that transglutaminase inhibitors blocked the internalization of a rhodamine-lactalbumin-EGF conjugate. The EGF derivative was synthesized from a commercial preparation of EGF that was later found to be a mixture of peptides. Therefore, these data (175) must be considered unreliable.

7. MOLECULAR MECHANISMS: EGF-STIMULATED PROTEIN KINASE

The cellular responses to the binding of EGF are extremely diverse and complex. In an attempt to obtain a more well-defined system in which to study the initial molecular event induced by EGF binding, Stanley Cohen's laboratory investigated the interaction of EGF with its receptor in isolated plasma membranes from A-431 cells. This cell line was chosen because it contains an extraordinarily high number of EGF receptors. They found that the membrane retained the ability to bind [125I]EGF *in vitro*, and the binding markedly enhanced the capacity of these membranes to phosphorylate endogenous proteins in the presence of γ-labeled [32P]ATP (176). The phosphorylation reaction required either Mg^{2+} or Mn^{2+} and was not influenced by cyclic nucleotides, and the stimulation by EGF was reversible by removing the hormone. Although EGF increased the phosphorylation of a number of membrane proteins, two components that appeared to be glycoproteins with molecular weights of 170 and 150 kilodaltons were primarily affected and were assumed to be the EGF receptor. The membranes could also phosphorylate certain exogenous soluble proteins such as histones, which suggests that cytosolic proteins could be phosphorylated *in vivo*. Membranes from NRK cells (177,178) and human placenta (179) also contain protein kinase activity that can be stimulated by EGF.

Both the EGF-binding activity and the EGF-stimulated protein kinase activity present in A-431 membranes could be solubilized with nonionic detergents (94). The solubilized EGF receptor was purified to near homogeneity on an EGF affinity column, and the purified receptor preparation retained the EGF-stimulated phosphorylation activity (94). This suggests that either the EGF receptor is itself a protein kinase or a protein kinase is closely associated with the EGF receptor.

An exciting new dimension to the problem recently emerged with the discovery by Ushiro and Cohen (180) that the EGF-stimulated kinase specifically phosphorylates tyrosine residues of proteins. The highly unusual property of phosphorylating tyrosine residues is shared with kinases from certain tumor viruses including polyoma virus (181), Rous sarcoma virus (182–184), and Abelson murine leukemia virus (185). The protein kinase activity of the Rous sarcoma virus, an RNA tumor virus, seems to be a property of the transformation-specific protein pp60^{src} that is encoded by the *src* gene and is essential for cellular transformation (186–190). A normal cellular homologue of viral pp60^{src}, designated pp60^{sarc} or pp60$^{proto-src}$, has also been identified and shown to have a protein kinase activity (191,192). The gene coding for viral pp60^{src} appears to share a common ancestral origin with the gene coding for normal cell protein pp60^{sarc} (193,194). It has been proposed that the protein kinase activity of cellular pp60^{sarc} regulates growth in normal cells, and inappropriate expression of the tyrosine-specific protein kinase of viral pp60^{src} results in neoplastic transformation (189,195). Indeed, it has been found that cellular levels of phosphotyrosine are increased by 10-fold following transformation by Rous sarcoma virus (190). One particularly attractive aspect of the above proposal is that it provides an explanation for the diverse phenotypic changes resulting from oncogenic transformation through the pleiotropic-substrate-specificity characteristic of most protein kinases. It should be noted that these studies do not suggest that there is a single mechanism for all types of oncogenic transformation; not all RNA tumor viruses contain genes for kinases, and studies of the proteins of the viruses that do code for tyrosine-specific kinases show that they have very diverse structures.

A cascade of tyrosine-specific protein kinases in Ehrlich ascites tumor cells that phosphorylate a number of cellular proteins recently has been described (see reference 196 for a review). The terminal kinase of the cascade is reported to phosphorylate the β subunit of the Na^+-K^+-dependent ATPase and render it inefficient, thereby explaining the Warburg effect. However, the validity of some of the reported data has been questioned (197).

The apparent similarities between the EGF receptor and the transforming protein of certain RNA tumor viruses prompted a more detailed investigation of the possibility that the proteins might be structurally related. Antisera specific for the transforming protein of Rous sarcoma virus, pp60[src], serve as substrates for phosphorylation by purified preparations of pp60[src]. Chinkers and Cohen (198) and Kudlow, Buss, and Gill (199) showed that an affinity-purified preparation of EGF receptor from A-431 cells also would phosphorylate antibodies directed against pp60[src] of Rous sarcoma virus. The interaction with anti-pp60[src] was specific, because the EGF-receptor/kinase would not phosphorylate a wide variety of antibodies including antisera that precipitated the tyrosine-specific kinases associated with polyoma virus, Abelson murine leukemia virus, and feline sarcoma virus. Although a specific relationship appears to exist between the EGF receptor and the transforming protein of Rous sarcoma virus, the two proteins are clearly not identical; the molecular weights of the two proteins are quite different, and antisera that precipitate pp60[src] do not precipitate the EGF-receptor/kinase (198,199).

The tyrosine-specific protein kinase in A-431 cells was stimulated by EGF in intact cultured cells as well as in membrane preparations (200). A fourfold increase in tyrosine phosphorylation was seen within 1 minute of the addition of EGF. Although there was an increase in phosphorylated tyrosine residues in the EGF receptor, the majority of the phosphotyrosine residues were on other proteins including an 81-kilodalton, membrane-bound phosphoprotein and a 39-kilodalton soluble phosphoprotein. The effect of EGF on phosphotyrosine levels was also seen in HeLa cells (200), but the increment of increase was much less than in A-431 cells, and this suggests that the effect can be readily studied in A-431 cells, because they have approximately 15 times more receptors. In summary, it is clear that *in vivo* the binding of EGF to its receptor stimulates a membrane-bound kinase. The role this kinase plays in the pleiotypic cellular response to EGF is not known. However, stimulation of this enzyme is the most rapid known cellular response to EGF and thus may be the initial molecular event following hormone binding.

DeLarco, Todaro, and co-workers have isolated low-molecular-weight polypeptide transforming growth factors from the media of cells transformed by various RNA tumor viruses (201,202, and chapter by De Larco in this volume). These factors share certain biological activities with EGF and appear to act by binding to the EGF receptor. Recently it has been shown that transforming growth factors, like EGF, increase the phosphotyrosine levels in A-431 cells in tissue culture and stimulate the phosphorylation of the EGF receptor in isolated A-431 membranes (203).

In summary, the following parallels can be drawn between EGF and certain RNA tumor virus: (1) although EGF is not tumorigenic, it shares with tumor viruses the property of causing the pleiotypic metabolic changes that lead to rapid cell division (1,204), (2) transformation of cultured cells by certain RNA tumor viruses leads to a dramatic reduction in the number of EGF-binding sites at the cell surface (205), (3) small polypeptide growth factors that specifically bind to the EGF receptor are produced by some transformed cells (202), (4) similar morphological changes occur in cultured cells following exposure to EGF (140) or transformation by Rous sarcoma virus (206), (5) it appears that both EGF and certain viruses exert their effects through tyrosine-specific protein kinases (180,195), and (6) the transforming protein of Rous sarcoma virus appears to be antigenically related, although not identical, to the EGF-receptor-associated kinase from A-431 cells (198,199).

The exact role the EGF-stimulated tyrosine-specific protein kinase plays in the cellular response to EGF is not known. However, it appears possible that both the naturally occurring polypeptide mitogen EGF and the transforming protein of Rous sarcoma virus exert their effects by phosphorylation of tyrosine residues on cellular regulatory proteins. The identification of such phosphoproteins and the role they play in cellular metabolism are problems of intense current interest. Although the kinase activity associated with Rous sarcoma virus probably is intrinsic to the 60-kilodalton phosphoprotein pp60^{src}, it is not known if the EGF receptor is itself a protein kinase or if this enzymatic activity resides in another protein that is closely associated with the EGF receptor. A detailed comparison of the mechanism by which EGF and Rous sarcoma virus control cellular replication via tyrosine-specific kinases promises to be a useful approach to the study of the molecular difference in the cellular control of normal versus malignant cell replication.

8. SUMMARY

Epidermal growth factor is a stable, well-characterized polypeptide hormone that can be obtained in milligram amounts from the submaxillary gland of the mouse. The exact physiological role EGF plays in metabolism and development remains to be established but promises to be an interesting area of research in the future.

A number of derivatives of EGF can be prepared that bind to cellular receptors in a highly specific manner and permit study of the interactions of EGF with its target cells at several different levels of resolution. Using these derivatives, it has been shown that EGF binds to specific receptors on the plasma membrane that are initially diffusely distributed. The hormone–receptor complex is rapidly clustered in specialized indentations on the plasmalemma that are coated on their cytoplasmic face with the protein clathrin. The clusters of EGF–receptor complexes are then specifically internalized into endocytic vesicles that eventually fuse with lysosomes. In the lysosomes, the EGF (probably along with its receptor) is degraded. The point in this pathway at which EGF generates its mitogenic signal is not known. However, at least one rapid effect of EGF, that is, stimulation of macropinocytosis, is caused by a transmembrane signal generated while EGF is on the cell surface.

The binding of EGF to its receptor in membrane preparations or in intact cells stimulates a tyrosine-specific protein kinase. The kinase activity is either tightly associated with, or is intrinsic to, the EGF receptor. Neither the primary physiological substrate of this enzyme nor the role the kinase plays in the pleiotypic effects of EGF are known. The kinase associated with the EGF receptor is immunologically related to the transforming protein of Rous sarcoma virus, which is also a tyrosine-specific protein kinase. Several parallels can be drawn between the reversible stimulation of growth by EGF and the irreversible stimulation of growth associated with transformation by certain tumor viruses, thereby providing an opportunity to compare normal and neoplastic growth.

ACKNOWLEDGMENTS

I thank Drs. Denise Van Horn-Haigler and Steve Wiley for critically reading this manuscript. Support from the Cancer Research Coordinating Committee Grant 555260 and U.S. Public Health Service Grant CA 31297 is acknowledged.

REFERENCES

1. Carpenter, G., and Cohen, S., *Annu. Rev. Biochem.*, **48**, 193 (1979).
2. Carpenter, G., in R. Baserga, Ed., *Tissue Growth Factors* (*Handbook of Experimental Pharmacology*), New York, Springer-Verlag, 1981, Vol. 57, pp. 89–123.
3. Gregory, H., in G. B. J. Glass, Ed., *Gastrointestinal Hormones* (in *Comprehensive Endocrinology*), New York, Raven, 1980, pp. 397–407.
4. Carpenter, G., and Cohen, S., in G. Litwack, Ed., *Biochemical Actions of Hormones*, New York, Academic, 1978, Vol. 5, pp. 203–247.
5. Adamson, E. D., and Rees, A. R., *Mol. Cell. Biochem.*, **34**, 129 (1981).
6. Cohen, S., *Proc. Natl. Acad. Sci. USA*, **46**, 301 (1960).
7. Cohen, S., *J. Biol. Chem.*, **237**, 1555 (1962).
8. Savage, C. R., Jr., and Cohen, S., *J. Biol. Chem.*, **247**, 7609 (1972).

9. Savage, C. R., Jr., Hash, J. H., and Cohen, S., *J. Biol. Chem.*, **248**, 7669 (1973).

10. Holladay, L. A., Savage, C. R., Jr., Cohen, S., and Puett, D., *Biochemistry*, **15**, 2624 (1976).

11. Taylor, J. M., Cohen, S., and Mitchell, W. M., *Proc. Natl. Acad. Sci. USA*, **67**, 164 (1970).

12. Taylor, J. M., Mitchell, W. M., and Cohen, S., *J. Biol. Chem.*, **249**, 3198 (1974).

13. Frey, P., Forand, R., Maciag, T., and Shooter, E. M., *Proc. Natl. Acad. Sci. USA*, **76**, 6294 (1979).

14. Greene, L. A., Shooter, E. M., and Varon, S., *Proc. Natl. Acad. Sci. USA*, **60**, 1383 (1968).

15. Thomas, K. A., Baglan, N. C., and Bradshaw, R. A., *J. Biol. Chem.*, **256**, 9156 (1981).

16. Cohen, S., and Carpenter, G., *Proc. Natl. Acad. Sci. USA*, **72**, 1317 (1975).

17. Gregory, H., *Nature*, **257**, 325 (1975).

18. Gregory, H., Bower, J. M., and Willshire, I. R., in K. W. Kastrup and J. H. Nielsen, Eds., *Growth Factors*, FEBS Colloquium B3, New York, Pergamon, 1978, Vol. 48, pp. 75–84.

19. Hollenberg, M. D., and Gregory, H., *Life Sci.*, **20**, 267 (1976).

20. Moore, J. B., Jr., *Arch. Biochem. Biophys.*, **189**, 1 (1978).

21. Birnbaum, J. E., Sapp, T. M., and Moore, J. B., Jr., *J. Invest. Dermatol.*, **66**, 313 (1976).

22. Cohen, S., and Elliott, G. A., *J. Invest. Dermatol.*, **40**, 1 (1963).

23. Bucher, N. L. R., Patel, U., and Cohen, S., *Adv. Enzyme Regul.*, **16**, 205 (1978).

24. Savage, C. R., Jr., and Cohen, S., *Exp. Eye Res.*, **15**, 361 (1973).

25. Frati, L., Daniele, S., Delogu, A., and Covelli, I., *Exp. Eye Res.*, **14**, 135 (1972).

26. Sundell, H., Grey, M. E., Serenius, F. S., Escabedo, M. B., and Stahlman, M. T., *Am. J. Pathol.*, **100**, 707 (1980).

27. Bower, J. M., Camble, R., Gregory, H., Gerring, E. L., and Willshire, I. R., *Experientia*, **31**, 825 (1975).

28. Gondalez, A., Garrido, J. D., and Vial, J. D., *J. Cell Biol.*, **88**, 108 (1981).

29. Catterton, W. Z., Escodebo, M. B., Gexson, W. R., Gray, M. E., Sundell, H. W., and Stahlman, M. T., *Pediatr. Res.*, **13**, 104 (1979).

30. O'Keefe, E., Hollenberg, M. D., and Cuatrecasas, P., *Arch. Biochem. Biophys.*, **164**, 518 (1974).

31. Nexo, E., Hollenberg, M. D., Figueroa, A., and Pratt, R. M., *Proc. Natl. Acad. Sci. USA*, **77**, 2782 (1980).

32. Adamson, E. D., Deller, M. J., and Warshaw, J. B., *Nature*, **291**, 656 (1981).

33. Barka, T., *J. Histochem. Cytochem.*, **28**, 836 (1980).

34. Elder, J. B., Williams, G., Lacey, E., and Gregory, H., *Nature*, **271**, 466 (1978).

35. Heitz, P. U., Kasper, M., Van Noorden, S., Polak, J. M., Gregory, H., and Pearse, A. G. E., *Gut*, **19**, 408 (1978).

36. Cohen, S., *Dev. Biol.*, **12**, 394 (1965).

37. Hoober, J. K., and Cohen, S., *Biochim. Biophys. Acta*, **138**, 357 (1967).

38. Savage, C. R., Jr., and Cohen, S., *Exp. Eye Res.*, **15**, 361 (1973).

39. Gospodarowicz, D., Mescher, A. L., Brown, K. D., and Birdwell, C. R., *Exp. Eye Res.*, **25**, 631 (1977).

40. Bradshaw, R. A., and Rubin, J. S., *J. Supramol. Struct.*, **14**, 183 (1980).

41. Armelin, H., *Proc. Natl. Acad. Sci. USA*, **70**, 2702 (1973).

42. Hollenberg, M. D., and Cuatrecasas, P., *Proc. Natl. Acad. Sci. USA*, **70**, 2964 (1973).

43. Aharonov, A., Pruss, R. M., and Herschman, H. R., *J. Biol. Chem.*, **253**, 3970 (1978).

44. Westermark, B., *Biochem. Biophys. Res. Commun.*, **69**, 304 (1976).

45. Rhienwald, J. G., and Green, H., *Nature*, **265**, 421 (1977).

46. Gospodarowicz, D., and Mescher, H. L., *J. Cell. Physiol.*, **93**, 117 (1977).

47. Bhargava, G., Rifas, L., and Markman, M. H., *J. Cell. Physiol.*, **100**, 365 (1979).

48. Gospodarowicz, D., Ill, C. R., and Birdwell, C. R., *Endocrinology*, **100**, 1108 (1977).

49. Osterman, J., and Hammond, J. M., *Horm. Metab. Res.*, **11**, 485 (1979).

50. Richman, R. A., Claus, T. H., Pilkis, S. J., and Friedman, D. L., *Proc. Natl. Acad. Sci. USA*, **73**, 3589 (1976).

51. Gospodarowicz, D., Brown, J. D., Birdwell, C. R., and Zetter, B. R., *J. Cell Biol.*, **77**, 774 (1978).

52. Yoneda, T., and Pratt, R. M., *Science*, **213**, 563 (1981).

53. Gerschenson, L. E., Conner, E. A., Yang, J., and Anderson, M., *Life Sci.*, **24**, 1337 (1979).

54. Holley, R. W., Armour, R., Baldwin, J. H., Brown K. D., and Yeh, Y. C., *Proc. Natl. Acad. Sci. USA*, **74**, 5046 (1977).

55. Carpenter, G., and Cohen, S., *J. Cell. Physiol.*, **88**, 227 (1976).

56. Haigler, H. T., and Carpenter, G., *Biochim. Biophys. Acta*, **598**, 314 (1980).

57. Shechter, Y., Hernaez, L., and Cuatrecasas, P., *Proc. Natl. Acad. Sci. USA*, **75**, 5788 (1978).

58. Rozengurt, E., and Heppel, L. A., *Proc. Natl. Acad. Sci. USA*, **72**, 4492 (1975).

59. Barnes, D., and Colowick, S. P., *J. Cell. Physiol.*, **89**, 633 (1976).

60. Hollenberg, M. D., and Cuatrecasas, P., *J. Biol. Chem.*, **250**, 3845 (1975).

61. Lembach, K. J., *J. Cell. Physiol.*, **89**, 277 (1976).

62. Schneider, J. A., Diamond, I., and Rozengurt, E., *J. Biol. Chem.*, **253**, 872 (1978).

63. Diamond, I., Legg, A., Schneider, J. A., and Rozengurt, E. J., *J. Biol. Chem.*, **253**, 866 (1978).

64. Rozengurt, E., in G. H. Sato and R. Rose, Eds., *Hormones and Cell Culture*, (Cold Spring Harbor Conferences on Cell Proliferation, Vol. 6) Cold Spring Harbor Laboratory, Cold Spring Harbor, N.Y., 1979, pp. 773–788.

65. Chen, L. B., Gudor, R. C., Sun, T.-T., Chen, A. B., and Mosesson, M. W., *Science*, **197**, 776 (1977).

66. Johnson, L. K., Baxter, J. D., Vlodavsky, I., and Gospodarowicz, D., *Proc. Natl. Acad. Sci. USA*, **77**, 394 (1980).

67. Benveniste, R., Speeg, K. V., Carpenter, G., Cohen, S., Lindner, J., and Rabinowitz, D., *J. Clin. Endocrinol. Metab.*, **46**, 169 (1978).

68. Ascoli, M., *J. Biol. Chem.*, **256**, 179 (1981).

69. Mondschein, J. S., and Schomberg, D. W., *Science*, **211**, 1179 (1981).

70. Sun, T.-T., and Green, H., *Nature*, **269**, 489 (1977).

71. Haigler, H., Ash, J., Singer, S. J., and Cohen, S., *Proc. Natl. Acad. Sci. USA*, **75**, 3317 (1978).
72. Fabricant, R. N., DeLarco, J. E., and Todaro, G. J., *Proc. Natl. Acad. Sci. USA*, **74**, 565 (1977).
73. King, A. C., Hernaez-Davis, L., and Cuatrecasas, P., *Proc. Natl. Acad. Sci. USA*, **77**, 3283 (1980).
74. Carpenter, G., and Cohen, S., *J. Cell Biol.*, **71**, 159 (1976).
75. Das, M., and Fox, C. F., *Proc. Natl. Acad. Sci. USA*, **75**, 2644 (1978).
76. Holley, R. W., Armour, R., Baldwin, J. H., Brown, K. D., and Yeh, Y., *Proc. Natl. Acad. Sci. USA*, **74**, 5046 (1977).
77. Vlodavsky, I., Brown, J. D., and Gospodarowicz, D., *J. Biol. Chem.*, **253**, 3744 (1978).
78. Brown, K. D., Yeh, Y., and Holley, R. W., *J. Cell. Physiol.*, **100**, 227 (1979).
79. Haigler, H. T., Maxfield, F. R., Willingham, M. C., and Pastan, I., *J. Biol. Chem.*, **255**, 1239 (1980).
80. Haigler, H. T., Willingham, M. C., and Pastan, I., *Biochem. Biophys. Res. Commun.*, **94**, 630 (1980).
81. Shimizu, N., Behzadian, M. A., and Shimizu, Y., *Proc. Natl. Acad. Sci. USA*, **77**, 3600 (1980).
82. Davies, R. L., Grosse, V. A., Kucherlapati, R., and Bothwell, M., *Proc. Natl. Acad. Sci. USA*, **77**, 4188 (1980).
83. Carpenter, G., Lembach, K. J., Morrison, M. M., and Cohen, S., *J. Biol. Chem.*, **250**, 4297 (1975).
84. Vlodavsky, I., Brown, J. D., and Gospodarowicz, D., *J. Biol. Chem.*, **253**, 3744 (1978).
85. Huff, K., End, D., and Guroff, G., *J. Cell Biol.*, **88**, 189 (1981).
86. Wrann, M., Fox, C. F., and Ross, R., *Science*, **210**, 1363 (1980).
87. Baker, J. B., Barsh, G. S., Carney, D. H., and Cunningham, D. D., *Proc. Natl. Acad. Sci. USA*, **75**, 1882 (1978).
88. Ivanovic, V., and Weinstein, I. B., *Nature*, **293**, 404 (1981).
89. Jetten, A. M., *Nature*, **284**, 626 (1980).
90. Carpenter, G., and Cohen, S., *Biochem. Biophys. Res. Commun.*, **79**, 545 (1977).
91. Pratt, R. M., and Pastan, I., *Nature*, **272**, 68 (1978).
92. Nexo, E., Hock, R. A., and Hollenberg, M. D., *J. Biol. Chem.*, **254**, 8740 (1979).
93. Hock, R. A., Nexo, E., and Hollenberg, M. D., *J. Biol. Chem.*, **255**, 10737 (1980).
94. Cohen, S., Carpenter, G., and King, L., Jr., *J. Biol. Chem.*, **255**, 4834 (1980).
95. Das, M., Miyakawa, T., Fox, C. F., Pruss, R. M., Aharonov, A., and Herschman, H., *Proc. Natl. Acad. Sci. USA*, **74**, 2790 (1977).
96. Hock, R. A., Nexo, E., and Hollenberg, M. D., *Nature*, **277**, 403 (1979).
97. Baker, J. B., Simmer, R. L., Glenn, K. C., and Cunningham, D. D., *Nature*, **278**, 743 (1979).
98. Linsley, P. S., Blifeld, C., Wrann, M., and Fox, C. F., *Nature*, **278**, 745 (1979).
99. Linsley, P. S., and Fox, C. F., *J. Supramol. Struct.*, **14**, 461 (1980).
100. O'Keefe, E. J., Battin, T. K., and Bennett, V., *J. Supramol. Struct.*, **15**, 15 (1981).

101. Comens, P. G., Simmer, R. L., and Baker, J. B., *J. Biol. Chem.*, **257**, 42 (1982).

102. Marchalonis, J. J., *Biochem. J.*, **113**, 299 (1969).

103. Kahn, C. R., *J. Cell Biol.*, **70**, 261 (1976).

104. Pappenheimer, A. M., Jr., *Annu. Rev. Biochem.*, **46**, 69 (1977).

105. Opresko, L., Wiley, H. S., and Wallace, R. A., *Cell*, **22**, 47 (1980).

106. Anderson, R. G. W., Brown, M. S., and Goldstein, J. L., *Cell*, **10**, 351 (1977).

107. Kaplan, J., and Nielsen, M. N., *J. Biol. Chem.*, **234**, 7329 (1979).

108. Willingham, M. C., Maxfield, F. R., and Pastan, I., *J. Cell Biol.*, **82**, 614 (1979).

109. Van Leuven, F., Cassiman, J. J., and Van den Berghe, H., *Exp. Cell Res.*, **117**, 273 (1978).

110. Kaplan, A. D., Achord, D. T., and Sly, W. S., *Proc. Natl. Acad. Sci. USA*, **74**, 2026 (1977).

111. Neufeld, E. F., Sando, G. N., Garvin, J., and Rome, L. H., *J. Supramol. Struct.*, **6**, 95 (1977).

112. Takahashi, K., Tauassoli, M., and Jacobsen, D. W., *Nature*, **288**, 18 (1980).

113. Tanabe, T., Pricer, W. E., Jr., and Ashwell, G., *J. Biol. Chem.*, **254**, 1038 (1979).

114. Wall, D. A., and Hubbard, A., *J. Cell Biol.*, **90**, 687 (1981).

115. Stockert, R. J., Howard, D. J., Morell, A. G., and Scheinberg, I. H., *J. Biol. Chem.*, **255**, 9028 (1980).

116. Helenius, A., Kartenbeck, J., Simons, K., and Fries, E., *J. Cell Biol.*, **84**, 404 (1980).

117. Marsh, M., and Helenius, A., *J. Mol. Biol.*, **142**, 439 (1980).

118. Willingham, M. C., and Pastan, I., *Cell*, **13**, 501 (1978).

119. Schlessinger, J., Shechter, Y., Cuatrecasas, P., Willingham, M. C., and Pastan, I., *Proc. Natl. Acad. Sci. USA*, **75**, 5353 (1978).

120. Schlessinger, J., Shechter, Y., Willingham, M. C., and Pastan, I., *Proc. Natl. Acad. Sci. USA*, **75**, 2659 (1978).

121. Gorden, P., Carpenter, J. L., Cohen, S., and Orci, L., *Proc. Natl. Acad. Sci. USA*, **75**, 5025 (1978).

122. Haigler, H. T., McKanna, J. A., and Cohen, S., *J. Cell Biol.*, **81**, 382 (1979).

123. McKanna, J. A., Haigler, H., and Cohen, S., *Proc. Natl. Acad. Sci. USA*, **76**, 5689 (1979).

124. Finegold, L., and Donnell, J. T., *Nature*, **278**, 443 (1979).

125. Karlin, A., in C. W. Cotman, G. Poste, and G. L. Nicolson, Eds., *The Cell Surface and Neuronal Function*, Amsterdam, North-Holland, 1980, pp. 192–242.

126. Willingham, M. C., and Pastan, I., *Cell*, **21**, 67 (1980).

127. Maxfield, F. R., Schlessinger, J., Shechter, Y., Pastan, I., and Willingham, M. C., *Cell*, **14**, 805 (1978).

128. Willingham, M. C., Rutherford, A. V., Gallo, M. G., Wehland, J., Dickson, R. B., Schlegel, R., and Pastan, I., *J. Histochem. Cytochem.*, **29**, 1003 (1981).

129. Goldstein, J. L., Anderson, R. G. W., and Brown, M. S., *Nature*, **279**, 679 (1979).

130. Fine, R. E., Goldenberg, R., Sorrentino, J., and Herschman, H. R., *J. Supramol. Struct.*, **15**, 235 (1981).

131. Rothman, J. E., and Fine, R., *Proc. Natl. Acad. Sci. USA*, **77**, 780 (1980).

132. Franke, W. W., Luder, M. R., Kartenbeck, J., Zorban, H., and Kennan, T. W., *J. Cell*

Biol., **69**, 173 (1976).

133. Jamieson, J. D., and Palade, G. E., *J. Cell Biol.*, **34**, 577 (1967).

134. Huet, C., Ash, J. F., and Singer, S., *Cell*, **21**, 429 (1980).

135. Bretscher, M. S., Thomason, J. N., and Pearse, B. M. F., *Proc. Natl. Acad. Sci. USA*, **77**, 4156 (1980).

136. Pastan, I., and Willingham, M., *Annu. Rev. Physiol.*, **43**, 239 (1981).

137. Salisbury, J. L., Condellis, J. S., and Satir, P., *J. Cell Biol.*, **87**, 132 (1980).

138. Silverstein, S. C., Steinman, R. M., and Cohn, Z. A., *Annu. Rev. Biochem.*, **46**, 669 (1977).

139. Haigler, H. T., McKanna, J. A., and Cohen, S., *J. Cell Biol.*, **83**, 82 (1979).

140. Chinkers, M., McKanna, J. A., and Cohen, S., *J. Cell Biol.*, **83**, 260 (1979).

141. Moehring, T. J., and Moehring, J. M., *Infect. Immun.*, **6**, 487 (1972).

142. Moehring, T. J., and Moehring, J. M., *Infect. Immun.*, **6**, 493 (1972).

143. Moehring, J. M., and Moehring, T. J., *Infect. Immun.*, **13**, 221 (1976).

144. Brown, K. D., Friedkin, M., and Rozengurt, E., *Proc. Natl. Acad. Sci. USA*, **77**, 480 (1980).

145. Maxfield, F. R., Davies, P. J. A., Klempner, L., Willingham, M. C., and Pastan, I., *Proc. Natl. Acad. Sci. USA*, **76**, 5731 (1979).

146. King, A. C., Hernaez-Davis, L., and Cuatrecasas, P., *Proc. Natl. Acad. Sci. USA*, **78**, 717 (1981).

147. Fox, C. F., and Das, M., *J. Supramol. Struct.*, **10**, 199 (1979).

148. Johnson, L. K., Vlodavsky, I., Baxter, J. D., and Gospodarowicz, D., *Nature*, **287**, 340 (1980).

149. Yankner, B. A., and Shooter, E. M., *Proc. Natl. Acad. Sci. USA*, **76**, 1269 (1979).

150. Goldfine, I. D., *Biochim. Biophys. Acta*, **650**, 53 (1981).

151. Delisi, C., *Nature*, **289**, 322 (1981).

152. Kahn, C. R., Baird, K. L., Jarrett, D. B., and Flier, J. B., *Proc. Natl. Acad. Sci. USA*, **75**, 4209 (1978).

153. Schechter, Y., Hernaez, L., Schlessinger, J., and Cuatrecasas, P., *Nature*, **278**, 835 (1979).

154. Cawley, D. B., Herschman, H. R., Gilliland, D. G., and Collier, R. J., *Cell*, **22**, 256 (1980).

155. Shimizu, N., Miskimins, W. K., and Schimizu, Y., *FEBS Lett.*, **118**, 274 (1980).

156. Scatchard, G., *Ann. N.Y. Acad. Sci.*, **55**, 660 (1949).

157. Rodbard, D., in B. W. O'Malley and A. R. Means, Eds., *Advances in Experimental Medicine and Biology*, Plenum, New York, Vol. 36, pp. 289–326.

158. Wiley, H. S., and Cunningham, D. D., *Cell*, **25**, 433 (1981).

159. Wiley, H. S., and Cunningham, D. D., *J. Biol. Chem.*, **257**, 4222 (1982).

160. Helenius, A., Marsh, M., and White, J., *Trends Biochem. Sci.*, **5**, 104 (1980).

161. Middlebrook, J. L. and Kohn, L. D., *Receptor-Mediated Binding and Internalization of Toxins and Hormones*, Academic, New York, 1981.

162. Brown, M. S., Kovanen, P. T., and Goldstein, J. L., *Science*, **212**, 628 (1981).

163. Ascoli, M., and Puett, D., *Proc. Natl. Acad. Sci. USA*, **75**, 99 (1978).

164. Kaplan J., *Science*, **212**, 14 (1981).

165. Krupp, M., and Lane, M. D., *J. Biol. Chem.*, **256**, 1689 (1981).

166. Hizuka, N., Gorden, P., Lesniak, M. A., Van Obberghen, E., Carpentier, J. L., and Orci, L., *J. Biol. Chem.*, **256**, 4591 (1981).

167. Kaplan, J., *Cell*, **19**, 197 (1980).

168. Van Leuven, F., Cassiman, J.-J., and Van den Berge, H., *Cell*, **20**, 37 (1980).

169. Gonzalez-Noriega, A., Grubb, J. H., Talkad, V., and Sly, W. S., *J. Cell Biol.*, **85**, 839 (1980).

170. Stahl, P., Schlesinger, P. H., Sigardson, E., Rodman, J. S., and Lee, Y. C., *Cell*, **19**, 207 (1980).

171. Willingham, M. C., Haigler, H. T., Dickson, R. B., and Pastan, I., *International Cell Biology*, 1980–1981, 613 (1981).

172. Davies, P. J. A., Davies, D. R., Levitzki, A., Maxfield, F. R., Milhaud, P., Willingham, M. C., and Pastan, I. H., *Nature*, **283**, 162 (1980).

173. Yarden, Y., Gabbay, M., and Schlessinger, J., *Biochim. Biophys. Acta*, **674**, 188 (1981).

174. Michael, H. J., Bishayee, S., and Das, M., *FEBS Lett.*, **117**, 125 (1980).

175. Maxfield, F. R., Willingham, M. C., Davies, P. J. A., and Pastan, I., *Nature*, **277**, 661 (1979).

176. Carpenter, G., King, L., Jr., and Cohen, S., *J. Biol. Chem.*, **254**, 4884 (1979).

177. Fernandez-Pol, J. A., *Biochemistry*, **20**, 3907 (1981).

178. Fernandez-Pol, J. A., *J. Biol. Chem.*, **256**, 9742 (1981).

179. Carpenter, G., Poliner, L., and King, L., Jr., *Mol. Cell. Endocrinol.*, **18**, 189 (1980).

180. Ushiro, J., and Cohen, S., *J. Biol. Chem.*, **255**, 8363 (1980).

181. Eckhart, W., Hutchinson, M. A., and Hunter, T., *Cell*, **21**, 829 (1979).

182. Hunter, T., and Sefton, B. M., *Proc. Natl. Acad. Sci. USA*, **77**, 1311 (1980).

183. Collett, M. S., Purchio, A. F., and Erickson, R. L., *Nature*, **285**, 167 (1980).

184. Neil, J. L., Ghysdael, J., Vogt, P. K., and Smart, J. E., *Nature*, **291**, 675 (1981).

185. Witte, D. N., Dasgupta, A., and Baltimore, D., *Nature*, **283**, 826 (1980).

186. Collett, M. S., and Erickson, R. L., *Proc. Natl. Acad. Sci. USA*, **75**, 2021 (1978).

187. Shefton, B. M., Hunter, T., and Beemon, K. J., *J. Virol.*, **33**, 220 (1980).

188. Levison, A. D., Oppermann, H., Levintow, L., Varmus, H. E., and Bishop, J. M., *Cell*, **15**, 561 (1978).

189. Erickson, R. L., Purchio, A. F., Erickson, E., Collett, M. S., and Brugge, J. S., *J. Cell Biol.*, **87**, 319 (1980).

190. Stefton, B. M., Hunter, T., Beemon, K., and Eckhart, W., *Cell*, **20**, 807 (1980).

191. Collett, M. S., Erickson, E., Purchio, A. F., Brugge, J. S., and Erickson, R. L., *Proc. Natl. Acad. Sci. USA*, **76**, 3159 (1979).

192. Oppermann, H., Levison, A. D., Varmus, H. E., Levintow, L., and Bishop, J. M., *Proc. Natl. Acad. Sci. USA*, **76**, 1804 (1979).

193. Wang, H.-L., Halpern, C. C., Nadel, M., and Hanafusa, H., *Proc. Natl. Acad. Sci. USA*, **75**, 5812 (1978).

194. Karess, R. E., Hayward, W. S., and Hanafusa, H., *Proc. Natl. Acad. Sci. USA*, **76**, 3154 (1979).

195. Hunter, T., *Cell*, **22**, 647 (1980).

196. Racker, E., and Spector, M., *Science*, **213**, 303 (1981).
197. Racker, E., *Science*, **213**, 1313 (1981).
198. Chinkers, M., and Cohen, S., *Nature*, **290**, 516 (1981).
199. Kudlow, J. E., Buss, J. E., and Gill, G. N., *Nature*, **290**, 519 (1981).
200. Hunter, T., and Cooper, J. A., *Cell*, **24**, 741 (1981).
201. Todaro, G. J., Fryling, C., and DeLarco, J. E., *Proc. Natl. Acad. Sci. USA*, **77**, 5258 (1980).
202. DeLarco, J. E., and Todaro, G. J., *Proc. Natl. Acad. Sci. USA*, **75**, 4001 (1978).
203. Reynolds, F. H., Jr., Todaro, G. J., Fryling, C., and Stephenson, J. R., *Nature*, **292**, 259 (1981).
204. Hanafusa, H., in H. Fraenkel-Conrat and R. P. Wagner, Eds., *Comprehensive Virology*, New York, Plenum, 1977, Vol. 10, pp. 401–483.
205. Todaro, G. J., DeLarco, J. E., and Cohen, S., *Nature*, **264**, 26 (1979).
206. Wang, E., and Goldbert, A. R., *Proc. Natl. Acad. Sci. USA*, **73**, 4065 (1976).

6

TUMOR PROMOTERS AND THEIR RELEVANCE TO ENDOGENOUS GROWTH FACTORS

Ann D. Horowitz
I. Bernard Weinstein

CONTENTS

Abbreviations

TPA	12-*O*-Tetradecanoyl phorbol-13-acetate
MEP	Major excreted protein
PDBu	Phorbol-12,13-dibutyrate
EGF	Epidermal growth factor
MSA	Multiplication-stimulating activity
gp 70	Murine type C ecotropic viral glycoprotein
PDD	Phorbol-12,13-didecanoate
2-DG	2-Deoxyglucose
BUdR	Bromodeoxyuridine
PA	Plasminogen activator
TS	Friend erythroleukemia subclones sensitive to phorbol esters
TR	Friend erythroleukemia subclones resistant to phorbol esters
DMSO	Dimethylsulfoxide
NEU	*N*-ethylnitrosourea
DMEM	Dulbecco's modified Eagle's medium
PBS	Phosphate-buffered saline
EDTA	Ethylene diamine tetraacetic acid
Plase	Phospholipase
AA	Arachidonic acid
PG	Prostaglandin

1. INTRODUCTION

Most naturally occurring cancers probably result from complex interactions
between endogenous (host) factors and exogenous (environmental) factors.
The carcinogenic process proceeds via several discrete steps and over a
time period that may occupy a considerable fraction of the lifespan of the
individual. Two stages in carcinogenesis, *initiation* and *promotion*, have
been experimentally well defined (1). Evidence that hepatocellular cancer,

bladder cancer, colon cancer, and breast cancer proceed via processes analogous to initiation and promotion has been reviewed in detail elsewhere
(2–4). Cell culture systems appear to be a valid model for analyzing multistage carcinogenesis, since malignant transformation of cells in culture
often proceeds by a multistep process (5–7) and can be enhanced by tumor
promoters (8–14).

Tumor promoters can be defined as compounds that lack significant carcinogenic activity when tested alone, but markedly enhance the yield of
tumors when applied after a low dose of an initiating carcinogen, for example,
benzo(a)pyrene. The most potent tumor promoters are macrocyclic diterpenes
of plant origin. The prototypes are 12-O-tetradecanoyl phorbol-13-acetate
(TPA) and related phorbol diesters produced by the *Euphorbiaceae* (3, 15–
17). A class of indole alkaloid tumor promoters of almost equal potency
have been isolated from *Streptomyces* (18) and the alga *Lyngbya majuscula*
(19). The major difference between initiating agents and tumor promoters
is that initiating agents usually generate electrophiles that bind covalently
to cellular DNA and cause mutations, whereas this is not the case for tumor
promoters. In addition, initiating agents are effective following a single
exposure, whereas tumor promotion requires repeated and prolonged exposure.

The cellular targets for the action of the phorbol ester tumor promoters
are not known with certainty, but recent studies in cell culture systems
have provided important clues. Some of the diverse effects of phorbol ester
tumor promoters on cells in culture are listed in Table 1. Early studies of
TPA action suggested that the cell surface membrane may be the initial and
major target of TPA action (15,20). Many of the most rapid effects of TPA
in cell culture occur at the cell membrane and are not blocked by inhibitors
of protein or RNA synthesis, for example, stimulation of release of [^{3}H]choline
from prelabeled phospholipids (21), enhancement of 2-deoxyglucose uptake
(22,23), altered membrane fluidity (24), altered cell adhesion (25), and
inhibition of binding of epidermal growth factor (EGF) to its receptor (26,27).
In addition, TPA produces morphological changes in enucleated chick embryo
fibroblasts (28) and induces aggregation of platelets, which lack a nucleus
(29,30). Several later effects of TPA, for example, induction of plasminogen
activator (PA) (31), synthesis of major excreted protein (MEP) glycoprotein
(32), and stimulation of arachidonic acid (AA) release and prostaglandin
(PG) synthesis (33–35), do require RNA and/or protein synthesis.

Other indirect evidence also suggests that TPA and related compounds
may act by usurping the function of a membrane-associated receptor normally
utilized by an endogenous growth factor (26,31). This evidence includes the
following: (1) TPA and related compounds act in a concentration range similar to that of several hormones and growth factors (i.e., 10^{-10}–10^{-8} M),

Table 1.   Effects of TPA on the Phenotype of Cell Cultures

EFFECT	REFERENCES
Cell-surface- and membrane changes	
Altered Na$^+$-K$^+$-ATPase	20
Increased uptake of 2-deoxyglucose, ^{32}P, ^{86}Rb	22, 23, 90, 91, 92
Increased membrane-lipid "fluidity"	24, 89
Increased release of AA, PGs	33–35, 52
Altered erythroleukemia cell adhesion	25, 153, 154
Increased pinocytosis	155
Altered fucose-glycopeptides	31, 156
Decreased LETS protein	157
"Uncoupling" of β-adrenergic receptors	69, 70
Inhibition of binding of EGF to receptors	26, 27, 44, 58–64
Inhibition of binding of thyrotropin-releasing hormone and somatostatin to receptors	44, 64
Decrease in acetylcholine receptors	71
Synergistic interaction with growth factors	114–119
Inhibition of metabolic cooperation	100, 101
Increased release and incorporation of choline	21, 79–81
Increased release of MEP glycoprotein from Balb/c 3T3 cells	32
Growth properties	
Increased saturation density	156
Altered morphology and cell orientation	20, 67, 90, 158, 159
Decreased serum requirement	97
Decreased calcium requirement	98, 108, 109
Decreased actin cables	99
Enzymatic	
Increased plasminogen-activator synthesis	122, 158, 160, 161
Increased ornithine decarboxylase	50, 51
Increased production of prolactin and growth hormone in GH$_4$C$_1$ cells	64
Modulation of differentiation (either inhibition or induction)	(For reviews, see 2, 3, 31, 66, 95, 96)
Enhancement of transformation	
Viral transformation	12, 14, 75, 97
Chemical or radiation-induced transformation	9–12, 102
Induction of anchorage-independent growth in partially transformed cells	6, 7, 97, 103, 113

(2) these compounds display similar structure–function requirements on cells of diverse origin, and (3) like known hormones, they induce highly pleiotropic effects, which vary considerably depending on the target cell. These effects include modulation of cellular responses to other growth factors (114–118). Initially, we attempted to demonstrate the existence of phorboid receptors in intact HeLa (36) or rat embryo cells (unpublished studies) using [^{3}H]TPA. However, a high background of nonspecific binding made these attempts unsuccessful. Recently, Blumberg and co-workers have used tritiated phorbol 12,13-dibutyrate (PDBu) to overcome this problem. Although PDBu is much less hydrophobic than TPA, it is also somewhat less potent as a tumor promoter. Saturable, high-affinity receptors for [^{3}H]PDBu have since been demonstrated in a wide variety of cell types and tissue preparations (37–45). In this paper we review in some detail studies from our own and other laboratories on the interactions of phorbol esters and other tumor promoters with phorboid receptors and their possible relation to the action of endogenous growth factors.

2. CELLULAR EFFECTS OF TUMOR PROMOTERS

2.1. Inhibition of Binding of Polypeptide Growth Factors

The tumor promoter TPA shares several effects on cells in culture with EGF. These include stimulation of proliferation of both epidermal and mesodermal cells, increase in deoxyglucose transport (22,23,46–49), induction of ornithine decarboxylase (50,51), stimulation of PG synthesis (33–35,52), induction of PA (31,53), and stimulation of release of MEP glycoprotein from Balb/c 3T3 cells (32,54). Epidermal growth factor has been reported to promote tumor induction (55), and it enhances viral and radiation-induced cell transformation *in vitro* (13). These data suggest that TPA might exert some of its effects via the EGF receptor. We examined the effect of TPA on binding of [^{125}I]EGF to its cell-surface receptors, and we found that TPA causes an immediate inhibition of EGF binding when added to HeLa cells simultaneously with [^{125}I]EGF (26). The inhibition of EGF binding by TPA occurs in the range of 10^{-8}–10^{-10} M TPA, the concentration range in which TPA exerts most of its other cellular effects. When TPA is added to cells to which EGF has previously been bound, a rapid decline in cell-bound EGF results (27,56).

We have also observed the inhibition of EGF binding by TPA in C3H 10T½ cells (57), in an early passage of rat embryo cells, and in established rat embryo fibroblast cell lines (40 and unpublished studies). The inhibition of EGF binding by TPA has been corroborated by a number of other investigators in various cell types (44,58–64). The inhibition is specific to EGF in most cell types tested, since TPA does not inhibit binding of concanavalin A, multiplication-stimulating activity (MSA), murine type C ecotropic viral glycoprotein (gp70) (58), or insulin (58,59) to receptors in 3T3, nor does it inhibit binding of MSA to rat kidney fibroblasts (58), nerve growth factor to human melanoma (58) or chick ganglia cells (60), or low-density lipoprotein to human foreskin cells in culture (58). However, it has recently been shown that TPA reduces the binding of thyrotropin-releasing hormone and soma-tostatin to their receptors in GH_4C_1 rat pituitary cells (44,64) in addition to reducing EGF binding. This appears to be directly related to the action of TPA on these cells, since TPA stimulates the production of prolactin and growth hormone in the same cell line (64).

Although our initial studies on the EGF receptor were motivated by the possibility that TPA might exert its action by occupying the EGF receptor, more detailed studies indicate that the effect of TPA on EGF receptors is an indirect one, perhaps related to TPA-induced changes in the lipid mi-croenvironment of EGF receptors (27,56). This is suggested by the obser-vations that TPA is unable to inhibit EGF binding when the assay is conducted at 4°C (27,56–58) or in a subcellular system (27,56). This interpretation is consistent with the synergistic action of EGF and TPA, which is discussed later. Studies with a variety of inhibitors (25,56) suggest that TPA inhibition of EGF binding does not require RNA or protein synthesis, energy metab-olism, or cytoskeletal changes. Thus the effect appears to be mediated directly at the level of the plasma membrane. Nor is the TPA inhibition of EGF binding due to increased degradation of EGF or increased internalization of the EGF-receptor complex (27,56). As a matter of fact, EGF degradation by cells is less in the presence of TPA than in its absence, apparently because in the presence of TPA, previously bound EGF is displaced into the medium (27,56).

With prolonged exposure to TPA, HeLa cells become refractory to TPA-induced inhibition of EGF binding (27,56). When HeLa cells were exposed to 33 ng/ml of TPA in serum-containing medium for 0–24 hours and at various times assayed for EGF binding, there was a progressive decrease in the inhibitory effect of TPA on EGF binding. By 24 hours the EGF-binding capacity had returned to 85% of that of parallel cultures not exposed to TPA (56). This was not due to exhaustion from the medium or degradation of TPA, since the addition of fresh TPA at 24 hours also failed to produce significant inhibition of EGF binding. On the other hand, if the cells were treated with TPA (33 ng/ml) for 60 minutes, rinsed once with serum-free medium, and incubated in serum-free medium for various periods of time, then the ability of the cells to bind [^{125}I]EGF remained significantly depressed for up to 9 hours. Even under these conditions, however, there was gradual recovery, so that 86% of the EGF-binding capacity was restored at 24 hours after the preincubation with TPA (56).

When HeLa cells were exposed to TPA over a more prolonged period (Table 2), the escape from TPA inhibition of EGF binding persisted for at least 4 days (56). Although TPA initially caused a marked decrease in EGF binding to its receptor, within 1 day of continuous exposure to TPA, the cells recovered the ability to bind EGF and became resistant to EGF-binding inhibition by freshly added TPA. The data obtained in this study by Lee and Weinstein (56) are shown in Table 2. In additional studies, it was found that 10 ng/ml of TPA was sufficient to produce the same ''escape'' effect.

The phenomenon of escape from the effects of TPA has been observed in other cell culture systems. These include TPA inhibition of melanogenesis in mouse melanoma B-16 cells (65), TPA inhibition of adipocyte differentiation (66), and TPA-induced morphological changes in 10T½ cell cultures (67). Since tumor promotion requires prolonged exposure to the promoting agents, the phenomenon of escape, occurring only after prolonged exposure, may be a significant factor in tumor promotion. It may be related to the observation of Barrett and Sisskind (68) that a single application of TPA induces a transient hyperplasia in hamster epidermis, whereas with repeated exposures this hyperplastic response diminishes rapidly.

As mentioned above, TPA has also been shown to inhibit binding of thyrotropin-releasing hormone and somatostatin to their receptors in GH_4C_1

Table 2. Cellular Escape From TPA-Induced Inhibition of EGF Binding During Growth in TPA[a]

GROWTH CONDITION	ASSAY CONDITION	[125I]EGF BOUND (cpm/10^6 Cells) ON DAY:				
		0	1	2	3	4
DMSO	DMSO	3486	2292	1322	979	930
DMSO	TPA	106	209	170	121	130
TPA	DMSO	106	1776	1342	1258	1246
TPA	TPA	106	1004	1085	1072	1171

Source: Reference 56.

[a] On day zero, HeLa cells were seeded at 7×10^5 per 5-cm dish in complete growth medium in the presence of TPA (20 ng/ml) or DMSO (0.002%) and grown at 37°C. During the subsesequent 4 days, replicate plates were used to determine cell counts and [125I]EGF binding. The binding assays were done for 55 minutes at 37°C with 11,900 cpm of [125I]EGF per plate (specific activity, 67 μCi/μg) plus or minus freshly added TPA (33 ng/ml) or DMSO (0.003%). By day 4 the cell counts in the DMSO-containing cultures were $5.3 \pm$ (SD) 0.3×10^6 cells per plate and those in TPA-containing cultures were $3.9 \pm 0.5 \times 10^6$ cells per plate. For additional details, see reference 56.

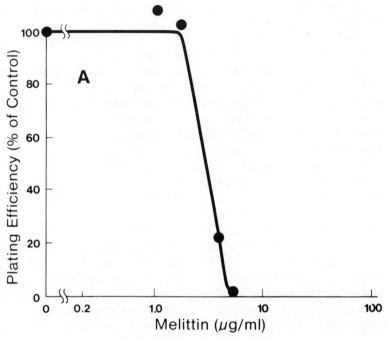

Figure 1. Effects of Melittin on CREF N Cells. (*A*) Toxicity. Cell survival was determined by plating efficiency. CREF N cells were grown in Dulbecco's modified Eagle's medium (DMEM) containing 10% calf serum in 5-cm tissue culture dishes. The cell monolayers were washed once with 5 ml of phosphate-buffered saline (PBS), then 2 ml of assay buffer (2 volumes of DMEM to 1 volume of PBS, plus 1 mg bovine serum albumin per milliliter) was added. Varying amounts of melittin (0–6 μg/ml) were added, and the cells were incubated for 3 hours at 37°C. The monolayers were washed carefully with PBS, then trypsinized and replated. The following day, the cultures were retrypsinized and counted in a Coulter counter. The plating efficiency is given as percentage of untreated control. There were 2 × 10^6 cells per dish;

rat pituitary cells (44,64). Additional effects of TPA on heterologous receptors include "uncoupling" of β-adrenergic receptors (69–70) and reduction in the number of acetylcholine receptors in chick myoblasts (71).

The diverse effects of TPA on cellular receptors suggest that its pleiotropic effects on cell function, growth, and differentiation may in part relate to its ability to affect membrane receptors and thereby alter the response of cells to extracellular signals. The variety of receptors affected by TPA also suggests that the effects may be caused indirectly through changes in membrane structure. In support of this hypothesis, we have found that a membrane-perturbing polypeptide from bee venom, melittin (73,74), can induce several

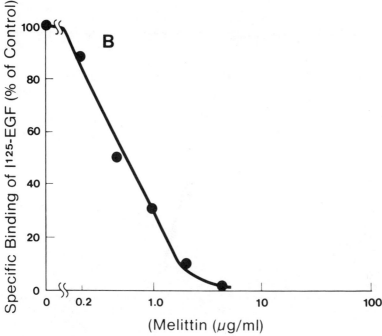

Figure 1. (*B*) Inhibition of [^{125}I]EGF binding. CREF N cells were prepared for the assay as described in (*A*). Following the addition of assay buffer, varying amounts of melittin and approximately 18,000 cpm of [^{125}I]EGF (84.7 Ci/μg, Collaborative Research) were added. Following a 50-minute incubation at 37°C, the monolayers were washed rapidly three times with 5-ml portions of ice-cold assay buffer, and 1 ml of solubilizing solution was added (0.8% Triton X-100, 0.25% trypsin, 0.02% EDTA in PBS). After at least 2 hours at 37°C, the plates were washed twice with 0.5-ml portions of 1% SDS, and the solution and washes were transferred to scintillation vials and counted in 15 ml of Hydrofluor (National Diagnostics);

effects similar to those of TPA, including inhibition of EGF binding (67,72) (Fig. 1). Melittin lyses cells by insertion into the phospholipid bilayer and stimulation of phospholipase A_2 activity (73,74). At concentrations well below the toxic dose (Fig. 1*A*) it inhibits binding of [^{125}I]EGF to cell monolayers at 37°C (Fig. 1*B*). This inhibition requires a higher concentration of melittin if the assay is done in a low-Ca^{2+} medium (unpublished studies). Like TPA, melittin is unable to inhibit EGF binding at 4°C or in a subcellular system, suggesting that the effect is indirect. Melittin does not produce this effect by binding to the phorboid receptor, since it does not inhibit [^{3}H]PDBu binding in a subcellular system (Fig. 1*C*). In cell monolayers melittin does inhibit [^{3}H]PDBu binding, but only at a concentration close to the toxic dose. The inhibition may be due, therefore, simply to toxicity (Fig. 1*C*).

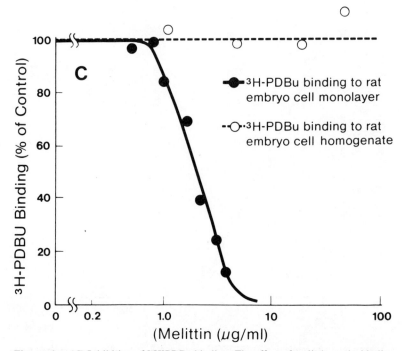

Figure 1. (C) Inhibition of [³H]PDBu binding. The effect of melittin on the binding of [³H]PDBu to CREF N monolayers (-●-) and to a crude membrane fraction from CREF N cells (-○-) was determined. The binding assay in CREF N monolayers was conducted as described in Fig. 1*B* of reference 40, except that the monolayer was incubated for 60 minutes at 37°C in assay buffer prior to the addition of melittin and 3 n*M* [³H]PDBu (6.4 Ci/mmol, Lifesystems Co.). After 30 minutes at 37°C, the monolayers were washed and solubilized as described in Fig. 1 (*B*) of reference 40. There were 1.1×10^6 cells per dish. The preparation of the crude membrane fraction and the binding assay were performed as described by Driedger and Blumberg (37), except that the total protein concentration in the homogenate was about 1 mg/ml. The final centrifugation was in an Eppendorf microfuge for 15 minutes, and the pellets were solubilized for scintillation counting in 1% SDS.

Like TPA, mellitin enhances adenovirus transformation of rat embryo cells (75).

Two other membrane-active compounds, δ-hemolysin and A_{23187} also produce several effects similar to those of TPA. The compound δ-hemolysin is a toxic polypeptide produced by *Staphylococcus aureus*. Like TPA, it inhibits EGF binding to its receptor and stimulates AA release and PG synthesis (76). Like TPA, the calcium ionophore A_{23187} stimulates PA synthesis (77) and AA release (21) and inhibits EGF binding (unpublished studies) to cultured cells. However, it does not stimulate release of choline from cellular phospholipids (21). It has recently been reported that the membrane-perturbing agent phospholipase C, but not phospholipase A, inhibits binding of EGF to its receptor (78).

2.2.   Effects of Phorbol Esters on Membrane Structure and Lipid Metabolism

One of the earliest effects of TPA is a change in membrane phospholipid metabolism. The TPA rapidly induces an increase in the incorporation of phosphate or choline into membrane phospholipids (79–83). In addition, TPA induces the release from membrane phospholipids of AA, and this is associated with increased PG synthesis (33–35). This effect is not blocked by actinomycin D, although it is blocked by inhibitors of protein synthesis (34).

Recently, we studied the release of water-soluble choline metabolites from C3H 10T½ cells prelabeled for 24 hours with [³H]choline (21). Within 5 minutes of exposure to TPA at 37°C, the release of [³H]choline metabolites was enhanced twofold and by 60–120 minutes the release was four to five times that of vehicle controls (Fig. 2). Choline-metabolite release was concentration dependent between 10 and 100 ng of TPA per milliliter. Phorbol-12,13-didecanoate (PDD) was also active, but 4-α-PDD, which is not a

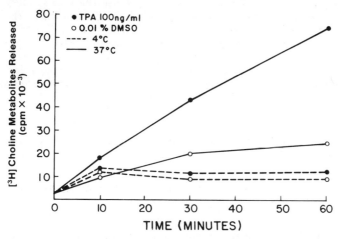

Figure 2.   Effect of TPA on the release of [³H]choline from prelabeled cells. The 10T½ cells were prelabeled with [³H]choline. At time 0, cultures were incubated at either 37°C or 4°C, 100 ng/ml TPA (●) or DMSO solvent (○) was then added, and the release of [³H]choline from the cells into the media was determined. For additional details see reference 21.

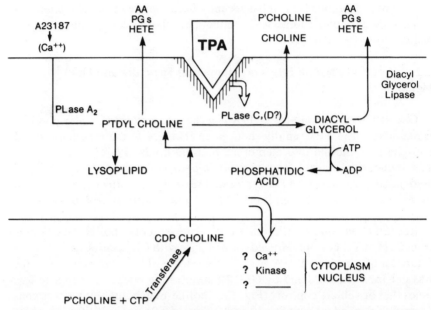

Figure 3. Schematic diagram of the effects of TPA and related compounds on phosphatidylcholine turnover. We postulate that the binding of TPA to specific cell-membrane receptors activates phospholipase (*Plase*) C and/or D, resulting in the conversion of phosphatidylcholine (*P'TDYL Choline*) to diacylglycerol plus choline. Arachidonic acid (*AA*) is then released by diacylglycerol lipase; prostaglandins (PGs) and other AA metabolites are also formed. The AA also may be released by the direct action of Plase A_2 on phosphatidylcholine. The calcium ionophore A_{23187} and melittin may induce AA release via the latter mechanism. Phosphatidylcholine may be resynthesized via CDP choline as shown. Presumably, during these biochemical transformations, a transmembrane signal to the cytoplasm and/or nucleus is generated, i.e., increased Ca^{2+} uptake or redistribution, activation of a protein kinase, or some other mediator. Phosphatidic acid, serving as a Ca^{2+} ionophore (86,106,107), or some other phosphatidylcholine metabolite may stimulate this process. For additional details see references 21, 134, and 135.

tumor promoter, was inactive. The radioactivity released by TPA was derived from phospholipids, since changes in the acid-soluble pool of choline metabolites were insufficient to account for the amount of material released. The released material was identified by chromatography as choline and phosphorylcholine. Neither cycloheximide (4–40 μg/ml) nor cordycepin (4–40 μg/ml) blocked the TPA-induced release. Like the effect of TPA on EGF binding, the release was temperature sensitive and did not occur at 4°C. TPA did not induce the release of [³H]inositol from prelabeled cells.

Different agonists induce qualitatively different responses in phospholipid metabolism when they interact with their membrane receptors. For example, certain growth factors, cholinergic agonists, and α-adrenergic agonists induce the turnover of phosphatidylinositol (for review see 84, also 85,86); β-adrenergic agonists, benzodiazepine agonists, and chemotactic peptides induce phospholipid methylation (for review, see 87,88), whereas TPA specifically induces the turnover of phosphatidylcholine (21,79–83,85,86).

We believe that TPA-induced choline release is due to activation of an endogenous phospholipase (Plase) C or D. It appears that TPA-induced choline release precedes TPA-induced AA release, TPA-induced incorporation of choline into membrane phospholipids, and TPA inhibition of EGF binding. A hypothetical scheme for the effects of TPA on phospholipid metabolism is given in Fig. 3. As discussed below, the initial interaction between TPA and cells appears to involve specific binding to cell-surface receptors. Presumably, this binding triggers activation of a Plase C or D as well as the other events shown in Fig. 3. It is not known how these membrane effects might induce signals or second messengers that mediate the subsequent cytoplasmic and nuclear events; however, we have obtained evidence suggesting that changes in membrane fluidity may be involved. In rat embryo cells, TPA can induce an increase in membrane fluidity (24). A similar effect of TPA has been reported in normal and malignant human lymphoblastoid cells (89). In rat embryo cells we have found that this effect is maximal after 3–4 hours of exposure to TPA. It is not blocked by cycloheximide or actinomycin D and does not occur with biologically inactive phorbol esters (24).

2.3. Stimulation of Membrane Transport by TPA

It has been shown that TPA and related compounds can exert a very rapid effect on membrane transport of 2-deoxyglucose (2-DG) (22,23). Transport of 2-DG is stimulated 12-fold in confluent 3T3 cells and 2.5-fold in HeLa cells (22). The effect is observable within 5 minutes and persists for at least 2 hours. Kinetic analysis showed that the increased 2-DG uptake is due to facilitated transport rather than simple diffusion. The ED_{50} for TPA-induced 2-DG uptake in HeLa cells is 0.2 nM (0.13 ng/ml), thus it is a very sensitive effect (22). The stimulation by TPA is not inhibited by cycloheximide or actinomycin D. Like many membrane effects of TPA, it is highly temperature dependent and does not occur at 4°C.

It has also been observed that TPA causes a rapid stimulation in cellular uptake of ^{32}P and ^{86}Rb (90–92). Rozengurt et al. (93,94) have emphasized the similarities between vasopressin and TPA in terms of effects on Na$^+$ and Rb$^+$ (a K$^+$ analog) uptake in cell culture.

2.4. Modulation of Differentiation

Since it is likely that carcinogenesis involves major disturbances in differentiation, it is of interest that TPA is a highly potent inhibitor or inducer of differentiation in a wide variety of cell systems (for reviews, see 2,3,31,66,95,96). The examples include a variety of programs of differentiation and cells from such diverse sources as birds, rodents, humans, and even echinoderms. It is possible that the ability of TPA to either induce or inhibit differentiation depends on the nature of membrane constituents of the target cells. Reciprocal effects of the same agent on differentiation, depending on the target cells, have been seen with other agents including glucocorticoid hormones, cyclic AMP, and bromodeoxyuridine (BUdR).

2.5. Mimicry of Transformation and Enhancement

The application of TPA induces several properties in normal cells that mimic those often seen in transformed cells. This mimicry includes changes in cell morphology, growth properties, cell-surface properties, and induction of PA, ornithine decarboxylase, and PG synthesis (2,3,31,66,95,96; see also Table 1). Recent findings that add to this growing list include TPA-induced decreases in growth requirements for serum (97) and Ca^{2+} (98), TPA-induced loss of actin cables (99), and TPA-induced loss of metabolic cooperation (100,101). All of these properties are frequently associated with cell transformation. It has also been shown that TPA can enhance the stable transformation of fibroblast cultures previously exposed to a chemical carcinogen, ultraviolet or X irradiation (9–12,102), an adenovirus (12,75,97), or Epstein-Barr virus (14). As described below, TPA can also induce the irreversible acquisition of anchorage-independent growth in "partially" transformed cells (6,7,103). These stable or irreversible effects of TPA indicate that "initiated" cells have a qualitatively different response to TPA than normal cells.

Enhancement of the transformed phenotype can be observed when transformed cells are exposed to phorbol esters. When TPA was applied to avian sarcoma virus–transformed chick embryo fibroblasts, which already synthesize a high level of PA, a further increase in PA synthesis was seen (31). However, recent studies show that TPA does not cause a significant increase in the amount or activity of the protein kinase (pp60[src]) that is a product of the avian sarcoma virus sarc gene, or the corresponding endogenous protein kinase (104,105). Further studies will be necessary to determine how TPA enhances the transformed phenotype in these cells.

Several findings suggest that alterations in Ca^{2+} uptake or intracellular distribution may play a role in mediating the cytoplasmic and nuclear events induced by TPA. As mentioned above, the calcium ionophore A_{23187} mimics some, though not all, of the actions of TPA. Michell et al. (84) have proposed that the effects of certain agonists on phosphatidylinositol turnover might be coupled to alterations in membrane Ca^{2+} flux, perhaps through the action of phosphatidic acid as an ionophore (86,106,107). As phosphatidic acid is also a product of phosphatidylcholine metabolism (Fig. 3), TPA might also alter Ca^{2+} flux. There is considerable evidence that Ca^{2+} plays an important role in modulating growth of normal fibroblasts and epithelial cells. In general, normal cells exhibit negligible or limited growth in media containing low Ca^{2+} concentrations (0.001–0.01 mM rather than 1.25 mM), and transformation by chemical carcinogens or viruses enhances the capacity of cells to grow in low-Ca^{2+} media (for reviews, see 98,108,109). Since TPA induces a number of phenotypic effects that mimic the properties of transformed cells (31) and since, as discussed above, EGF, TPA, and the membrane-active polypeptide melittin share a number of phenotypic effects, it is of interest that TPA (98,108,109), EGF (108,110–112), and melittin (108) can enhance the growth of either normal or transformed cells in media containing low amounts of Ca^{2+}.

The effects of TPA on adenovirus transformation of rat embryo cells include an enhancement of the efficiency of transformation (12,108), induction of anchorage-independent growth in early-passage adenovirus-transformed cells that cannot grow in agar in the absence of TPA (7,97,113), and enhancement of anchorage-independent growth of late-passage adenovirus-transformed cells (7,97,113). Melittin and EGF are also effective in these assays (6,67,108). This data has been recently reviewed (75).

2.6. Interactions with Polypeptide Growth Factors

As mentioned earlier, TPA produces several effects similar to those of known growth factors, notably EGF. It acts synergistically with serum (114-116) and plasma (117) in stimulating DNA synthesis. In addition, TPA acts synergistically with polypeptide growth factors in a number of systems. The polypeptides platelet-derived growth factor (117), EGF (117,118), fibroblast growth factor (117), fibroblast-derived growth factor (118), insulin (117,118), and multiplication-stimulating activity (117) all act synergistically with TPA to stimulate DNA synthesis in 3T3 cells. And TPA is also synergistic with EGF, insulin, fibroblast-derived growth factor, and serum in stimulating 2-DG uptake and ornithine decarboxylase activity in 3T3 cells (93). Vasopressin also acts synergistically with these growth factors in inducing 2-DG uptake and ornithine decarboxylase activity, and in stimulating DNA synthesis (93,119). But vasopressin and TPA are not synergistic with each other, suggesting that they may act through a common mechanism (93,94). However, they do not appear to share the same receptor system (40, and Table 6).

3.   RECEPTOR BINDING OF THE PHORBOL ESTERS

3.1.   Distribution and Characteristics of Phorboid Receptors

Diverse lines of evidence suggest that the tumor-promoting phorbol esters may bind to and utilize cellular receptors for some endogenous hormone or growth factor. With [³H]PDBu (37) it is possible to study the characteristics of the phorboid receptors in tissues and cultured cells. In the course of our studies, we have determined the binding constants and receptor numbers in a wide variety of cell types (Table 3). In general, one or two classes of receptor are found in each cell type. In most cases, the high-affinity site, with a K_D in the range of 3–17 nM is present at $0.2 \times 10^5 - 4 \times 10^5$ sites per cell. Where a second, lower-affinity site is observed, the K_D is 300 nM or greater, and the number of sites is greater than 1×10^6 per cell. Some variation in receptor number occurs within a cell line depending on the growth state of the cells at the time of assay. When only one binding site is detected, the affinity for PDBu appears to be lower (K_D of 12–41 nM), but the number of sites is, in general, higher. In the case of cell lines of glial origin (B-15 and B-92, Table 4) as many as 2×10^6 high-affinity sites per cell are present. This observation is in accord with the results of Nagle et al. (120), showing that brain tissue contains a very large number of phorboid receptors. It suggests that the cells in brain that have large numbers of receptors may be glial rather than neuronal cells. We have also demonstrated PDBu receptors in human keratinocytes (45), normal and transformed human melanocytes (45), C3H 10T½ cells, and HeLa cells (unpublished data).

Most of our studies have been conducted in a rat embryo cell line (CREF N) derived in this laboratory by Dr. Paul B. Fisher (75). Binding of [³H]PDBu is rapid and reversible in these cells (40). When CREF N cell monolayers were incubated with 3 nM [³H]PDBu at 37°C, specific binding occurred rapidly and reached a maximum within 10 minutes (Fig. 4A). Specific binding decreased slightly (24%) by 20 minutes, but remained constant thereafter for at least 3 hours at 37°C. The decrease between 10 and 20 minutes was observed repeatedly, but its significance is not known. At 4°C, specific [³H]PDBu binding was considerably slower, requiring 3 hours to reach a maximum (Fig. 4A). The plateau value at 4°C was similar to that obtained at 37°C. Nonspecific binding was determined in the presence of a

Table 3. Characterization of Phorboid Receptors in Various Cell Types

Cell Type	$K_{D,1}$ (nM)	Number/Cell	$K_{D,2}$ (nM)	Number/Cell
CREF N Rat embryo fibroblast[a]	7.6[b]	1.6 × 10^5	710[b]	2.8 × 10^6
CREF A Rat embryo fibroblast	7	3.8 × 10^5	1700	4 × 10^6
CREF A2 Variant of CREF A	18	1 × 10^6	—[c]	—[c]
E-11 Adenovirus-transformed rat embryo fibroblast[a]	11	1.5 × 10^5	1100	1.4 × 10^6
K-22 Rat liver epithelial[d]	26	2.5 × 10^5	1450	9.4 × 10^6
TS19-0 TPA-sensitive Friend erythroleukemia cells[e]	8[f]	3 × 10^4	800[f]	3 × 10^6
TR19-4 TPA-resistant Friend erythroleukemia cells[e]	8[f]	3 × 10^4	800[f]	3 × 10^6
B-35 NEU[i]-transformed rat neuronal cell[g]	25	4.1 × 10^5	—[c]	—[c]
B-103 NEU-transformed rat neuronal cell[g]	36	4.5 × 10^5	—[c]	—[c]
B-49 NEU-transformed rat cell with neuronal and glial characteristics	8.7	1.6 × 10^5	330	5.4 × 10^6
B-15 NEU-transformed rat glial cell[g]	40	1.5 × 10^6	—[c]	—[c]
B-92 NEU-transformed rat glial cell[g]	37	1.4 × 10^6	—[c]	—[c]
SC-9 RSV-transformed rat cerebellar cells[h]	15	1.8 × 10^5	700	4.4 × 10^6
WC-5 RSV-transformed rat cerebellar astrocyte[h]	3	2 × 10^4	380	1.3 × 10^6

We thank Dr. G. J. Giotta of the Salk Institute for cell lines B-35 through WC-5. Lines B-35 through B-92 were isolated by Dr. D. Schubert of the Salk Institute.

[a] Reference 75.
[b] Reference 40.
[c] Only a single class of binding sites observed.
[d] Reference 162.
[e] Reference 128.
[f] Reference 41.
[g] Reference 163–165.
[h] Reference 166.
[i] NEU is N-ethylnitrosourea.

Table 4. Inhibition of PDBu and EGF Binding by Various Compounds

Compound	PDBu Binding[e] ID_{50}(ng/ml) CREF N	EGF Binding[e]		
		CREF N	ID_{50}[e](ng/ml) C3H 10T½	HeLa
TPA	4[a,d]	0.7[c]	0.5	2.5[b]
PDBu	12.5[c]	4[c]	—	—
Teleocidin B[f]	2.7[a]	—	1.0[a]	—
Lyngbyatoxin A[f]	3.3[c]	—	—	—
Mezerein	20[d]	—	—	4.7[b]
Gnidipalmin	>1000[c]	500	—	>100[b]
Gnilatimacrin	16[c]	1.2	—	4.5[b]
Gnidilatin	48[c]	5.7	—	21.5[b]
Phorbol	NI[d]	—	—	NI[b]
4-α-PDD	NI[d]	—	—	NI[b]

Source: From reference 130.

[a] Reference 57.

[b] Reference 26.

[c] A. D. Horowitz and I. B. Weinstein, unpublished data.

[d] Reference 40.

[e] Abbreviations: ID_{50}: concentration inhibiting binding by 50%; NI: not inhibitory.

[f] Teleocidin B and lyngbyatoxin kindly provided by Dr. T. Sugimura.

vast excess (50 μM) of unlabeled PDBu and was subtracted from the total binding to obtain the specific binding. Nonspecific [³H]PDBu binding was complete within 30 minutes, and accounted for less than one third of the total cell-associated radioactivity.

When binding of [³H]PDBu at 37°C was allowed to reach a plateau and the cell monolayer was then transferred to buffer lacking [³H]PDBu, the bound radioactivity rapidly dissociated from the cells (Fig. 4B), demonstrating the reversibility of binding. The dissociation was slower at 4°C than at 37°C.

In CREF N cells, we found two classes of binding sites for [³H]PDBu (40) (Table 3 and Fig. 5). The high-affinity site has a K_D of 7.6 nM, with 1.6×10^5 binding sites per cell. The weaker binding site has a K_D of 710 nM, at 2.8×10^6 sites per cell. The significance of the low-affinity binding sites is not known. Some variation in the number of binding sites per cell occurred, depending on the growth state of the cells, but the overall binding varied no more than threefold. Figure 5 shows a Scatchard analysis of

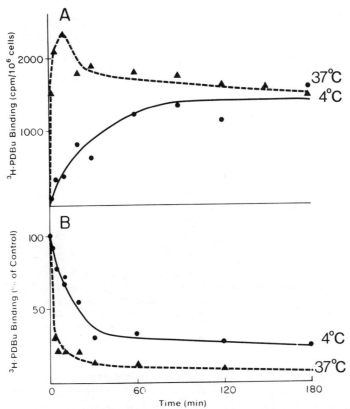

Figure 4. (A) Time course of the specific binding of [³H]PDBu to CREF cells. The [³H]PDBu binding was conducted at 37°C (▲) or 4°C (●). All values have been corrected for nonspecific binding, which was determined in parallel assays. The assay was performed as described in the legend to Fig. 1(C) and reference 40. (B) Dissociation of [³H]PDBu from CREF cells. The [³H]PDBu was allowed to bind to monolayers of CREF cells (2 × 10⁶ cells per dish) at 37°C for 30 minutes as in (A). The assay buffer was then rapidly replaced with fresh assay buffer, and the monolayers were incubated for varying time intervals at 37°C (▲) or 4°C (●). All values have been corrected for nonspecific binding. From reference 40.

specific binding of [³H]PDBu in CREF N cells. Data from two different experiments are shown. This curve was obtained after a 30-minute incubation with [³H]PDBu at 37°C, but identical results are obtained if binding is conducted at 4°C for 3 hours (40). Specific receptor binding can also be demonstrated in a crude membrane fraction from CREF N cells using methods described by Driedger and Blumberg (37).

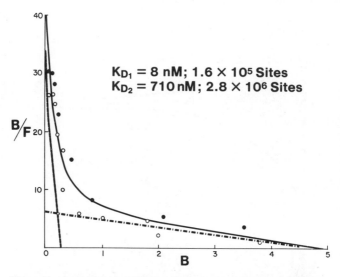

Figure 5. Scatchard plot of the specific binding of PDBu to CREF N cells. The assay was performed as described in Fig. 1*C*. Results of two separate assays are shown. Nonspecific binding has been subtracted from all points. Bound PDBu (*B*) is in picomoles. Free PDBu (*F*) is in moles per liter. The dashed lines show the binding to each of the two classes of binding sites. From reference 40.

3.2. Macrocyclic Inhibitors of Phorbol Ester Binding

The biological responses to phorbol esters show great specificity according to the stereochemistry of the ring system and to the ester functions attached to it (17,31,121). In CREF N cells, binding of [³H]PDBu shows similar specificity. It is not inhibited by the inactive compounds phorbol or 4-α-phorbol didecanoate, but it is strongly inhibited by TPA, and more weakly by PDBu and mezerein (Table 4) (40). Other laboratories have studied the binding of additional phorbol esters to the phorboid receptor and find a full correlation with biological activity (37,42). There are several tumor promoters and antileukemic compounds derived from various natural sources that do not have the phorbol ring system and yet induce many of the same effects in cell culture as the phorbol ester tumor promoters (26,31,57,122). We have measured the ability of these compounds to inhibit [³H]PDBu binding in CREF N cell monolayers, expressing the results as ID_{50}, that is the dose required to produce a 50% inhibition. The results are shown in Table 4. In addition, we have listed the ED_{50} (50% effective dose) for inhibition of [¹²⁵I]-EGF binding by the same compounds, where these data are available. Some of these data were obtained with different cell types, but they are included for comparison. The indole alkaloid teleocidin B is derived from *Streptomyces* 2A 1563 (123). It is a potent tumor promoter (18) and is strongly inhibitory of [^{125}I]EGF binding in C3H 10T½ cells (57). It also inhibits [^{3}H]PDBu binding quite strongly (57, and Table 4). A structurally similar toxin, lyngbyatoxin A (19), is derived from a blue-green alga (*Lyngbya majuscula* Gomont). Lyngbyatoxin A is also a potent inhibitor of [^{3}H]PDBu binding to its receptor (Table 4). We have also studied some plant diterpenes that have structures similar to those of the phorbol esters and have been reported to have antileukemic activity (124–126). Of these compounds, gnidilatin and gnilatimacrin have been previously reported to stimulate induction of PA (122) and to inhibit binding of [^{125}I]EGF to HeLa cells (26), whereas gnidipalmin was much less active. In the [^{3}H]PDBu-binding assay, gnidilatin and gnilatimacrin were potent inhibitors, whereas gnidipalmin was inactive up to 250 ng/ml. It is striking that compounds having such diverse chemical structures can apparently bind with high affinity to the same receptors. They are all somewhat amphipathic molecules, suggesting that the phorboid receptor may contain both hydrophobic and hydrophilic domains. Among the phorbol compounds the amphipathic feature is also required for maximum activity, since phorbol itself and phorbol-12,13-diacetate compete weakly or not at all for the phorboid receptor, whereas TPA and PDD, which have long-chain fatty esters at C-12, have high affinity for these receptors (37,42). Model-building studies suggest that the region of the phorbol esters containing the C-3 carbonyl residue and the region of the indole alkaloids that also has a carbonyl residue may share somewhat similar conformations, thus explaining their ability to bind to the same receptors (unpublished studies).

3.3. Phorboid Receptors and Cellular Responsiveness to Phorbol Esters

Subclones of Friend erythroleukemia cells that are resistant to the action of the phorbol ester tumor promoters have been isolated (127,128). Among the actions of TPA observed in the sensitive (TS), but not the resistant (TR), clones are inhibition of differentiation, induction of cell adherence to plastic tissue culture dishes, and release of AA and PGs E$_2$ and F$_{2\alpha}$ (25,35,127,128). We studied these cell lines to see whether the defect in the TR cells was in the number or affinity of receptors. As can be seen in Table 5 there was no significant difference between TS 19-10 and TR 19-4 in receptor affinity or number (41). We did observe, however, a difference between the two lines in membrane fluidity, as measured by fluorescence anisotropy of a diphenylhexatriene probe. The probe diphenylhexatriene was less mobile in the membrane of TR cells than in TS cells. We were able to cause an apparent decrease in the membrane fluidity of the TS cells by treating them with cholesterol hemisuccinate (41), since this resulted in an increase in fluo-

Table 5. Fluorescence Anisotropy of Diphenylhexatriene in TR and TS Friend Erythroleukemia Cells (25° C)

Cell Type	Agent	Treatment Time (hours)	$DPH[(r_0/r) - 1]^{-1}$ (mean $\pm$ SE)[a]
TR 19-4	None	0	2.45 $\pm$ 0.04
	DMSO[b]	4	2.12 $\pm$ 0.01
	TPA[c]	4	2.01 $\pm$ 0.03
TR 19-19	None	0	2.15 $\pm$ 0.03
	DMSO	4	2.02 $\pm$ 0.03
	TPA	4	2.06 $\pm$ 0.02
TS 19-6	None	0	1.92 $\pm$ 0.02
	DMSO	4	1.78 $\pm$ 0.07
	TPA	4	1.74 $\pm$ 0.02
TS 19-10	None	0	1.62 $\pm$ 0.02
	DMSO	4	1.42 $\pm$ 0.05
	TPA	4	1.47 $\pm$ 0.03

[a] Cells were loaded with diphenylhexatriene and fluorescence anisotropy estimated as described in reference 41. Data are the mean values $\pm$ SE of duplicate samples.
[b] Exposure to 0.01% dimethylsulfoxide (DMSO) vehicle alone for 4 hours at 37°C.
[c] Exposure to 100 ng/ml of TPA in 0.01% DMSO for 4 hours at 37°C. For additional details see reference 41.

rescence anisotropy of the diphenylhexatriene probe. Treatment with cholesterol hemisuccinate also reduced the adherence of TS cells in response to TPA to the level of that of TR cells. These data support the hypothesis that cellular responses to TPA are intimately involved with, and influenced by, perturbations of the membrane structure. It has also been observed that certain TPA-resistant variants of the HL-60 human promyelocytic leukemia cell line retain receptors for the binding of phorboids, although these variants displayed alterations in down-regulation of the phorboid receptors (43). Taken together these data suggest that phorbol ester resistance may frequently arise as a change in a step in the cellular response to phorbol esters subsequent to phorbol ester binding. Membrane structure appears to be important in one or more of these steps. Thus loss of phorboid receptors is not required for TPA resistance.

3.4. Down-Regulation of the Phorboid Receptor

When CREF N cells are cultured in the continuous presence of PDBu, and [³H]PDBu binding is measured after removal of all bound and free

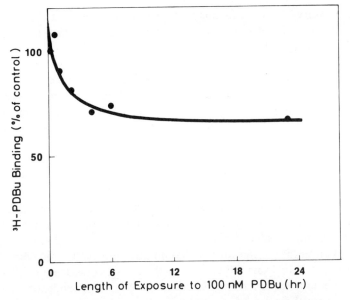

Figure 6. Time course of down-regulation of PDBu receptors. CREF N cells in 5-cm culture dishes were grown in DMEM plus 10% calf serum, plus or minus 100nM PDBu. At the end of the incubation period, cell monolayers were washed with PBS and incubated in fresh assay buffer at 37°C for 30 minutes to allow all bound PDBu to dissociate. The monolayer was washed again in PBS, and fresh assay buffer and [³H]PDBu were added. Specific binding of [³H]PDBu is given as percentage of control binding. The control plates were not pretreated with 100 nM PDBu. From reference 130.

PDBu, a decrease in the binding of [³H]PDBu is observed (Fig. 6). This decrease arises from a decrease in the number of available receptors as determined by Scatchard analysis, and therefore is referred to as *down-regulation*. The 50% effective dose for down-regulation is 8 nM, which is the K_D of the high-affinity binding site in these cells (40). At a concentration of PDBu higher than that at which the high-affinity site is saturated, no further down-regulation of phorboid receptors is seen. The down-regulation reaches only about 50% of the control binding in these cells. It is maximal within 6 hours in the presence of 100 nM PDBu. Down-regulation of phorboid receptors has also been reported in other cell types (43,44). In their susceptibility to down-regulation, the phorboid receptors behave like other known cellular receptors. However, following a 50% down-regulation of the phorboid receptors, CREF N cells, unlike HeLa cells (27), remain sensitive to the inhibition of EGF binding by PDBu (Horowitz and Weinstein, unpublished observations). This suggests that at least 50% of the phorboid receptors in CREF N cells are spare receptors, that is, they are not required for the full biological response to PDBu.

Thus our data show that the phorboid receptors behave in a manner consistent with our knowledge of other cellular receptors: they show high affinity (8–30 nM K_D), the binding constants of various ligands correlate well with relative biological activity, ligand binding is reversible, and partial down-regulation of these receptors occurs in the continued presence of the ligand.

3.5.   Inhibition of PDBu Binding by a Factor from Human Serum

We believe that the phorboid receptors may normally be occupied and used by an endogenous ligand. The search for an endogenous ligand of the phorboid receptor led us to test numerous growth factors and physiological fluids for their ability to inhibit PDBu binding. The results are summarized in Tables 6 and 7. In Table 6 diverse growth factors, corticosteroids, lectins, and other compounds are listed. None of these showed inhibitory activity at the concentrations tested. Epidermal growth factor at a concentration sufficient to saturate its cellular receptors did not inhibit [³H]PDBu binding. Neither did fibroblast growth factor, platelet-derived growth factor, nor concanavalin A, all of which have been reported to act synergistically with TPA (117,118,129, and P. B. Fisher and I. B. Weinstein, unpublished data). Although it has been suggested that vasopressin acts by a common mechanism with the phorbol esters (93,94), neither arginine nor lysine vasopressin competed with [³H]PDBu for binding to the phorboid receptors. Prosta-glandins E, E_2, and $F_{2\alpha}$ have been tested in other laboratories and have been found to have no effect (37,42). The sera and other physiological fluids that we have tested are listed in Table 7. We have found that sera from several species, including human serum, and human amniotic fluid were potent inhibitors of [³H]PDBu binding. Human serum albumin was slightly inhib-itory, but much less so than the corresponding concentration of serum.

We have partially purified, by two chromatographic steps, an inhibitory factor from human serum. It is labile to heating at 70°C for 10 minutes, precipitable by 80% ethanol, anionic at neutral pH, and has a molecular weight of about 60,000 (40). We have characterized its effect on PDBu binding in a variant of CREF cells (CREF A2) that has only a single binding site for [³H]PDBu (Table 3), since this facilitated binding studies. A double-reciprocal plot of PDBu binding in the presence of 0, 13, and 27 μg/ml of the partially purified serum factor is shown in Fig. 7 (130, and Horowitz, Nicolaides, Woodward, and Weinstein, manuscript in preparation). The serum factor reduced the number of available phorboid receptors from

Table 6. Substances That Did Not Inhibit [³H]PDBu Binding to CREF Cells

SUBSTANCES	CONCENTRATION TESTED (μg/ml)
Phorbol	1.0
4-α-phorbol didecanoate	1.0
Epidermal growth factor	0.05
Fibroblast growth factor	0.10
Platelet-derived growth factor	0.10
T-cell growth factor	CM[a]
Arginine vasopressin	0.15
Lysine vasopressin	0.30
Luteinizing hormone releasing hormone	0.50
Thrombin	2.5 (units/ml)
Fetuin	1000
Transcortin	5.0
Human chorionic gonadotropin	100
Thymopoietin	50
Ubiquitin	50
T$_3$	0.33
Ganglioside GM$_1$	0.15
Total brain gangliosides	0.15
Neurotensin	25
Hepatic-proliferation inhibitor[b]	100
Cortisol	5.0
Fluocinolone acetonide	45
Diazepam	30
Cytochalasin B	1.0
Concanavalin A	0.10
Wheat germ agglutinin	0.10
4-α-Methylglucoside	3×10^4

Source: From references 40, 130.

[a] Conditioned medium from normal peripheral blood lymphocytes stimulated with phytohemagglutinin was a gift from Dr. R. Mertelsmann. It was tested at a dilution of 1:4.

[b] Hepatic proliferation inhibitor was derived from rat liver (167).

Table 7. Inhibition of [^{3}H]PDBu Binding by Various Physiological Fluids

Test Substance	Approximate ID$_{50}$[a] (mg/ml)
Calf serum	11
Fetal bovine serum	11
Pooled human serum	4
Pregnant human serum	2
Platelet-depleted human serum	4
Lipoprotein-depleted human serum	4
Rhesus monkey serum	8
Rat serum	1
Human amniotic fluid	2
Rat embryo homogenate	0.3
Rat liver homogenate	1
Human cerebrospinal fluid	—[b]
Rhesus monkey cerebrospinal fluid	—
Pregnant human urine (10X)	—
Human milk	—
Human serum albumin	25

Source: From references 40, 130.
[a] The ID$_{50}$ is defined as the concentration of test substance required to produce 50% inhibition of specific [^{3}H]PDBu binding to rat embryo cells.
[b] Designates no activity detected when tested at a final concentration of 50% physiological fluid in the binding-assay buffer. Cerebrospinal fluid was used as such. Urine was first dialyzed and then concentrated 10-fold by evaporation.

4.6×10^5 to 3.6×10^5 and 2.9×10^5 per cell, respectively, without altering their apparent affinity. This type of behavior is typical of noncompetitive inhibition. In further experiments, the inhibition of PDBu binding by the serum factor was found to be rapid and reversible at 4°C (131). The inhibition reached an equilibrium value rapidly, which makes it unlikely that it acts by enzymatically destroying the PDBu. Nor does the serum factor act by irreversible inactivation of the phorboid receptors, but probably by physically blocking access of PDBu to the receptor.

We were concerned that the serum factor might act by binding or trapping [^{3}H]PDBu, thereby preventing it from binding to the phorboid receptor. However, in a gel-filtration assay, we were unable to detect any binding of

[³H]PDBu by partially purified serum factor. Unfractionated serum did, however, bind [³H]PDBu (Horowitz, Greenebaum, Nicolaides, Woodward, and Weinstein, manuscript in preparation). It appears, therefore, that the serum factor acts by interacting with phorboid receptors or with sites on the membrane that influence the activity of the phorboid receptors.

We have also investigated the influence of the serum factor on certain cellular responses to PDBu. By itself, the serum factor is inactive in stimulating AA or choline release from C3H 10T½ cells (130, and Horowitz, Okin, and Weinstein, unpublished observations), or in inhibiting [¹²⁵I]EGF binding to CREF N cells (130). In all three of these assays, however, whole human serum is quite effective. Since the serum factor blocks PDBu binding, we would expect it to antagonize the cellular effects of TPA such as inhibition of EGF binding. We also studied the effect of purified human serum factor on the inhibition of [¹²⁵I]EGF binding by PDBu. When we studied the

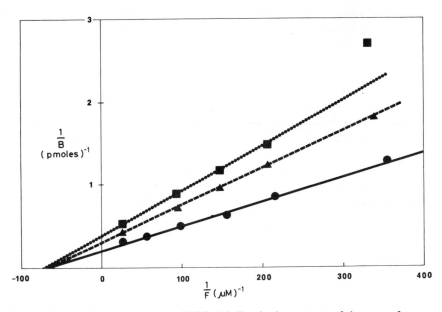

Figure 7. Double-reciprocal plot of PDBu binding in the presence of the serum factors. Binding was determined in the presence of 0 (-●-), 13 (-▲-), and 27 (··■··) μg/ml of serum factor. A tracer amount of 3 nM [³H]PDBu was used. The assay was conducted in assay buffer (2 volumes of DMEM to 1 volume of PBS plus 1 mg of bovine serum albumin per milliliter) as described in Fig. 1 of reference 40 on 5.6 × 10⁶ CREF A2 cells per dish, at 37°C. Nonspecific binding was that observed in the presence of 50μM PDBu, and has been subtracted from all points. From reference 130.

inhibition of EGF binding in the presence or absence of the serum factor, we found that a higher concentration of PDBu was required when the serum factor was present (130). Thus in the absence of serum factor 50% inhibition of EGF binding was obtained with 10 nM PDBu, whereas in the presence of 150 µg/ml serum factor, 50 nM PDBu was required to produce the same inhibition. These results are consistent with what we calculate to be the amount of PDBu receptor binding that occurs in the presence of this concentration of serum factor.

In summary, although we have isolated a substance from human sera that strongly inhibits phorbol ester binding in a noncompetitive manner, the putative endogenous ligand for the phorboid receptor remains elusive. In analogy with the transforming growth factors isolated by Todaro and co-workers (132,133), which bind to EGF receptors, one might speculate that tumor-promoting growth factors may eventually be isolated from transformed cells. At the present time it is not clear whether or not the serum factor we have isolated plays a role in host susceptibility to carcinogenesis. If so, our findings suggest that it may have a protective rather than an enhancing role. On the other hand, very little is known about the normal biological role of the phorboid receptors.

4.   RELEVANCE OF TUMOR PROMOTION TO HUMAN CANCER; PROBABLE ROLE OF HORMONES AND GROWTH FACTORS

What might be the normal function of phorboid receptors and their putative endogenous ligand? We postulate that this effector system could play a role during embryogenesis by enhancing the outgrowth of new stem-cell populations. In the adult this same system might enhance expansion of stem-cell populations during hyperplasia, wound healing, and regeneration. In all of these situations it might be necessary to inhibit, transiently, terminal differentiation so as to expand the proliferative population and then, at a later time, to turn off this effector system to allow terminal differentiation to proceed and thus return to a stable state of tissue renewal. Thus the inhibitory effects on differentiation and the growth stimulation produced by the phorbol esters in experimental systems might occur, under host control, via the phorboid effector system during normal development and physiological states. What could be unusual during two-stage carcinogenesis is that initiating carcinogens might generate aberrant stem cells by producing genomic changes, either through mutation, gene transposition, or modification of the signals that normally control gene expression (for detailed discussion, see 31,95,96,134–136). The subsequent continuous application of a potent exogenous agonist (TPA) would cause excessive stimulation of the phorboid receptor system, thus allowing outgrowth of the abnormal cells. This model has obvious implications in terms of the normal control of proliferation of stem-cell populations and the possible role of endogenous host factors as promoters of the carcinogenic process. If our hypothesis is correct, then it might also be possible to develop analogs of the phorbol esters that could be used as pharmacological agents to stimulate normal tissue repair and to enhance the repletion of tissues with stem cells following trauma, radiation, or drug toxicity.

We have previously reviewed the possible relevance of tumor promotion to human cancers (4) and, in particular, breast cancer (2). Mammary carcinogenesis is a multistep process resulting from a complex interaction between multiple and diverse factors extending over a considerable fraction of the lifespan of the individual. The known risk factors for human breast cancer and some of their implications in terms of etiology have been reviewed in detail by others (137–140). In the discussion that follows we attempt to fit these aspects into a model of tumor initiation and promotion.

Let us first consider the phase of mammary carcinogenesis that might be the equivalent of initiation on mouse skin. It is well known that in humans an early age of menarche and a late age of first pregnancy markedly increase the risk of breast cancer. The protective effect of first pregnancy is greatest when it occurs within the first decade or so after menarche (138,139). There is evidence from studies on survivors of Hiroshima and Nagasaki (141) and from women exposed to extensive radiation for diagnostic reasons (142,143) that women exposed to radiation during adolescence are at a higher risk of breast cancer than those exposed at later periods of life. Yet in the irradiated women, breast cancer did not appear until decades after radiation exposure. Taken together, these findings suggest that in mammary carcinogenesis, the phase of initiation is most likely to occur during the first decade after menarche. This is the time when there is the first extensive outgrowth into the mammary tissue of a ductal network. Perhaps this provides an expanding population of replicating ''stem'' cells that are highly susceptible to initiating carcinogens. We have discussed this theory in more detail elsewhere (2). The protective effect of an early age of first pregnancy might be explained by the fact that it causes stem cells in the previously established ductal network to undergo extensive terminal differentiation into lactating alveolar tissue. This is later followed by involution and degeneration.

According to our model, the phases of tumor promotion and progression occur mainly in adult life and can extend over several decades. We would assume that during these phases, hormonal factors and nutritional and other exogenous factors may exert a promoting role on initiated cells in the mammary gland. Evidence that hormonal factors may act during mid or late adult life to enhance mammary carcinogenesis includes the following: (1)

the decreased risk of breast cancer in women who have had surgical or radiation ablation of ovarian function (138), (2) the increased risk in women who have a late age of menopause (138), and (3) the increased risk in women who receive postmenopausal estrogens for 15 or more years (144).

Since we postulate that hormones may serve as promoters, we must ask to what extent these hormones share the three types of epigenetic effects observed with the phorbol ester tumor promoters: (1) mimicry of transformation, (2) modulation of differentiation, and (3) membrane changes that affect nutrient transport, receptors for growth factors, and cell–cell interactions. With respect to mimicry, it is of interest that like TPA, steroidal hormones are potent modulators of PA in cell culture (145,146), and marked changes in PA accompany mammary-tissue development, both normal and neoplastic (145). Prolactin, steroidal hormones, insulin, and other hormones are potent modulators of mammary-tissue differentiation, growth, and involution (140,145,147). Which of the latter effects prevail depends upon complex interactions. It is also possible that one or more of these hormones induces alterations in the structure and function of cellular membranes analogous to those produced by TPA, and this remains to be examined.

There is evidence that increased body weight and/or a high-fat diet are associated with an increased incidence of breast cancer, endometrial cancer, colon cancer, and certain other cancers. In the case of breast cancer, it has been postulated that this may relate to the conversion of androstenedione to estrone in body fat stores (138–140), or an enhanced secretion of pituitary prolactin (148). The lipid composition and physical properties of cellular membranes are influenced by dietary factors, both in the intact animal and in cell culture (149–151). Essential fatty acids in the growth medium of cells in culture also influence a number of functional properties, particularly those related to the cell surface (for review see 152 and 2). It is possible, therefore, that dietary lipids could directly influence tumor promotion. It would be of interest to see to what extent the lipid composition of cell-culture media might alter growth properties and influence cell transformation induced by chemical carcinogens or viruses. The paradigm of initiation and promotion can also be applied to other human cancers, as has been discussed elsewhere (2,4).

5. CONCLUSIONS

The relationship of the tumor-promoting phorbol esters and related compounds to endogenous growth factors has several facets. In their ability to bind to receptors in animal cells in a specific manner, their pleiotropic effects, including effects on cell proliferation and differentiation, and their synergism with a number of growth factors, the phorbol esters resemble known growth factors. In addition, the phorbol esters affect regulation of heterologous growth-factor receptors. Therefore, it appears that the phorbol esters may exert their effects by usurping the role of an endogenous growth factor. The development of a binding assay for phorbol ester receptors permits one to explore this possibility by looking for an endogenous substance that competes with [³H]PDBu for receptor binding.

The multistage nature of carcinogenesis *in vivo* suggests that tumor promotion may be an important factor in determining cancer incidence. Although tumor promotion may frequently be the result of exposure to specific environmental (exogenous) factors, endogenous factors such as hormones and growth factors, many of which may remain to be discovered, may also have a promoting effect because of their effects on cell proliferation and differentiation. Thus carcinogenesis may reflect a complex interaction between environmental and host factors. An unraveling of these complex interactions could offer more effective measures for cancer prevention.

ACKNOWLEDGMENTS

These studies were supported by DHS, NCI grants CA 26056 and CA 21111, and a research fellowship from the Dupont Company. The authors acknowledge the valuable contributions made to these studies by several colleagues, including Drs. Paul Fisher, Alan Mufson, Lih Syngh Lee, Jeffrey Laskin, Ellen Greenebaum, Kazuo Umezawa, Maria Nicolaides, and Kimball Woodward. Several of the studies on the indole alkaloid tumor promoters described in this paper were done in collaboration with Drs. Takashi Sugimura and Hirota Fujiki. We thank Val Stinson for valuable assistance in preparing this manuscript.

REFERENCES

1. Berenblum, I., in F. F. Becker, Ed., *Cancer*, Plenum, New York, 1975, p. 323.

2. Weinstein, I. B., in C. McGrath, Ed., *Systematics of Mammary Cell Transformation*, Academic Press, New York, pp. 425–450.

3. Slaga, T. J., Sivak, A., and Boutwell, R. K., Eds., *Mechanisms of Tumor Promotion and Cocarcinogenesis*, Raven, New York, 1978, Vol. 2.

4. Greenebaum, E., and Weinstein, I. B., in C. M. Fenoglio and M. Wolff, Eds., *Progress in Surgical Pathology*, Masson, New York, 1981, pp. 27–43.

5. Barrett, J. C., and T'so, P. O. P., *Proc. Natl. Acad. Sci. USA*, **75**, 3761 (1978).

6. Fisher, P. B., Bozzone, J. H., and Weinstein, I. B., *Cell*, **18**, 695 (1979).

7. Fisher, P. B., and Weinstein, I. B., in R. Montesano, H. Bartsch, and L. Tomatis, Eds., *Molecular and Cellular Aspects of Carcinogen Screening Tests*, International Agency for Research on Cancer Scientific Publication No. 27, Lyon, 1980, pp. 113–131.

8. Lasne, C., Gentil, A., and Chouroulinkov, I., *Nature*, **247**, 490 (1974).

9. Mondal, S., Brankow, D. W., and Heidelberger, C., *Cancer Res.*, **36**, 2254 (1976).

10. Mondal, S. and Heidelberger, C., *Nature*, **260**, 710 (1976).

11. Kennedy, A., Mondal, S., Heidelberger, C., and Little, J. B., *Cancer Res.*, **38**, 439 (1978).

12. Fisher, P. B., Weinstein, I. B., Eisenberg, D., and Ginsberg, H. S., *Proc. Natl. Acad. Sci. USA*, **75**, 2311 (1978).

13. Fisher, P. B., Mufson, R. A., Weinstein, I. B., and Little, J. B., *Carcinogenesis*, **2**, 183 (1981).

14. Yamamoto, N., and zurHausen, H., *Nature*, **280**, 244 (1979).

15. Van Duuren, B. L., *Progr. Exp. Tumor Res.*, **11**, 31 (1969).

16. Boutwell, R. K., *CRC Crit. Rev. Toxicol.*, **2**, 419 (1974).

17. Hecker, E., in T. J. Slaga, A. Sivak, and R. K. Boutwell, Eds., *Mechanisms of Tumor Promotion and Cocarcinogenesis*, Raven, New York, 1978, Vol. 2, pp. 11–48.

18. Fujiki, H., Mori, M., Nakayasu, M., Terada, M., Sugimura, T., and Moore, R. E., *Proc. Natl Acad. Sci. USA*, **78**, 3872 (1981).

19. Cardellina, J. H., Marner, F. J., and Moore, R. E., *Science*, **204**, 193 (1979).

20. Sivak, A., and Van Duuren, B. L., *Science*, **157**, 1443 (1967).

21. Mufson, R. A., Okin, E., and Weinstein, I. B., *Carcinogenesis*, **2**, 1095 (1981).

22. Lee, L. S., and Weinstein, I. B., *J. Cell. Physiol.*, **99**, 451 (1979).

23. Lillehaug, J. R., Mondal, S., and Heidelberger, C., *Proc. Am. Assoc. Cancer Res.*, **17**, 194 (1978).

24. Fisher, P. B., Flamm, M., Schachter, D., and Weinstein, I. B., *Biochem. Biophys. Res. Commun.*, **86**, 1063 (1979).

25. Yamasaki, H., Weinstein, I. B., Fibach, E., Rifkind, R. A., and Marks, P. A., *Cancer Res.*, **39**, 1989 (1979).

26. Lee, L. S., and Weinstein, I. B., *Science*, **202**, 313 (1978).

27. Lee, L. S., and Weinstein, I. B., *Carcinogenesis*, **1**, 669 (1980).

28. Nagle, D. S., and Blumberg, P. M., *Cancer Res.*, **40**, 1066 (1980).

29. Mufson, R. A., Kulkarni, P., Eakins, K. E., and Weinstein, I. B., *Cancer Res.*, **39**, 3602 (1979).

30. Zucker, M. B., Troll, W., and Belman, S., *J. Cell Biol.* **60**, 325 (1974).

31. Weinstein, I. B., Wigler, M., and Pietropaolo, C., in H. H. Hiatt, J. D. Watson, and J. A. Winston, Eds., *Origins of Human Cancer*, Cold Spring Harbor Laboratory, Cold Spring Harbor, New York, 1977, pp. 751–772.

32. Gottesman, M. M., and Sobel, M. E., *Cell*, **19**, 449 (1980).

33. Levine, L., and Hassid, A., *Biochem. Biophys. Res. Commun.*, **79**, 477 (1977).

34. Mufson, R. A., DeFeo, D., and Weinstein, I. B., *Mol. Pharmacol.*, **16**, 569 (1979).

35. Yamasaki, H., Mufson, R. A., and Weinstein, I. B., *Biochem. Biophys. Res. Commun.*, **89**, 1018 (1970).

36. Lee, L. S., and Weinstein, I. B., *J. Environ. Pathol. Toxicol.*, **1**, 627 (1978).

37. Driedger, P. E., and Blumberg, P. M., *Proc. Natl. Acad. Sci. USA*, **77**, 561 (1980).

38. Delclos, K. B., Nagle, D. S., and Blumberg, P. M., *Cell*, **19**, 1025 (1980).

39. Dunphy, W. G., Delclos, K. B., and Blumberg, P. M., *Cancer Res.*, **40**, 3635 (1980).

40. Horowitz, A. D., Greenebaum, E., and Weinstein, I. B., *Proc. Natl. Acad. Sci. USA*, **78**, 2315 (1981).

41. Fisher, P. B., Cogan, U., Horowitz, A. D., Schachter, D., and Weinstein, I. B., *Biochem. Biophys. Res. Commun.*, **100**, 370 (1981).

42. Shoyab, M., and Todaro, G., *Nature*, **288**, 451 (1980).

43. Solanki, V., Slaga, T. J., Callahan, M., and Huberman, E., *Proc. Natl. Acad. Sci. USA*, **78**, 1722 (1981).

43a. Solanki, V., and Slaga, T. J., *Proc. Natl. Acad. Sci. USA*, **78**, 2549 (1981).

44. Jaken, S., Tashjian, A. H., and Blumberg, P. M., *Cancer Res.*, **41**, 2175 (1981).

45. Greenebaum, E., Nicolaides, M., Eisinger, M., Vogel, R. H., and Weinstein, I. B. (manuscript in preparation).

46. Hoober, J. K., and Cohen, S., *Biochim. Biophys. Acta*, **138**, 347 (1967).

47. Cohen, S., *Dev. Biol.*, **12**, 394 (1965).

48. Barnes, D., and Colowick, S. P., *J. Cell. Physiol.*, **89**, 633 (1976).

49. Stasny, M., and Cohen, S., *Biochim. Biophys. Acta*, **204**, 578 (1970).

50. Yuspa, S. H., Lichti, U., Ben, T., Patterson, E., Hennings, H., Slaga, T. J., Colburn, N., and Kelsey, W., *Nature*, **262**, 402 (1976).

51. O'Brien, T. G., and Diamond, L., in T. J. Slaga, A. Sivak, and R. K. Boutwell, Eds., *Mechanisms of Tumor Promotion and Cocarcinogenesis*, Raven, New York, 1978, Vol. 2, pp. 273–287.

52. Levine, L., and Hassid, A., *Biochem. Biophys. Res. Commun.*, **76**, 1181 (1977).

53. Lee, L. S., and Weinstein, I. B., *Nature*, **274**, 696 (1978).

54. Nilsen-Hamilton, M., Hamilton, R. T., Allen, W. R., and Massaglia, S. L., *Biochem. Biophys. Res. Commun.*, **101**, 411 (1981).

55. Rose, S. P., Stahn, R., Passovoy, D. S., and Herschman, H., *Experientia*, **32**, 913 (1976).

56. Lee, L. S., and Weinstein, I. B., *Proc. Natl. Acad. Sci. USA*, **76**, 5168 (1979).

57. Umezawa, K., Weinstein, I. B., Horowitz, A., Fujiki, H., Matsushima, T., and Sugimura, T., *Nature*, **290**, 411 (1981).

58. Shoyab, M., DeLarco, J. E., and Todaro, G., *Nature*, **279**, 387 (1979).

59. Brown, K. D., Dicker, P., and Rozengurt, E., *Biochem. Biophys. Res. Commun.*, **86**, 1037 (1979).

60. Ishii, D. N., *Cancer Res.*, **38**, 3886 (1978).

61. Lockyer, J. M., Bowden, G. T., Matrisian, L. M., and Magun, B. E., *Cancer Res.*, **41**, 2308 (1981).

62. Magun, B. E., Matrisian, L. M., and Bowden, G. T., *J. Biol. Chem.*, **255**, 6373 (1980).

63. Murray, A. W., and Fusenig, N. E., *Cancer Lett.*, **7**, 71 (1979).

64. Osborne, R., and Tashjian, A. H., *Endocrinology*, **108**, 1164 (1981).

65. Mufson, R. A., Fisher, P. B., and Weinstein, I. B., *Cancer Res.*, **39**, 3915 (1979).

66. Diamond, L., O'Brien, T. G., and Rovera, G., *Nature*, **269**, 247 (1977).

67. Mufson, R. A., Laskin, J. D., Fisher, P. B., and Weinstein, I. B., *Nature*, **280**, 72 (1979).

68. Barrett, J. C., and Sisskin, E. E., in B. Pullman, P. O. P. T'so, and H. Gelboin, Eds., *Carcinogenesis: Fundamental Mechanisms and Environmental Effects*, D. Reidel, Boston, 1980, pp. 427–439.

69.   Mufson, R. A., Simsiman, R. C., and Boutwell, R. K., *Cancer Res.*, **37**, 665 (1977).

69a. Grimm, W., and Marks, F., *Cancer Res.*, **34**, 3128 (1974).

70.   Garte, S. J., and Belman, S., *Proc. Am. Assoc. Cancer Res.*, **20**, 52 (1979).

71.   Miskin, R., Easton, T. G., Maelicke, A., and Reich, E., *Cell*, **15**, 1287 (1978).

72.   Horowitz, A. D., Greenebaum, E., and Weinstein, I. B., *J. Cell Biol.*, **87**, 174a (1980).

73.   Verma, S. P., Wallach, D. F. H., and Smith, I. C. P., *Biochim. Biophys. Acta*, **345**, 129 (1974).

74.   Mollay, C., Kreil, G., and Berger, H., *Biochim. Biophys. Acta*, **426**, 317 (1976).

75.   Fisher, P. B., Dorsch-Hasler, K., Weinstein, I. B., and Ginsberg, H. S., *Teratogen, Carcinogen, Mutagen*, **1**, 245 (1980).

76.   Umezawa, K., Weinstein, I. B., and Shaw, W. V., *Biochem. Biophys. Res. Commun.*, **94**, 625 (1980).

77.   Chou, S. N., Roblin, R. O., and Black, P. H., *J. Biol. Chem.*, **252**, 6256 (1977).

78.   Shoyab, M., and Todaro, G., *Arch. Biochem. Biophys.*, **206**, 222 (1981).

79.   Kinzel, V., Kreibich, G., Hecker, E., and Suss, R., *Cancer Res.*, **39**, 2743 (1979).

80.   Suss, R., Kreibich, G., and Kinzel, V., *Eur. J. Cancer*, **8**, 299 (1972).

81.   Wertz, P. W., and Mueller, G. C., *Cancer Res.*, **28**, 2900 (1978).

82.   Rohrschneider, L. R., and Boutwell, R. K., *Cancer Res.*, **33**, 1945 (1973).

83.   Rohrschneider, L. R., O'Brien, D. H., and Boutwell, R. K., *Biochim. Biophys. Acta*, **280**, 57 (1972).

84.   Michell, R. H., Jafferji, S. S., and Jones, L. M., in N. G. Bazan, R. R. Brenner, and N. M. Giusto, Eds., *Function and Biosynthesis of Lipids*, Plenum, New York, 1977, pp. 447–464.

85.   Fain, J. W., and Beridge, M. J., *Biochem. J.*, **178**, 45 (1979).

86.   Salmon, D. M., and Honeyman, T. W., *Nature*, **284**, 344 (1980).

87.   Hirata, F., and Axelrod, J., *Science*, **209**, 1082 (1980).

88.   Cassileth, P. A., Suholet, D., and Cooper, R. A., *Blood*, **58**, 237 (1981).

89.   Castagna, M., Rochette-Egly, C., Rosenfeld, C., and Mishal, Z., *FEBS Lett.*, **100**, 62 (1979).

90.   Driedger, P. E., and Blumberg, P. M., *Cancer Res.*, **37**, 3257 (1977).

91.   Moroney, J., Smith, A., Tomel, L. D., and Wenner, C. E., *J. Cell. Physiol.*, **95**, 287 (1978).

92.   Dicker, P., and Rozengurt, E., *Biochem. Biophys. Res. Commun.*, **100**, 433 (1981).

93.   Dicker, P., and Rozengurt, E., *Nature*, **287**, 607 (1980).

94.   Dicker, P., and Rozengurt, E., *J. Supramol. Struct.*, **11**, 79 (1979).

95.   Weinstein, I. B., Lee, L. S., Fisher, P. B., Mufson, R. A., and Yamasaki, H., in P. Emmelot and E. Kriek, Eds., *Environmental Carcinogenesis*, Elsevier, North-Holland, Amsterdam, 1979, pp. 265–285.

96.   Weinstein, I. B., Lee, L. S., Fisher, P. B., Mufson, R. A., and Yamasaki, H., *J. Supramol. Struct.*, **12**, 195 (1979).

97.   Fisher, P. B., Goldstein, N. I., and Weinstein, I. B., *Cancer Res.*, **39**, 3051 (1979).

98.   Fisher, P. B., and Weinstein, I. B., *Cancer Lett.*, **10**, 7 (1980).

99.   Rifkin, D. B., Crowe, R. M., and Pollack, R., *Cell*, **18**, 361 (1979).

100. Murray, A. W., and Fitzgerald, D. J., *Biochem. Biophys. Res. Commun.*, **91**, 395 (1979).

101. Yotti, L. P., Chang, C. C., and Trosko, J. E., *Science*, **206**, 1089 (1979).

102. Kennedy, A. R., Murphy, G., and Little, J. B., *Cancer Res.*, **40**, 1915 (1980).

103. Colburn, N. H., Former, B. F., Nelson, K. A., and Yuspa, S. H., *Nature*, **281**, 589 (1979).

104. Laskin, J. D., Pietropaolo, C., and Erikson, R. L., *Proc. Am. Assoc. Cancer Res.*, **21**, 116 (1980).

105. Goldberg, A. R., Delclos, K. B., and Blumberg, P. M., *Science*, **208**, 191 (1980).

106. Tyson, C. A., Zande, H. V., and Green, D. E., *J. Biol. Chem.*, **251**, 1326 (1976).

107. Putney, J. W., Weiss, S. J., VandeWalle, C. M., and Haddas, R. A., *Nature*, **284**, 345 (1980).

108. Fisher, P. B., and Weinstein, I. B., *Carcinogenesis*, **2**, 89 (1981).

109. Boynton, A. L., and Whitfield, J. F., *Cancer Res.*, **40**, 4541 (1980).

110. Boynton, A. L., Whitfield, J. F., and Trembley, R. J., *J. Cell. Physiol.*, **87**, 25 (1975).

111. Lechner, J. F., and Kaighn, M. E., *Exp. Cell Res.*, **123**, 432 (1979).

112. McKeehan, W. L., and McKeehan, K. A., *Exp. Cell Res.*, **123**, 397 (1979).

113. Fisher, P. B., Dorsch-Hasler, K., Weinstein, I. B., and Ginsberg, H. S., *Nature*, **281**, 591 (1979).

114. Yuspa, S. H., Lichti, U., Hennings, H., Ben, T., Patterson, E., and Slaga, T. J., in T. J. Slaga, A. Sivak, and R. K. Boutwell, Eds., *Mechanisms of Tumor Promotion and Cocarcinogenesis*, Raven, New York, 1978, pp. 245–256.

115. Sivak, A., *J. Cell. Physiol.*, **80**, 167, (1972).

116. Boynton, A. L., Whitfield, J. E., and Isaacs, R. J., *J. Cell. Physiol.*, **87**, 25 (1976).

117. Frantz, C. N., Stiles, C. D., and Scher, C. D., *J. Cell. Physiol.*, **100**, 413 (1979).

118. Dicker, P., and Rozengurt, E., *Nature*, **276**, 723 (1978).

119. Rozengurt, E., Legg, A., and Pettican, P., *Proc. Natl. Acad. Sci. USA*, **76**, 1284 (1979).

120. Nagle, D. S., Jaken, S., Castagna, M., and Blumberg, P. M., *Cancer Res.*, **41**, 89 (1981).

121. Yamasaki, H., Weinstein, I. B., and VanDuuren, B. L., *Carcinogenesis*, **2**, 537 (1981).

122. Wigler, M., Defeo, D., and Weinstein, I. B., *Cancer Res.*, **38**, 1434 (1978).

123. Fujiki, H., Mori, M., Nakayasu, M., Terada, M., and Sugimura, T., *Biochem. Biophys. Res. Commun.*, **90**, 976 (1979).

124. Kupchan, S. M., and Baxter, R. L., *Science*, **187**, 652 (1975).

125. Kupchan, S. M., Shizure, Y., Summer, W. C., Jr., Haynes, H. R., Leighton, A. P., and Sickles, B. R., *J. Org. Chem.*, **41**, 3850 (1976).

126. Kupchan, S. M., Uchidi, I., Branfman, A. R., Daily, R. G., and Fei, B. Y., *Science*, **191**, 571 (1976).

127. Yamasaki, H., Fibach, E., Weinstein, I. B., Nudel, U., Rifkind, R. A., and Marks, P. A., in Y. Ikawa and T. O. Kada, Eds., *Oncogenic Viruses and Host Cell Genes*, Academic, New York, 1979, p. 365.

128. Fibach, E., Yamasaki, H., Weinstein, I. B., Marks, P. A., and Rifkind, R. A., *Cancer Res.*, **38**, 3685 (1978).

129. Mastro, A. M., and Mueller, G. C., *Exp. Cell Res.*, **88**, 40 (1974).

130. Horowitz, A. D., and Weinstein, I. B., in T. J. Powles, R. Bockman, K. Hann, and

P. Ramwell, *Proceedings of the International Conference on Prostaglandins and Cancer*, Alan R. Liss, New York, 1982 (in press).

131. Horowitz, A. D., Greenebaum, E., and Weinstein, I. B., *72nd Annual Meeting of the American Association of Cancer Research*, Abstract, 1981, p. 136.

132. DeLarco, J. E., and Todaro, G. J., *J. Cell. Physiol.*, **102**, 267 (1980).

133. Roberts, A. B., Lamb, L. C., Newton, D. L., Sporn, M. B., DeLarco, J. E., and Todaro, G. J., *Proc. Natl. Acad. Sci. USA*, **77**, 3494 (1980).

134. Weinstein, I. B., Horowitz, A. D., Mufson, R. A., Fisher, P. B., Ivanovic, V., Laskin, J., and Greenebaum, E., in H. Gelboin and P. O. P. T'so, Eds., *Polycyclic Hydrocarbons and Cancer*, Academic, New York, 1981, Vol. 3., pp. 293–315.

135. Weinstein, I. B., Mufson, R. A., Lee, L. S., Fisher, P. B., Laskin, J., Horowitz, A., and Ivanovic, V., in B. Pullman, P. O. P. T'so, and H. Gelboin, Eds., *Carcinogenesis: Fundamental Mechanisms and Environmental Effects*, Reidel, Amsterdam, 1980, pp. 543–563.

136. Weinstein, I. B., Yamasaki, H., Wigler, M., Lee, L. S., Fisher, P. B., Jeffrey, A., and Grunberger, D., in A. C. Griffin and C. R. Shaw, Eds., *Carcinogens: Identification and Mechanisms of Action*, Raven, New York, 1979, pp. 399–418.

137. Lippman, M. E., Ed., John E. Fogorty Int'l. Center Conf. on Hormones and Cancer, *Cancer Res.* **38** (part 2), 3982 (1978).

138. MacMahon, B., Cole, P., and Brown, J., *J. Natl. Cancer Inst.*, **50**, 21 (1973).

139. MacMahon, B., *Nutr. Cancer*, **1**, 38 (1979).

140. Sherman, B. M., and Korenman, S. G., *Cancer*, **33**, 1306 (1974).

141. Wanebo, C. K., Johnson, K. G., and Sato, K., *N. Engl. J. Med.*, **279**, 667 (1968).

142. Mackenzie, I., *Br. J. Cancer*, **19**, 1 (1965).

143. Myrden, J. A., and Hiltz, J. E., *Can. Med. Assoc. J.*, **100**, 1032 (1969).

144. Hoover, R., Gray, L. A., Cole, P., and MacMahon, B., *N. Engl. J. Med.*, **295**, 401 (1976).

145. Ossowski, L., Biegel, D., and Reich, E., *Cell*, **16**, 929 (1979).

146. Wigler, M., Ford, J. P., and Weinstein, I. B., in E. Reich, D. B. Rifkin, and E. Shaw, Eds., *Proteases and Biological Controls*, Cold Spring Harbor Laboratory, Cold Spring Harbor, New York, 1975, pp. 849–856.

147. Topper, Y. J., Oka, T., Vonderhaar, B. K., in J. G. Hardman, and B. W. O'Malley, Eds., *Methods in Enzymology*, Academic, New York, Vol. 39, 1975, pp. 443–454.

148. Chan, P., Head, J. F., Cohen, L. A., and Wynder, E. L., *J. Natl. Cancer Inst.*, **59**, 1279 (1977).

149. Burns, C. P., Luttenegger, D. G., Dudley, D. T., Buettner, G. R., and Spector, A. A., *Clin. Res.*, **27**, 289A (1979).

150. Hill, D. J., and Borysenko, J. Z., *J. Cell Biol.*, **83**, 218 (1979).

151. Schaeffer, B. E., and Curtiss, A. S. G., *J. Cell Science*, **26**, 47 (1977).

152. Kidwell, W. P., Manaco, M. E., Wicha, M. S., and Smith, G. S., *Cancer Res.*, **38**, 4091 (1978).

153. Lowe, M. E., Pacifici, M., and Holtzer, H., *Cancer Res.*, **38**, 2350 (1978).

154. Castagna, M., Rochette-Egly, C., and Rosenfeld, C., *Cancer Lett.*, **6**, 227 (1979).

155. Haigler, H., McKanna, J. A., and Cohen, S., *J. Cell Biol.*, **83**, 82 (1979).

156. Weinstein, I. B., Wigler, M., Fisher, P., Sisskin, E., and Pietropaolo, C., In T. J.

Slaga, A. Sivak, and R. K. Boutwell, Eds., *Mechanisms of Tumor Promotion and Cocarcinogenesis*, Raven, New York, 1978, Vol. 2, pp. 313–333.

157. Blumberg, P. M., Driedger, P. E., and Rossow, P. W., *Nature*, **264**, 446 (1976).

158. Wigler, M., and Weinstein, I. B., *Nature*, **259**, 232 (1976).

159. Goldfarb, R. H., and Quigley, J. P., *Cancer Res.*, **38**, 4601 (1978).

160. Loskutoff, D. J., and Edgington, T. S., *Proc. Natl. Acad. Sci. USA*, **74**, 3093 (1977).

161. Vassalli, J. D., Hamilton, J., and Reich, E., *Cell*, **8**, 271 (1977).

162. Weinstein, I. B., Yamaguchi, N., Gebert, R., and Kaighn, M. E., *In Vitro*, **11**, 130 (1975).

163. Schubert, D., Heinemann, S., Carlisle, W., Tarikas, H., Kimes, B., Patrick, T., Steinbach, J. H., Culpano, W., and Brandt, B. L., *Nature*, **249**, 224 (1974).

164. Stallcup, W. B., *Cell. Neurobiol.*, p. 165 (1977).

165. Stallcup, W. B., and Cohn, M., *Exp. Cell Res.*, **98**, 285 (1978).

166. Giotta, G. J., Heitzmann, H., and Cohn, M., *Brain Res.*, **202**, 445 (1980).

167. McMahon, T. B., and Iype, P. T., *Cancer Res.*, **40**, 1249 (1980).

7

SARCOMA GROWTH FACTOR AND THE TRANSFORMING GROWTH FACTORS

Joseph E. DeLarco

CONTENTS

Abbreviations

EGF	Epidermal growth factor
AIG	Anchorage-independent growth
RSV	Rous sarcoma virus

OSF   Overgrowth-stimulating factor

RCM   Rous conditioned medium

BHK   Baby hamster kidney

TF   Transforming factor

MoSV   Moloney murine sarcoma virus

SGF   Sarcoma growth factor

KiMSV   Kirsten murine sarcoma virus

NRK   Normal rat kidney

KNRK   NRK cells transformed by wild type Kirsten murine sarcoma virus

TGF   Transforming growth factor

HPLC   High-performance liquid chromatography

SDS   Sodium dodecyl sulfate

FGF   Fibroblast growth factor

MSA   Multiplication-stimulating activity

1. INTRODUCTION

Under normal conditions, the final density of untransformed cells in tissue culture is dependent upon the concentration of growth factors that are either supplied in the serum supplement or added to the medium as partially or totally purified components. Quiescent cells can often be stimulated to undergo mitosis by adding either fresh serum or purified growth factor to the existing medium. Transformed cells tend to grow to a much higher density than their untransformed counterparts. Quite often this leads to overgrowing and the formation of multiple cell layers. The cells may lose their aligned pattern and begin to crisscross over one another in what appears to be total disorganization. The transformed cells usually have a much lower serum requirement than their untransformed controls. One of the more stringent criteria of transformation is anchorage-independent growth (AIG) as seen by either growth in a semisolid medium, such as soft agar, or growth in suspension.

There are several possible models that could help explain the altered growth behavior displayed by transformed cells. It is possible that transformed cells no longer require growth factors, and their physiology is such that they continue to divide until either their nutrients are depleted or their metabolic by-products reach a toxic level. If this were the case these cells would only need the serum for the trace elements and nutrients not supplied in the medium. Another possibility is that transformed cells are much more sensitive to growth factors; that is, they have a much lower requirement and yield a much greater response per unit of growth factor. Cells with lower serum requirements grow to higher densities before they deplete the serum growth factors and may actually deplete their nutrients (i.e., essential amino acids, energy sources, trace elements, etc.) before the growth factors in their media are depleted. A third possibility is that the transformed cells produce and release their own growth factors. If these cells are responsive to the growth factors they produce and release, they are potentially independent of an external source of growth factors and could be grown in serum-free medium as long as their essential nutrients are supplied by this medium.

It is the last model that is examined briefly in this chapter: the production by transformed cells of peptide factors that can stimulate untransformed indicator cells to grow to a higher density and possibly cause them to display a transformed phenotype. The morphological effects caused by these factors, unlike those displayed by genetically transformed cells, are transient and depend on the continued presence of the factors. If the treated cells are subcultured in the absence of these factors, they regain their untransformed morphology with respect to both saturation density and AIG.

2. ORIGINAL OBSERVATIONS

In 1970 Rubin (1) observed that most of the cells in a culture that was infected with Rous sarcoma virus (RSV) acted as if transformed by day 4 or 5 after the initial infection, even though only a small percentage of the cells in the culture were genetically transformed by the RSV. This suggested to him that the RSV-transformed cells were releasing a factor that stimulated the continued overgrowth of the crowded cells, those not transformed by the RSV as well as the transformants. He assayed the media for the overgrowth-stimulating factor (OSF) by measuring the overgrowth in secondary cultures of chick fibroblasts that had been treated with dialyzed Rous conditioned media (RCM). The incorporation of [^{3}H]thymidine into cells that had been overlayed with agar was used to quantitate the activity present. The rate of incorporation was three to six times higher in cultures treated with RCM than in the controls. Confluent cultures doubled their cell numbers by 65 hours in the treated cultures while the control cultures remained constant. These treated cells began to round up and lose their swirled fibroblastic pattern, and began to form multiple layers. This was not an irreversible change in the growth pattern of these cells. Unlike the cells that had been genetically transformed by the RSV, the cells treated with RCM regained their normal morphology and intercellular arrangement by

100 hours after overlay. The compound responsible for the OSF activity was nondialyzable and heat labile. It or a similar activity could be found in the cytosol of normal chick embryo cells disrupted by sonication (2). The intracellular activity increased threefold to fourfold by 3 days after infection. The factor or factors had little or no effect on the rate of growth of sparse, rapidly growing cultures.

In 1973 Burk showed (3,4) that a baby hamster kidney line (BHK 21/13) transformed by SV-40 (SV-28) produced and released an activity (migration factor) into its medium that differed chromatographically from the serum migration factor that had been described by Lipton et al. (5). This factor stimulated tissue-culture cells to migrate into a wound in a monolayer. High doses produced a uniform stimulation of the treated monolayers to undergo cell division; at limiting concentrations, however, only the cells on the edge of the wound were stimulated to go through mitosis. Burk (6,7) and co-workers later separated this activity into two distinct components using isoelectric focusing. These activities, A and B, acted additively in the stimulation of migration. Both were able to stimulate cells to grow beyond their normal density when added in the presence of 10% calf serum. Both A and B were released by the SV-28, whereas the untransformed parental line BHK 21/13 produced only B. The activity in peak A was able to stimulate cell migration, cell growth, and a morphological effect in tissue-culture monolayers. The activity in peak B was able to stimulate both migration and cell division, but did not accentuate the morphological effects seen with A. A possible interpretation of these results is that prior to viral transformation, the BHK 21/13 line produces a nontransforming growth factor that is capable of stimulating cell division and migration. After SV-40 transformation, these cells produce an additional factor that can stimulate migration and mitosis and produce a morphological change in treated monolayers. This factor, A, can act either alone or together with B to produce the transformed phenotype.

Kaplan et al. (8) very recently have reported the ability of conditioned media from SV-40-transformed rat embryo fibroblasts to stimulate AIG. They found that concentrates of conditioned media stimulated rat cell lines to form colonies in soft agar. Secondary cultures of rat embryo fibroblasts did not, however, respond to the conditioned media while in soft agar. These authors referred to the activity present in the conditioned media as transforming factor (TF). Without characterization of their TF it would be difficult to conclude that the activity these authors describe is the equivalent of Burk's A. It does, however, appear to be a possibility, since both are derived from SV-40-transformed cells and both are able to stimulate the indicator cells to display a transformed morphology.

In 1978 DeLarco and Todaro (9) reported on a murine line transformed by Moloney murine sarcoma virus (MoSV) that produced, and released into serum-free media, a series of growth-stimulating activities. The untransformed controls did not release measurable quantities of these growth activities. From the data on gel-permeation chromatography (BioGel P-60) of MoSV-conditioned media concentrates, there appeared to be several distinct peaks of activity, indicating different apparent molecular weights. These activities were able to stimulate mitogenesis in untransformed indicator cells using either serum-depleted cultures (0.1% serum) or density-inhibited cultures in media containing 10% serum. Also these activities had the ability to stimulate phenotypic changes in the morphology of indicator cells. In the presence of these factors, the cells exhibited the morphology of MoSV-transformed cells. In the presence of 10% serum and 10 μg of crude activity per milliliter, these cells grew to a density that was four times greater than that of controls. The cells crisscrossed over one another and formed multiple layers. The same activity also was able to stimulate AIG in the untransformed indicator cells. In a highly passaged culture of indicator cells, the response to these factors was heterogeneous and dose dependent; some cells gave a good response at low concentrations, while others required higher doses to give a good AIG response. If a cell gave a large AIG response at low concentrations of growth factor and was picked from the soft agar, the progeny from this clone gave a uniformly good response for the next several passages. As with the activity described by Rubin, the effects of these factors were reversible or phenotypic rather than genetic. Once the factor was removed from the growth media, the "transformed" indicator cells reverted to the untransformed phenotype.

3. SARCOMA GROWTH FACTOR AND THE EGF RECEPTOR

Previous studies (10,11) had shown that MoSV-transformed cells either lacked or had a greatly decreased number of available epidermal growth factor (EGF) receptors, whereas most untransformed lines, as well as the DNA-tumor-virus-transformed and most chemically transformed lines, retained a full complement of EGF receptors (10). Epidermal growth factor is a potent peptide mitogen acting through plasma-membrane receptors (12,13) (see Chapter 5). It is a heat-stable peptide with a molecular weight of approximately 6000, and its activity is sensitive to disulfide-reducing agents. To determine if the activities released by this MoSV-transformed line were either EGF or EGF-related factors, fractions from the sizing column were tested for their ability to compete in a radioimmune assay and a radioreceptor assay for EGF. There was no detectable competing activity in the radioimmune assay. There were, however, several peaks of activity that competed in the EGF-radioreceptor assay, and these competing activities coeluted with the mitogenic and AIG-stimulating activities. These factors, like EGF, were shown to be heat-stable peptides that were sensitive to disulfide-reducing agents.

The initial results, then, showed that there were several peaks of activity released by the MoSV-transformed cells that appeared to be EGF-like. These materials competed with radiolabeled EGF in a radioreceptor assay and were potent mitogens. One of these peaks of activity, the peak that eluted with an apparent molecular weight of approximately 10,000 (9), was chosen for further studies since it gave the greatest AIG response. The activity in this peak was named sarcoma growth factor (SGF), since it was derived from a sarcoma virus-transformed cell. A more appropriate name, however, would have been sarcoma-derived growth factor, since it was derived from a sarcoma virus-transformed line, and its mitogenic or growth factor activity was not restricted to sarcoma cells, as its name might imply, but was exerted on most cells tested.

A cell line instrumental in the further studies was an epidermoid carcinoma line (A-431) with an unusually large number of EGF receptors (14,15). This cell line had approximately 2×10^6 EGF receptors per cell. The cells retained the ability to bind EGF even after being permanently attached to tissue-culture dishes with a 5% formaldehyde solution. These fixed cells were used as an affinity matrix to purify molecules that bind to the EGF receptor from a complex radiolabeled peptide mixture (14). The EGF or EGF-like material in a grossly impure preparation was bound to the EGF receptors on the fixed cells, the unbound material removed, the monolayers washed with a neutral salts solution to remove the remaining unbound material, and the bound peptides eluted from the EGF receptors by washing the fixed cells in dilute acetic acid. This process could be repeated using the same matrix and the preparation selectively enriched for radiolabeled peptides that were EGF-like. The specific binding rose from 0.12% of the input for the uncycled radiolabeled peptide pool to 24% of the input for twice-cycled material. Unlabeled EGF was able to block this specific binding. The uncycled radiolabeled peptide pool did not have a discrete isoelectric point. The major portion of the radiolabeled material had an acidic pI; the twice-cycled material had a sharp, discrete pI of 6.8. Radiolabeled, cycled EGF had a pI of 4.4. When recycled, labeled material was analyzed by isoelectric focusing in the presence of the crude, unlabeled material, most of the biological activity also focused at a pI of 6.8. The fixed A-431 cells were also very efficient at adsorbing out and releasing the biological activity in a crude BioGel P-60 pool. These results are consistent with a model in which SGF binds to, and is eluted from, the EGF receptor.

An EGF-receptorless line isolated from a highly passaged culture of a murine 3T3 line (16) was used to determine if the EGF receptor is necessary for the phenotypic transformation brought about by this factor. The SGF pool from the BioGel P-60 was tested for both morphological and mitogenic effects. The parental line (3T3/8) formed large agar colonies after treatment with SGF, whereas the EGF-receptorless clone (NR 6/6) remained as single cells in the presence of SGF. The results on mitogenesis are seen in Table 1. The 3T3/8 parent line responded well in terms of [³H]thymidine incorporation to all growth factors tested, whereas the NR 6/6 responded to all growth factors except EGF and SGF. These results are consistent with the model in which SGF works through, and requires, the EGF receptor to bring about its effects. Also consistent with this model are the observations of Carpenter (personal communication) that antibody to the EGF receptor can block the mitogenic effect of SGF as well as EGF.

Ozanne et al. (17) found that rat cells transformed by Kirsten murine sarcoma virus (KiMSV) released a factor(s) into their serum-free media that had an activity similar to that released by the MoSV-transformed murine cells. All the KiSV transformants released the TF, whereas untransformed cells and revertants failed to release appreciable quantities of TF. This activity was partially purified from the conditioned media by dialysis and DEAE-cellulose chromatography. Under their conditions of chromatography most of the proteins bound to the column, whereas the TF activity either passed directly through the column unbound or was eluted during the first

Table 1. Effect of Various Growth Factors on the Induction of DNA Synthesis in Resting Murine 3T3 Cells and an EGF-Receptorless Clone

	[³H]Thymidine Incorporation (cpm × 10⁻³)	
ADDITIONS	3T3/8 (EGF-R⁺)	NR 6/6 (EGF-R⁻)
None	2.4	2.8
EGF (10 ng/ml)	33.5	3.1
SGF (1 μg/ml)	63.7	2.9
Calf serum (600 μg/ml)	55.3	63.7
FGF (10 ng/ml)	31.5	47.3
MSA (10 ng/ml)	18.2	14.3

wash step. This procedure yielded about a sixfold purification of the activity. The TF was shown to be a heat- and acid-stable peptide or protein that was sensitive to reducing agents. It could compete with EGF for plasma-membrane receptors and caused a transient phenotypic transformation. The TF caused a marked change in the morphology of cells in monolayers as well as the stimulation of large colony formation in an AIG assay using soft agar as the semisolid media. These alterations were not genetic, and the cells regained their untransformed phenotype shortly after treatment with TF was discontinued.

To determine if either RNA and/or protein synthesis was required for this effect, indicator cells were treated with either actinomycin D (to block RNA synthesis) or cycloheximide (to block protein synthesis) prior to or at the time TF was added. Both drugs blocked TF-mediated morphological transformation. These results indicated that both new RNA and protein synthesis were necessary before the TF-induced "transformation" could be seen. Actinomycin D blocked the morphological effects only if added shortly after the addition of TF. If it was added more than 4 hours after the initiation of TF treatment, it failed either to block or to reverse the morphological changes. Protein synthesis inhibitors, in contrast, blocked or reversed the "transformation" of the TF-treated cells at any time.

Transforming factor induced the dissociation of actin fibers in treated cells. Within 3 hours there was a marked dissociation of actin cables, and this effect was nearly complete by 12 hours. The dissociation of the actin fibers required both RNA synthesis and protein synthesis. This dissociation, similar to the morphological effects, was rapidly reversed by cycloheximide, but not by actinomycin D.

It is well known that virally transformed cells transport glucose and glucose derivatives at a much higher rate than their nontransformed indicator cells. Ozanne et al. (17) found that TF activity caused a marked increase in this transport system as measured by the uptake of 2-deoxy-D-glucose in treated cells. The treated cells accumulated 2-deoxy-D-glucose at nearly five times the rate of the untreated cells. The rate of transport in the treated cells approximated that seen in their sarcoma-virus-transformed counterpart.

4.   ORIGIN OF THE SARCOMA GROWTH FACTOR GENE

The release of these growth factors by virally transformed cells raises a fundamental question. Are these factors direct products of the viral genome, or are they host-cell gene products whose expression is either controlled by a viral gene or a viral gene product? If the growth factors that are able to confer the transformed phenotype on untransformed cells are viral gene products, one might expect them to be temperature sensitive when obtained from cells that are transformed by a sarcoma virus that is temperature sensitive with respect to transformation. If they are products of the host cell, they would be no more temperature sensitive than the growth factors isolated from cells transformed by the wild-type virus. The regulation of their expression would, however, be temperature dependent, and at the nonpermissive temperature, the ts-sarcoma gene product would be inactivated and therefore unable to stimulate the host's expression of these growth factors.

To answer this question, investigators used cells that had been transformed by sarcoma viruses that are temperature sensitive with respect to transformation. At the nonpermissive temperature the transformed cells reverted to the untransformed morphology; they no longer displayed AIG nor did they produce the "transforming" growth factors (17–19), and their number of available EGF receptors increased toward the number present on the untransformed parent (18,19). Growth factors released from normal rat kidney (NRK) cells transformed by either a wild-type KiMSV (KNRK) or a KiMSV variant that is temperature sensitive with respect to transformation (ts-371) (20) were obtained from serum-free conditioned media collected at the permissive temperature (32°C). These factors were partially purified using gel-permeation chromatography (19). The main SGF-like peaks from both transformed clones eluted with an apparent molecular weight of approximately 8500 and contained the AIG-stimulating activity and the EGF-radio-receptor-competing activity, as well as the mitogenic activity, measured by the stimulation of [³H]thymidine incorporation into serum-depleted NRK cells.

To determine if the major SGF-like activity released by ts-371 is itself temperature sensitive and therefore potentially responsible for the ts properties of this transformant, the pooled activity from the BioGel P-60 column was heated and the biological activities tested. These results were compared with the equivalent pool of activity released by the KNRK cells. The results from this experiment are seen in Table 2. When the ts-371 heated and unheated samples are compared for their ability to stimulate thymidine incorporation, it appears there were no significant differences at either dilution. The soft-agar-growth-stimulating activity was also insensitive to this heat-treatment step. The results from the heat treatment of an equivalent pool from KNRK cells were quite similar. Since the SGF-like factor released by the ts-371 cells was as heat stable, under the assay conditions, as the SGF-like factor released by cells transformed by the wild-type sarcoma virus, it appears that these growth factors are not direct products of the sarcoma viral gene, but rather products of host genes that are normally suppressed.

5. EGF-DEPENDENT TRANSFORMING GROWTH FACTORS

Roberts and co-workers have published a series of papers on the characterization of transforming growth factors (TFGs) obtained by extracting

Table 2. Effects of Heating on the Biological Activity of Growth Factors Released by Cells Transformed by Either KiMSV or ts-371

Source of Growth Factor	Dilution	Stimulation of [³H]Thymidine Incorporation (cpm above control)	Dilution	Percentage of NRK Cells That Formed Soft-Agar Colonies[a]
ts-371	1:4	30,651	1:1	75
	1:16	4,758	1:4	62
ts-371 heated[b]	1:4	28,588	1:1	76
	1:16	6,119	1:4	61
KNRK	1:3	125,721	1:3	70
	1:15	28,892	1:15	52
			1:75	4
KNRK heated[b]	1:3	129,766	1:3	66
	1:15	26,552	1:15	40
			1:75	8

[a] Colonies were scored 10 days after seeding. Those colonies larger than approximately 20 cells were scored as positive.
[b] Heat treatment was carried out for 120 minutes in a water bath maintained at 65°C. The samples were adjusted to pH 7.0 before heating.

either MoSV-transformed cells or tumors produced by these cells (21–23). The cells, the same as those used to produce SGF, or tumors derived from these cells, were extracted using a cold-ethanol–HCl procedure that is a modification of one used to extract insulin from the pancreas (24). The ethanol-HCl-soluble activities obtained using this procedure were shown to reside in heat-stable, disulfide-containing peptides. The authors showed that the specific activity of the peptides obtained from the MoSV-transformed cells was 10-fold higher than that obtained by extracting a chemically induced tracheal carcinoma line. The ethanol-HCl extract was passed over a BioGel P-60 column that had been equilibrated in, and eluted with, 1 M acetic acid. The activities eluted as peptides with apparent approximate molecular weights of 7000 and 10,000. There was a broad peak of EGF-competing activity as measured in a radioreceptor assay. Coeluting with these activities were factors that were able to confer the transformed phenotype on untransformed indicator cells as measured by AIG in soft agar.

After further purification of these materials it was found that there were two distinct classes of activities that were referred to as TGFs. The first class was similar to the SGFs already described (9); the factors competed with EGF for the membrane receptors and stimulated AIG in the absence of additional growth factors. A second class of TGFs was described that when further purified did not compete with radiolabeled EGF in a radioreceptor assay and was not able to stimulate AIG. In the presence of EGF, however, these second kinds of TGFs were potent stimulators of AIG and were referred to as EGF-dependent TGFs. If the AIG assays were performed in the absence of EGF, the SGF-like growth factor present in the cell extract accounted for greater than 90% of the activity; if these assays were performed in the presence of 2 ng of EGF per milliliter, then the EGF-dependent TGF accounted for approximately 90% of the total colony-forming units. Epidermal growth factor had no apparent effect on the dose response of the SGF-like TGF in an AIG assay, whereas it increased the response of the indicator cells to the EGF-potentiated class of TGF by between 100-fold and 800-fold, as measured by colony formation. Epidermal growth factor or the EGF-like peptides were the only growth factors tested that were able to potentiate the TGF properties of this class of TGFs. The factors tested without effect were platelet-derived growth factor, nerve growth factor, insulin, and the insulin-like growth factors.

Similar EGF-dependent TGFs can be extracted from untransformed cells, as well as from normal tissues from adult mice, using the ethanol-HCl extraction procedure (22). The tissues examined and found to contain these TGFs were submaxillary gland, kidney, liver, muscle, heart, and brain.

When extracts of tissues containing high levels of endogenous EGF, such as kidney and submaxillary glands, were assayed for AIG-stimulatory activity, their EGF-dependent TGFs were fully potentiated and therefore had higher apparent specific activities than the extracts from tissues with low levels of EGF such as liver, muscle, brain, and heart. In the presence of optimal concentrations of EGF, the specific activity of the ethanol-HCl extracts of these tissues were all similar to one another, as well as to that of the extract from MoSV-transformed cells.

This EGF-dependent TGF was further purified to apparent homogeneity by the same group using BioGel P-60 chromatography and reverse-phase high-performance liquid chromatography (HPLC) (25). By extracting 1.5 kg of MoSV-transformed 3T3 cells using the ethanol-HCl procedure, the authors obtained 580 μg of purified EGF-dependent TGF. The purified peptide had an apparent molecular weight of approximately 13,000 as determined by sodium dodecyl sulfate (SDS) polyacrylamide gel electrophoresis. In the presence of optimal concentrations of EGF (2 ng/ml) this peptide stimulated AIG at concentrations in the nanogram range (10 ng/ml gave a response that was approximately ⅓ of the maximal response).

The two main activities extracted from these cells were compared with EGF by HPLC. The SGF-like activity eluted earlier than the EGF marker, whereas the EGF-dependent TGF eluted noticeably after EGF from a C_{18} column developed with an acetonitrile gradient. The EGF-dependent TGF was further purified on a second HPLC column, a cyano column developed with an n-propanol gradient. The activity was preferentially retained on this column and did not elute until 48% n-propanol was reached.

This family of apparently ubiquitous peptides, the EGF-dependent TGFs, can indeed be called biological-response modifiers. Their mode of action is not yet fully understood. The intriguing interaction between EGF and this family of peptides cannot help but raise many fundamental questions about their mode of action and their physiological role in the control of cell function or proliferation. Do these EGF-dependent TGF peptides possess intrinsic mitogenic activity or are they totally dependent upon EGF for their action? Do they have their own membrane receptors or do they have to interact first with EGF before they can interact with the cell? Which cellular component gives rise to these factors and would they be released using a neutral-aqueous-buffer system or is the ethanol-HCl step required for their extraction? Are these TGFs normally extracellular and, if so, how are their plasma levels controlled?

6. TRANSFORMING GROWTH FACTORS FROM CHEMICALLY TRANSFORMED CELLS

Moses and co-workers (26) have been characterizing the TGFs released from a chemically transformed murine clone. The activities are sensitive to both trypsin and dithiothreitol and are heat stable. These properties suggest that the activities are associated with heat-stable, disulfide-containing peptides. When a concentrate of the conditioned media was chromatographed over a BioGel P-60 column, the activities eluted in the molecular-weight range of 10,000–12,000. These peptides were able to stimulate AIG in untransformed AKR cells. As with the previous factors, this was a phenotypic transformation rather than a genetic event. The further purification of the peptides eluted from the BioGel P-60 column, using carboxymethylcellulose column chromatography, revealed three peaks of AIG-stimulating activity. The first peak that eluted from the column contained both AIG-stimulating activity and EGF-radioreceptor-competing activity. The AIG activity present in this fraction was minor compared with that present in the two later-eluting peaks. The two major peaks of AIG-stimulating activity eluted close to one another near the end of the gradient. Neither of these peaks of AIG activity contained measurable EGF-radioreceptor-competing activity.

The major difference between the activities released by these chemically transformed cells and the factors released by MoSV-transformed cells is that the major activities released by chemically transformed cells did not appear to compete with EGF, whereas the MoSV-transformed cells released several factors with strong EGF-competing activity. Also the specific activity of the factors released by the MoSV-transformed cells was noticeably higher.

These data from chemically transformed cells are consistent with the idea that the growth factors are of host origin rather than viral gene products; they also indicate that peptides need not interact through the EGF-receptor system to confer the transformed phenotype on untransformed indicator cells as determined by AIG. They raise an important series of questions regarding the origin and function of these peptides. Since they appear to be independent of the EGF-receptor system, what receptor recognizes them? With the purification and production of antibodies to these factors, it is hoped that one can study the levels in normal tissue as well as tissue distribution of these factors. Development of radioreceptor binding assays using these purified mitogens will allow the detection and purification of competing peptides from this family of growth factors.

7. CLINICAL STUDIES

Recently, cancer patients with heavy tumor loads have been examined for the presence of TGFs in their serum or urine (27). The urine from these patients was assayed for the ability to stimulate AIG in an untransformed indicator line. Transforming growth factor activity was found in the urine samples of all the untreated cancer patients examined, and none was found in the noncancer-patient controls. The activity present in the urine was dependent upon tumor load and type. After surgical removal of the tumors, the activity could no longer be detected. These results are consistent with the hypothesis that TGFs contribute to the uncontrolled growth in the neoplastic state.

8.   EFFECTS OF RETINOIC ACID

What is the function of these growth factors in the expression and control of neoplasia? One might suggest that either the control of their production or the modulation of their effect on their target cells could potentially control the expression of the neoplastic state. This has been addressed in a limited way using retinoids, compounds that block the effects of many tumor promoters. It was shown that in nontoxic doses retinoids could partially block the effects of SGF on NRK cells (28). When suboptimal concentrations of SGF were used, the AIG effects were blocked by the retinoids. At higher concentrations of SGF, the blocking effect of the retinoids was totally overcome. In more recent experiments, a transformed clone isolated from a murine embryoid body was shown to produce and release an SGF-like peptide that was heat stable and contained disulfide bonds, and could confer AIG on an untransformed indicator cell, as well as compete with [^{125}I]EGF for binding in a radioreceptor assay (29). Treatment of this clone with a nontoxic dose of retinoic acid caused a reversible expression of the transformed phenotype. These effects were unlike those seen with embryonal carcinoma cells (30), since the effects were reversible, and there did not appear to be a change in the state of differentiation. Treated monolayers grew to confluence, stopped dividing, and maintained their media at a neutral pH; the untreated sister cultures reached confluence, continued to divide, overgrew into multiple layers, and their media became acidic. The untreated cells were efficient in forming colonies when seeded in soft agar; if they were seeded in the presence of 10^{-6} M retinoic acid, however, they did not form colonies.

The untreated cells had few, if any, membrane receptors available to bind [^{125}I]EGF. After 3 days of retinoic acid treatment, the number of available receptors increased dramatically. Serum-free conditioned media was collected from retinoic-acid-treated and untreated cells. The medium from the untreated cells had an SGF-like activity that had all of the properties expected of an SGF-like molecule. All of the activities coeluted from a BioGel P-60 column. They included the ability to stimulate [^{3}H]thymidine incorporation, compete with [^{125}I]EGF in a radioreceptor assay, and stimulate AIG in an untransformed indicator cell line. When the conditioned medium collected from cells that had been treated with retinoic acid was examined, it contained little or no measurable SGF-like activity. These results are consistent with the model in which retinoic acid regulates the expression of an SGF-like molecule that is partially responsible for the transformed phenotype expressed by these cells. This treatment showed little or no toxicity to the cells, but only prevented the cells from expressing the transformed phenotype. Such treatments might allow the arrest of the growth of neoplastic cells but are not themselves cures for the disease, since the drug is not selectively toxic to tumor cells.

9. CONCLUSION

The experiments discussed here have answered some questions, but they have certainly raised many more. The questions raised are the beginnings of new investigations. One of the obvious goals for future research is the complete purification of these factors and the determination of their amino acid sequences. Efforts along these lines are currently under way in several laboratories. The peptide sequences may indicate homologies that are not obvious at the moment. With the sequence information available, synthetic peptides can be made for immunization and antibody production. These sequences will also allow the synthesis of DNAs for the isolation of mRNAs and the eventual cloning of the TGF genes. With either antibodies to these peptides or clones of the genes in hand, several basic questions can be answered. What is the tissue distribution of these factors? Are they expressed during development and, if so, is it only during development or are they normally expressed in the adult? What are their physiological functions and controlling elements? What happens to their expression during tumor progression and in different forms of neoplasia? Experiments along these lines may lead to the discovery of yet-unknown hormones, growth factors, or differentiating agents.

ACKNOWLEDGMENTS

I thank my co-workers for their patience and Mrs. Virginia Frye for excellent secretarial assistance.

REFERENCES

1. Rubin, H., *Science*, **167**, 1271 (1970).
2. Rubin, H., *Proc. Natl. Acad. Sci. USA*, **67**, 1256 (1970).

3. Burk, R. B., *Exp. Cell Res.*, **101**, 293 (1976).
4. Burk, R. B., *Proc. Natl. Acad. Sci. USA*, **70**, 369 (1973).
5. Lipton, A., Klinger, I., Paul, D., and Holley, R. W., *Proc. Natl. Acad. Sci. USA*, **68**, 2799 (1971).
6. Burk, R. B., in L. Jimenez de Asua, R. Levi-Montalcini, R. Shields, and S. Iacobelli, Eds., *Control Mechanisms in Animal Cells*, Raven, New York, 1980, pp. 245–257.
7. Leuthard, P., Steck, G., Burk, R. B., and Otto, A., in L. Jimenez de Asua, R. Levi-Montalcini, R. Shields, and S. Iacobelli, Eds., *Control Mechanisms in Animal Cells*, Raven, New York, 1980, pp. 259–268.
8. Kaplan, P. L., Topp, W. C., and Ozanne, B., *Virology*, **108**, 484 (1981).
9. De Larco, J. E., and Todaro, G. J., *Proc. Natl. Acad. Sci. USA*, **75**, 4001 (1978).
10. Todaro, G. J., De Larco, J. E., and Cohen, S., *Nature*, **264**, 26 (1976).
11. De Larco, J. E., and Todaro, G. J., *J. Cell. Physiol.*, **94**, 335 (1978).
12. Hollenberg, M. D., and Cuatrecasas, P., *Proc. Natl. Acad. Sci. USA*, **70**, 2964 (1973).
13. Carpenter, G., and Cohen, S., *J. Cell. Physiol.*, **88**, 227 (1976).
14. De Larco, J. E., Reynolds, R., Carlberg, K., Engle, C., and Todaro, G. J., *J. Biol. Chem.*, **255**, 3685 (1980).
15. Haigler, H., Ash, J. F., Singer, S. V., and Cohen, S., *Proc. Natl. Acad. Sci. USA*, **75**, 3317 (1978).
16. Pruss, R. M., and Herschman, H. R., *Proc. Natl. Acad. Sci. USA*, **74**, 3918 (1977).
17. Ozanne, B., Fulton, R. J., and Kaplan, P. L., *J. Cell. Physiol.*, **105**, 163 (1980).
18. De Larco, J. E., and Todaro, G. J., *Cold Spr. Harb. Symp. Quant. Biol.*, **44**, 643 (1980).
19. De Larco, J. E., Preston, Y. A., and Todaro, G. J., *J. Cell. Physiol.*, **109**, 143 (1981).
20. Shih, T. Y., Weeks, M. O., Young, M. A., and Scolnick, E. M., *J. Virol.*, **31**, 546 (1979).
21. Roberts, A. B., Lamb, L. C., Newton, D. L., Sporn, M. B., De Larco, J. E., and Todaro, G. J., *Proc. Natl. Acad. Sci. USA*, **77**, 3494 (1980).
22. Roberts, A. B., Anzano, M. A., Lamb, L. C., Smith, J. M., and Sporn, M. B., *Proc. Natl. Acad. Sci. USA*, **78**, 5339 (1981).
23. Roberts, A. B., Anzano, M. A., Lamb, L. C., Smith, J. M., Marquardt, H., Todaro, G. J., and Sporn, M. B., *Nature*, **295**, 417 (1982).
24. Davoren, P. R., *Biochim. Biophys. Acta*, **63**, 150 (1962).
25. Anzano, M. A., Roberts, A. B., Smith, J. M., and Sporn, M. B., *Anal. Biochem.*, **125**, 217 (1982).
26. Moses, H. L., Branum, E. L., Proper, J. A., and Robinson, R. A., *Cancer Res.*, **41**, 2842 (1981).
27. Twardzik, D. R., Sherwin, S. A., Ranchalis, J. E., and Todaro, G. J., *J. Natl. Cancer Inst.*, **69**, 793 (1982).
28. Todaro, G. J., De Larco, J. E., and Sporn, M. B., *Nature*, **276**, 272 (1982).
29. De Larco, J. E., and Preston, Y. A., manuscript in preparation.
30. Strickland, S., and Mahdavi, V., *Cell*, **15**, 393 (1978).

8

COLONY-
STIMULATING FACTOR

Adel A. Yunis
Ming-Chi Wu
Alan M. Miller

CONTENTS

Abbreviations

CFU-GM	Colony-forming unit–granulocyte-macrophage
CSF	Colony-stimulating factor
NGF	Nerve growth factor
EP	Erythropoietin
CFU-E	Colony forming unit-erythroid precursor
PGE	Prostaglandin E
cAMP	Adenosine 3′,5′-monophosphate
PG	Prostaglandin
PGF	Prostaglandins, F series
CIA	Colony inhibitory activity
cALL	Common acute lymphocytic leukemia
CFU-Eos	Colony forming unit-eosinophils
CFU-D	Colony forming unit-Diffusion chamber—Pre CFU-GM
CFU-S	Colony forming unit-progenitor stem cell
DMEM	Dulbecco's modified Eagle's medium
HLCM	Human-lung-conditioned medium
DME-SF	Dulbecco's modified Eagle's medium, serum free
ConA	Concanavalin A
MGI	Macrophage-granulocyte inducer
IEF	Isoelectric focusing
PAS	Periodic acid-Schiff

BFU-E	Burst-forming unit–erythroid precursor
BPA	Burst-promoting activity
RIA	Radioimmunoassay
TM	Tunicamycin
SDS	Sodium dodecyl sulfate
D-factor	Differentiation factor
GARG	Goat anti-rabbit-globulin
AML	Acute myelogenous leukemia
MGI	Macrophage-granulocyte inducer protein
ATG	Anti-thymocyte globulin

1. INTRODUCTION

Recent progress in our understanding of hematopoiesis has clearly indicated that the different cell lines are derived from a common precursor pool and that the control of their production is regulated by chemically similar stimulator molecules. In the marrow, the noncommitted compartment is composed of multipotential stem cells that are capable of self-replication as well as giving rise to committed stem cells that are the progenitors for megakaryocytes, erythrocytes, or granulocytes and macrophages (1).

The study of the mechanisms involved in the regulation of granulocyte and macrophage production has been facilitated by the development of an *in vitro* cloning method, independently by Pluznick and Sachs (2) and by Bradley and Metcalf (3). When marrow cells are cultured in this semisolid assay system, the granulocyte-macrophage progenitor cells proliferate and differentiate to form colonies composed of granulocytes and/or macrophages, hence the term colony-forming unit– granulocyte-macrophage or CFU-GM. The formation and development of these colonies requires the continuous presence of a protein factor that has been termed colony-stimulating factor (CSF). The use of this culture system with various modifications in the past 15 years has allowed extensive investigations to be made on CSF, its target cell the CFU-GM, their interaction, and the various modulators involved. As a result, much insight has been gained into some of the *in vitro* regulatory mechanisms in granulopoiesis and differentiation, the nature of CSF, the CFU-GM, and various modulator molecules (stimulators and inhibitors), and some clinically relevant alterations in the characteristics of CFU-GM and its growth patterns. In spite of this near-explosive progress, however, the field is still in its infancy, with many uncertainties remaining, particularly regarding the role of CSF *in vivo*. Further progress will ultimately depend on the availability of highly purified systems including the hormone CSF and its target cell the CFU-GM. In this review we attempt to summarize current knowledge in this area with particular emphasis on CSF, CFU-GM, and their interaction. Several reviews on CSF and related subjects have recently appeared (4–7).

2.   CSF AND *IN VITRO* COLONY FORMATION

The earliest reports of systems for clonal growth of CFU-GM described the need for stimulators provided by leukocyte feeder layers (2,3,8). It was subsequently shown that the monocytes are the primary source of CSF in these feeder layers. However, soluble crude preparations of CSF can be obtained from a variety of cell- and tissue-conditioned media and extracts (*vide infra*). When CFU-GM are cultured in the presence of CSF they proliferate and differentiate to form colonies composed of macrophages and/ or granulocytes. The formation and development of colonies is absolutely dependent on CSF (2,3,9,10), and the dose response follows a sigmoidal pattern (10). The cells within a colony can be either granulocytes, macrophages, or a mixture of both. The type of colony formed from normal marrow depends on the source and concentration of CSF (10) as well as on the presence or absence of inhibitors (11). Mouse marrow CFU-GM form primarily macrophage colonies under stimulation by mouse L-cell or pregnant mouse uterine extract CSF (12), whereas at high concentration, mouse-lung-conditioned media (4) and pancreatic-carcinoma-cell-conditioned media (13) yield high percentages of granulocyte colonies. At lower concentrations, these same sources stimulate mouse macrophage colonies. Similarly, human marrow CFU-GM form more macrophage colonies with leukocyte-conditioned medium or urinary CSF (14), but yield granulocyte colonies in the presence of conditioned medium prepared from human lung, pancreatic carcinoma cells, or fibroblasts (7,13,15,16).

The type of colonies is also influenced by lipoprotein inhibitors that are present in normal serum. Preincubation of CFU-GM with these inhibitors followed by culture in their absence yields high proportions of macrophage colonies (11). Marrow cells from Balb/c, a mouse strain with high levels of serum inhibitor, tend to produce macrophage colonies *in vitro*, whereas marrow cells from the low-inhibitor strain C57/BL produce a higher proportion of granulocytes or mixed colonies.

In addition to its role in colony growth, CSF is required for the survival *in vitro* of CFU-GM. Culture of CFU-GM in the absence of CSF leads to their rapid death or loss of their capacity to proliferate (10,17), and in this CSF resembles nerve growth factor (NGF), which is necessary for survival of nerve cells (18), and erythropoietin (EP), which is required for the survival of the colony-forming unit-erythrocyte (CFU-E) (19).

Whereas the action of CSF is directed mainly at its target cell, the CFU-GM, it appears to exert various effects on the differentiated progeny as well. These include stimulation of phagocytic and cytocidal activity by mouse peritoneal macrophages (20), enhancement of plasminogen-activator release by mononuclear cells (21), and modification in the rate of synthesis of a number of proteins in polymorphonuclear leukocytes (4). Here too, CSF is similar to EP, which in addition to stimulating erythropoietic cell proliferation, also stimulates hemoglobin synthesis.

Perhaps the most thoroughly studied noncolony-stimulating activity of CSF has been the stimulation of prostaglandin E (PGE) synthesis by mature monocytes and macrophages (22–25). Kurland et al. have postulated that this CSF-induced PGE synthesis serves as a negative-feedback mechanism in colony formation; in the presence of high CSF levels, monocytes and macrophages produce PGE, which in turn inhibits further colony formation by its action on the CFU-GM (22).

3. SOURCES AND PRODUCTION OF CSF

Colony-stimulating activity has been found in a wide variety of tissues and body fluids. In mouse, it has been found in submaxillary glands and thymus (26), uterus (27), kidney (27), spleen (26,28), embryo (27,29), and lung (26,27,30). In man, it has been reported in lung (31–33) placenta (34–36), embryonic kidney and fibroblasts (37,38), spleen (39), and pulmonary macrophages (40). Virtually every tissue that has been examined contains some CSF activity. Media conditioned by these tissues also stimulate *in vitro* granulopoiesis. Serum (26), urine (41), and amniotic fluid (Wu, unpublished results) also contain CSF.

Production of CSF has been demonstrated in macrophages (42–44), mitogen-stimulated lymphocytes (45–48), and endothelial cells (49,50), as well as established cell lines such as cultured human lung (51), and mouse L cells (52,53). Hybridomas derived from the fusion of mitogen-stimulated spleen cells and HAT-sensitive T-lymphoma cells (54) produce CSF indistinguishable from CSF-GM isolated from mouse-lung-conditioned medium (55).

In addition, a number of established tumor cell lines have been shown to produce CSF. Examples are the mouse leukemia cell line WEHI-3 (56), Yoshida sarcoma cell line (57), human squamous cell carcinoma T3M-1 (58), T-lymphocyte cell line (Mo) derived from hairy cell leukemia (59), and others. Svet-Moldavsky et al. (60) have screened 50 cultured human tumor cell lines and found that most of them produce CSF activity. In our laboratory several tumor cell lines have been examined, including two human pancreatic carcinomas, MIA PaCa-2 (61) and PANC-1 (62), a squamous cell carcinoma (63), a human breast carcinoma, and several melanomas. All of them have been found to secrete CSF activity in varying amounts.

4. *IN VIVO* ROLE OF CSF

Because of its essential role in granulocyte-macrophage colony formation *in vitro*, CSF has been postulated to be the primary regulator of granulocyte production *in vivo*. Although there is no direct experimental evidence to indicate that CSF functions as a granulopoietin, data derived from both murine and human studies suggest that CSF may play an important role in the regulation of granulopoiesis. The indirect evidence is similar to that obtained for EP, namely an inverse relationship of serum stimulator level to cell count, for example, increasing EP levels with decreasing hemoglobin concentrations. Variations in CSF levels are seen corresponding to changes in peripheral granulocyte count whether these changes are induced experimentally or found in certain pathological states. Increased serum CSF levels are found at the nadir granulocyte count in alkylating-agent-induced granulocytopenia (64) or granulocytopenia induced by the injection of anti-neutrophilic serum (65). The injection of endotoxin in mice results in a 50–200-fold increase in the serum CSF level within hours, followed by an increased peripheral granulocyte count and then a fall in the CSF level (66). In a series of studies, Quesenberry et al. have provided evidence that endotoxin-induced granulocytosis is CSF mediated and not due to a change in serum inhibitor levels (67–69). Furthermore, endotoxin does not exert its effects directly on the CFU-GM (70). Zidar and Shadduck demonstrated low CSF levels during endotoxin-induced neutrophilia and high CSF levels in cyclophosphamide-induced granulocytopenia, but in both cases the serum inhibitor level remained unchanged (64,71). Hinterberger et al. demonstrated a similar effect of endotoxin in normal human subjects: a sharp rise in serum CSF levels in six subjects following the administration of low doses of endotoxin (72). These observations have led to speculations that one determinant of the normal granulocyte pool may involve intermittent low-level endotoxemia, providing a steady CSF level needed for sustained granulopoiesis (72). Additional evidence for a CSF role in *in vivo* granulopoiesis has come from observations made in certain disorders of granulopoiesis. In both the genetically determined cyclic neutropenia in grey collie dogs (73) and in cyclic neutropenia in man (74), CSF levels were found to be inversely related to the granulocyte count, with the highest levels coinciding with the nadir neutrophil count (73,74). Peak CSF levels are followed by neutrophil recovery. Elevation in serum and/or urine CSF levels can be demonstrated in mice with spontaneous, viral-induced, or transplanted leukemia (75) as well as in a high percentage of patients with acute granulocytic and monocytic leukemia (76). When cells from a squamous cell carcinoma were transplanted into athymic nude mice, the animals developed neutrophilia associated with high level of CSF in cyst fluid (77). Stimulation of granulopoiesis in nude mice transplanted with a human lung tumor that produced CSF activity has also been described (78). However, in none of these studies can the conclusion be made that the observed effect was due to CSF, and alternative mechanisms cannot be excluded (4).

The *in vivo* activity of EP has been established by the injection of active material into animals in whom endogenous erythropoiesis and EP production has been suppressed by inducing a polycythemic state (79). Such animals do not incorporate radioactive iron into new erythroid cells, but can be induced to do so by the administration of EP. Clearly, similar experiments with CSF are not readily accomplished for lack of methods for either quantitating or shutting off endogenous granulopoiesis and because of unavailability heretofore of highly purified CSF. In one series of experiments, McGarry et al. (80) demonstrated *in vivo* stimulation of eosinophil production in mice after suppression of endogenous eosinophilopoiesis with hydrocortisone. The injection of these mice with conditioned media of splenic lymphocytes secondarily challenged with schistosome egg antigen resulted in a specific increase in bone marrow eosinophils. To date similar experiments with CSF have not been reported. Nevertheless both CSF and antibody to CSF have been injected into animals in attempts to demonstrate *in vivo* granulopoietic activity (81–85). The intravenous injection into neonatal mice of partially purified human urinary CSF (81,82) resulted in monocytosis and neutrophilic granulocytosis within 48 hours, whereas in adult mice only a monocytosis was evident. A mean serum half-life of 3 hours was calculated for the injected CSF. A serum half-life of less than 4 hours was reported for L-cell CSF (83), with no preferential accumulation in any organ, and a half-life of 7.3 hours has been recorded for purified CSF from mouse-lung-conditioned medium (85). The injection of anti-CSF sera failed to produce leukopenia or suppress marrow granulopoiesis, but some suppression of granulopoiesis was observed in intraperitoneal diffusion chambers (84). Clearly none of these studies allow a definite conclusion to be made regarding the *in vivo* role of CSF. The short half-life of CSF suggests that the observed effects from injected material are not due to CSF itself, but may be nonspecific. The answer must ultimately come from the availability of highly purified CSF and specific monoclonal antibodies. Only then can one perform controlled CSF infusion and neutralization studies to resolve this issue. It should also be noted that the biochemical and immunochemical heterogeneity of CSF (*vide infra*) calls for use of antibodies specific to the CSF that is being tested.

5. MODULATORS OF CSF ACTION

Although CSF is a requirement for colony growth, a variety of substances, particularly low-molecular-weight compounds, are capable of enhancing or inhibiting CSF-induced colony formation. Cyclic adenosine 3:5'-monophosphate (cAMP), theophylline, epinephrine, and prostaglandin E inhibit colony growth in both in mouse and human marrow (86,87). Cyclic GMP enhances colony formation, an effect opposite to that of cAMP (88). The effect of prostaglandin (PG) on CFU-GM growth has been studied rather extensively (22–25,89). Concentrations of PGE as low as 10^{-10} M inhibit CFU-GM proliferation. This inhibition is associated with decreased responsiveness of the CFU-GM to CSF and can be countered by raising the CSF concentration (23–25,89). Kurland et al. proposed that PGE produced locally within the bone marrow environment or in sites of inflammation may serve to limit the proliferation of CFU-GM cells (25), and that this is accomplished via a feedback loop involving the mononuclear phagocytes. In situations requiring granulocyte-macrophage production, for example, inflammation, these cells produce and release CSF. As the number of cells and CSF level increase, mononuclear phagocytes release PGE, which dampens the CFU-GM responsiveness to CSF, thereby slowing down its proliferation. Thus the mononuclear phagocyte plays a biphasic role in granulomonocytopoiesis, alternating between stimulation and inhibition according to need. It has further been shown that the inhibitor activity of macrophages can be overcome by the addition of indomethacin, an inhibitor of PG synthesis, lending further support to the modulating role of PG in granulopoiesis (25,90). Miller et al. examined the role of the F series of PG (PGF) (91). Concentrations of 0.1×10^{-9}–2×10^{-9} M PGF$_{2\alpha}$ enhanced colony growth by as much as 50%. And PGF$_{2\alpha}$ and PGE$_1$ had counteracting effects when added together, and this suggested that the PGF:PGE ratio may play a determining role in granulocyte proliferation. It is of interest in this regard that the PGF:PGE ratio was twofold to threefold greater in myeloid hyperplastic rat marrow than in normal marrow and was 18-fold higher than normal in rat chloroleukemic tumor cells (92). This alteration in ratio appeared to be due primarily to increased conversion of PGE to PGF via the NADH-dependent PGE$_2$ 9-ketoreductase rather than increased PGF synthesis (92,93). What may be a related observation was recently made by Taetle and Mendelsohn, who demonstrated lack of inhibition or paradoxical stimulation by PGE of the CFU-GM from chronic myelocytic leukemia, acute leukemia, and myeloid metaplasia (94). Although several explanations for these findings are possible, the data of Ziboh et al. (92) suggest possible conversion of PGE to PGF or some other intermediate in these myeloproliferative disorders.

Lithium was associated with an increased granulocyte count *in vivo* (95–97), and the increase was shown not to be due to redistribution (98–101).

It was subsequently shown that lithium enhances granulopoiesis *in vitro* (100–104). In human marrow the mechanism appears to be enhancement of endogenous CSF production (102–105). Thus the effect of lithium can be abolished by prior removal of CSF-producing cells (adherent cell population) from the marrow (102). Additionally, lithium is able to protect the CFU-GM from inhibition by drugs such as chloramphenicol and chlorpromazine in a manner similar to that provided by increased CSF concentrations (102,106). There is evidence that in murine bone marrow, lithium acts not by increasing CSF production but rather directly on the CFU-GM (Miller, unpublished). Thus enhancement of colony growth is observed with lithium with or without removal of the adherent cell (CSF-producing) population, and lithium does not protect against inhibition by chloramphenicol or chlorpromazine as observed in human marrow. A non-CSF-mediated role of lithium in mouse marrow has been reported by Levitt and Quesenberry (107). Using long-term marrow cultures, these workers demonstrated accelerated recruitment of CFU-GM cells from more-premature progenitors in the presence of lithium, suggesting yet another level of action for lithium. Some of the confusion that has existed regarding the mechanism of action of lithium may be attributable to species differences.

Reports on the effects of corticosteroids on hematopoiesis have been contradictory. Golde et al. demonstrated that dexamethasone potentiates both murine and human erythropoiesis *in vitro* in the presence of EP (108). Subsequently, a number of investigators reported inhibition of erythroid colony growth by corticosteroids in mouse (109–111), and rat marrow (112). Urabe et al. (111) found that in contrast with the cells of mouse marrow precursors, human marrow erythroid precursors are stimulated by similar dexamethasone concentrations. Inhibition by corticosteroid of CFU-GM from mouse (110,113,114) and human (115) marrow has also been reported, although the levels necessary were generally greater than those required for erythroid inhibition. Our findings are at variance with these. In a series of marrow samples from nine human volunteers, dexamethasone consistently enhanced CFU-GM growth (Miller, unpublished). The stimulation was not due to increased endogenous CSF production, but appeared to result from a direct action on the progenitor cell. Other corticosteroids were equally effective. Progesterone, which competes with dexamethasone for binding, can block this enhancing effect. The increased granulocyte proliferation in the presence of dexamethasone may contribute to the chronic neutrophilia observed in patients receiving corticosteroids.

Broxmeyer recently described two inhibitors of granulopoiesis; the first is produced by normal granulocytes, and was originally named colony-inhibitory activity or CIA (116–118) but later identified as lactoferrin (117). Lactoferrin is an iron-binding glycoprotein concentrated in the secondary granules of mature granulocytes (119,120). It exerts its inhibitory action on colony formation by inhibiting the production and/or release of CSF from monocytes (118) by an unknown mechanism. The release of lactoferrin from granulocytes might thus serve as a negative-feedback mechanism, inhibiting further production of granulocytes. Although lactoferrin inhibits baseline synthesis of CSF by monocytes, it does not block endotoxin-stimulated CSF synthesis, thus presumably allowing for uninterrupted production of granulocytes in the face of continuing demand, such as persistent infection.

The second inhibitor, derived from leukemic cells (leukemia-inhibiting activity) (121,122), has been identified as acidic isoferritin (122) and appears to act directly on the CFU-GM. Perhaps more significant is that the leukemic CFU-GM appears to be relatively insensitive to inhibition by acidic isoferritins (121,122), suggesting that a product of leukemic cells can preferentially inhibit normal granulopoiesis, possibly contributing to the pathogenesis of leukemia.

Low-molecular-weight substances called chalones (123) derived from mature granulocytes have been reported to inhibit granulocytic proliferation, but their role in the regulation of granulopoiesis remains uncertain.

Both inhibitory (124–126) and stimulatory non-CSF serum factors (125–127) have been described. Inhibition of colony growth by interferons has recently been observed (128). Augmentation of *in vitro* growth by certain antigens (129), and red cell lysates (130) has also been reported.

A plethora of substances with various properties appear to have a modulating effect on CSF-induced CFU-GM growth *in vitro*. The significance of this modulation remains uncertain and may in some instance be simply an *in vitro* artifact, but a better definition of these interactions must await the further elucidation of the molecular mechanisms underlying CFU-GM proliferation and differentiation.

6. CHARACTERIZATION OF CFU-GM

The definition and characterization of the CFU-GM was made possible largely through the application of the *in vitro* cloning assay. It has been clearly demonstrated in these cultures by cell-transfer experiments that colonies of granulocytes and monocytes are derived from a single cell (131). The CFU-GM is distinct from the multipotential stem cell or CFU-S (132–142) and differs from it in several respects. The CFU-GM has a higher proliferative rate (132,133,136) and little capacity for self-replication (143). In its morphology the CFU-GM resembles a transitional lymphocyte (131) and appears to reside in the null cell fraction as determined by cytochemical and cell-surface-marker studies (144,145). The human CFU-GM possesses allotypic HLA-A,B antigenic determinants as demonstrated with cytotoxic HLA typing sera (146) and Ia-like antigens as confirmed by monoclonal antibodies (147) but lacks T-lymphocyte antigen (148,149), the common acute lymphocytic leukemia (cALL) antigen (150), and ABO antigens (151).

In studying the CFU-GM, it became apparent quite early that these cells are heterogeneous with respect to a number of parameters. In 1971 Janoshwitz et al. separated mouse marrow CFU-GM according to density into subpopulations that would preferentially form granulocytes or macrophages; those forming macrophage colonies had a higher density (152). Subsequent studies confirmed this heterogeneity according to density and further demonstrated heterogeneity in their sensitivity to different CSF sources (12,153). It was also observed that as density increased, the maturation rate increased, but the proliferative capacity decreased (12). Das et al. and Morley et al. distinguished the CFU-GM that gave rise to granulocytes and macrophages from the colony-forming unit–eosinophils (CFU-Eos), which produced eosinophilic colonies (154,155); neutrophilic colonies appeared earlier and lysed more rapidly than eosinophilic colonies.

Recently, three groups of workers independently observed heterogeneity of human CFU-GM as analyzed by sedimentation velocity (156–158). In all cases the CFU-GM could be separated into two distinct populations, one sedimenting at 8 mm/hour and forming colonies by day 7 of culture, and another sedimenting at 6.5 mm/hour and yielding colonies by day 12–14. In addition, the rapidly sedimenting population was more sensitive to CSF (156), responding to certain CSF better than to others (158) and possessing a greater fraction of cells in cycle than the slowly sedimenting population (157,159). We have also reported that 14-day CFU-GM were more sensitive to inhibition by the drug chloramphenicol (160). It appears from these studies that the slow-sedimenting and the fast-sedimenting CFU-GM have a parent–progeny relationship, as proposed by Jacobsen et al., the 14-day CFU-GM giving rise to the more differentiated 7-day CFU-GM (157).

In addition, it has been demonstrated that granulocytes arising in diffusion chambers implanted intraperitoneally in mice are derived from a progenitor stem cell (CFU-D) that sediments at 5 mm/hour and has a smaller cycling fraction (7%) than either of the two CFU-GM classes (161). When fractions containing CFU-D without CFU-GM are cultured in diffusion chambers, both types of CFU-GM can be subsequently recovered (161). It would thus appear that the CFU-D is the precursor of both the fast- and the slow-sedimenting CFU-GM, that is, $\text{CFU-S} \rightarrow \text{CFU-D} \rightarrow \text{CFU-GM}_{14d} \rightarrow \text{CFU-GM}_{7d}$. Differentiation in this order is accompanied by increase in cell size and density (156–158), percentage of cycling cells (157–159), and perhaps greater specificity with regard to CSF response and to the type of mature cells formed.

7.   PREPARATION OF CSF FROM TISSUES

Murine CSF with relatively highly specific activity (2×10^4 colonies/ mg) can be prepared from medium conditioned with lung tissue obtained from endotoxin-treated mice as described by Burgess et al. (55). It exhibits heterogeneity in charge and size, probably due to variation in sialic acid content; treatment with neuraminidase followed by chromatography on a Sepharose 6BL column in $6 M$ guanidine hydrochloride yields a single molecular species (162).

Human CSF has been similarly prepared from autopsy human lung, and the procedure has been described by Fojo et al. (31). Lung tissue obtained at autopsy is minced in small pieces, suspended in serum-free Dulbecco's modified Eagle's medium (DMEM) (0.1 g of tissue per milliliter), and incubated at 37°C for 3 days. The medium is then cleared by centrifugation, dialyzed against water, and sterilized by filtration. The human-lung-conditioned medium (HLCM) thus prepared has CSF activity in the range of 1000–4000 colonies/ml as assayed on mouse marrow and 600–3000 colonies/ ml as assayed on human marrow. Human CSF can also be obtained from placental tissue according to procedures described by Wu and Fischer (36) and Nicola et al. (163).

8.   PREPARATION OF CSF FROM CULTURED CELL LINES

Although mouse and human CSF can be prepared from tissue-conditioned media, the media are usually heavily contaminated with tissue and serum proteins, thereby rendering the purification of CSF more difficult. Serum-free conditioned media of cultured cell lines offer larger quantities of CSF at much higher specific activity, hence providing better starting materials for purification. The preparation of mouse L-cell CSF from cell culture has been described in detail by Stanley et al. (52) and by Shadduck et al. (53). The L-cells can be grown both in spinner and in monolayer culture. A CSF with a specific activity of 3×10^5 colonies/mg protein can be obtained from these conditioned media (52).

There are at least three cultured human cell lines (59,164,165) that provide excellent sources of human CSF. In the preparation of CSF from human pancreatic carcinoma MIA PaCa-2 cells (165), cells are grown in DMEM supplemented with 2.5% fetal bovine serum, 5% newborn-calf serum, and 3% horse serum, either in Petri dishes, flasks, or roller bottles. When cultures have reached near confluence, the medium is aspirated, and the plates are rinsed three times with Hank's balanced salt solution. Serum-free DMEM is then added to each plate, and the incubation is continued for 3 days, after which the conditioned serum-free DMEM (DMEM-SF) is harvested and centrifuged to remove any cell debris (166). The specific activity of CSF from the DMEM-SF is about 5×10^4–10×10^4 colonies/mg as assayed in mouse marrow and 1–5×10^4 colonies/mg as assayed in human marrow.

9. ISOLATION AND PURIFICATION OF CSF

Although CSF has been found in a wide variety of tissues, body fluids, and different types of cells, only a few of CSFs have been highly purified and characterized.

9.1. Partially Purified CSF From Human Sources

Conditioned medium prepared from human peripheral leukocytes contains CSF that can replace the leukocyte feeder layer used in the early assay system (167,168). Price et al. (168) have fractionated and purified CSFs from conditioned media by methods including ammonium sulfate precipitation, DEAE-cellulose, hydroxyapatite, and gel filtration. Three species of CSF have been purified with molecular weights of 93,000, 36,500, and 14,700. However, Shah et al. (42) have reported that conditioned media prepared from peripheral blood monocyte and mitogen-stimulated lymphocytes contains essentially only two CSF activities that can be separated by gel filtration on Sephadex G-150: a high-molecular-weight CSF ($>$150,000 daltons) that stimulates mouse marrow and a lower-molecular-weight CSF (35,000 daltons) that stimulates both human and mouse marrow.

Human-placenta-conditioned medium contains two types of CSF: one active in mouse marrow and another active in both mouse and human marrow (36). Burgess et al. (35) have partially purified the human active CSF 1800-fold to a specific activity of 2.5×10^5 colonies/mg with 5% yield. The purified CSF has a molecular weight of 30,000 daltons and stimulates macrophage and granulocyte colony formation in human marrow. Furthermore, this preparation of 30,000-dalton CSF contains two types of CSF activities that can be separated on a phenyl-Sepharose column. One of the activities stimulates only neutrophil colonies, whereas the other one stimulates both neutrophil and eosinophil colony growth (169).

Conditioned medium prepared from autopsy human lung tissue (HLCM) also provides a good source of CSF (31). Fojo et al. (32) have purified CSF from HLCM 2250-fold to a specific activity of 2.7×10^6 colonies/mg.

DiPersio et al. (170) have purified CSFs from a human monocyte cell line GCT. Three differing species of CSF were found. A high-molecular-weight CSF (150,000 daltons) is only active on mouse marrow and produces macrophage colonies, and two lower-molecular-weight CSFs (35,000 daltons) can be separated by isoelectric focusing (IEF) and gradient polyacrylamide gel electrophoresis. One of these is active in mouse marrow and the other in human marrow. The mouse and human active low-molecular-weight CSF were purified about 1000-fold to specific activities of 0.55 and 1.12×10^6 colonies/mg, respectively, with only 3% yield. The human active CSF from the GCT cell line stimulates both neutrophil and eosinophil colony formation.

Golde et al. (59) have reported that a human T-lymphocyte cell line (Mo) derived from a T-lymphocyte variant of hairy-cell leukemia produces CSF activity that can be stimulated by concanavalin A (ConA). In subsequent studies, Lusis et al. (171) purified the Mo-CSF to a specific activity of 3.5 $\times 10^6$ colonies/mg with 31% yield. In contrast with CSFs produced by other cell lines, the Mo cell line produces only a human-active CSF with a molecular weight of 34,000 daltons. It stimulates both macrophage and granulocyte colony formation in human marrow with only little activity in mouse marrow.

A fibroblast-like cell line derived from autopsy human lung tissue also produces CSF in serum-free conditioned medium. Yunis et al. (51) have partially purified this CSF over 1000-fold to a specific activity of 1.8×10^7 colonies/mg with 12% yield as assayed on mouse marrow and a specific activity of 1.2×10^7 colonies/mg with 18% yield as assayed on human marrow.

9.2. Highly Purified Murine CSF

Mouse CSF has been purified to apparent homogeneity from medium conditioned by endotoxin-stimulated mouse lung by Burgess et al. (55) using standard protein-purification methods including calcium phosphate gel, DEAE-cellulose, ConA-Sepharose affinity column, gel filtration, and preparative gel electrophoresis. A 3500-fold purification has been achieved with 8% yield and a specific activity of 7×10^7 colonies/mg for the purified CSF. The CSF thus purified has a molecular weight of 23,000 daltons as determined by sodium dodecyl sulfate (SDS) gel electrophoresis and stimulates both granulocyte and macrophage colony formation. Another mouse CSF has also been purified to apparent homogeneity from serum-free conditioned medium of mouse L cells independently by two laboratories (52,53). Stanley and Heard (52) have used procedures including DEAE-cellulose, gel filtration on Sephadex G-200, ConA-Sepharose, and gradient gel electrophoresis to purify this CSF 1100-fold to apparent homogeneity as shown on SDS-gel electrophoresis. The yield was 25% and the specific activity 3.5×10^8 colonies/mg. The purified CSF has a molecular weight of 70,000 daltons and consists of two subunit components of 35,000 daltons each.

Similarly, Waheed and Shadduck (53) have applied methods including alcohol precipitation, DEAE-cellulose, and ConA-Sepharose to fractionate serum-free conditioned medium prepared from mouse L cells. Two activities could be separated by a ConA-Sepharose column, one that was not adsorbed to the column (peak I) and one that was (peak II). Both activities were further purified by gel filtration on Sephadex G-150 and density-gradient centrifugation to apparent homogeneity with 1000-fold purification and 50–70% yield. The specific activities for the purified CSFs were 21.2×10^6 and 51.9×10^6 colonies/mg for peaks I and II, respectively. Although they have different affinity for ConA-Sepharose, both have a molecular weight of 70,000 daltons and both consist of two subunit components of 35,000 daltons each. Both purified CSFs show strong periodic-acid Schiff (PAS) staining for carbohydrate and a change in electrophoretic mobility after neuraminidase treatment.

The specific activities of mouse L-cell CSF reported from these two laboratories are somewhat different; the molecular weights and all other properties are similar or identical. The discrepancy in specific activity can be explained by the differences in assay conditions.

The purification of yet another murine CSF was reported by Guez and Sachs (172). These authors isolated and purified from the culture medium of a cloned mouse cell line a protein that could induce macrophage and granulocyte colony formation from undifferentiated hematopoietic cells of embryonic liver, hence the name macrophage-granulocyte inducer, or MGI. It has a molecular weight of 68,000 daltons. Interestingly enough, the purified factor is inactive; however, adenine or adenine-containing nucleotides can fully restore its biological activity (173). The specific activity of the purified MGI was about 2×10^6 colonies/mg as determined in their assay system. Although it is similar in molecular weight to mouse L-cell CSF, amino acid and sugar analysis indicated that MGI has no cystine, cysteine, glucosamine, or any other sugars.

9.3. Highly Purified Human CSF

From human urine, CSF activity was reported early in the study of *in vitro* myelopoiesis (41,174) and was highly purified by Stanley et al. (175) using conventional protein-purification methods including DEAE-cellulose, hydroxyapatite, gel filtration, ConA-Sepharose, and preparative gel electrophoresis. They have purified urinary CSF 110,000-fold to a specific activity of 1.6×10^8 colonies/mg with 14% yield. Although the preparation appears as a single PAS-stained band, it has several protein bands when stained with Coomassie blue. Neuraminidase treatment reduces its electrophoretic mobility on gel electrophoresis, indicating that urinary CSF is a sialic-acid-containing glycoprotein. Suprisingly, the purified urinary CSF stimulates only macrophage colony formation in mouse marrow and has only "cluster formation" activity in human marrow (176). Motoyoshi et al. (177) have reported the purification of urinary CSF 4000-fold to a specific activity of 10^6 and 6.7×10^5 colonies/mg on mouse and human marrow cells, respectively. The purification methods included concentration with polyethylene glycol, ammonium sulfate precipitation, chromatography on DEAE-cellulose, gel filtration, and preparative gel electrophoresis. The CSF thus purified has a molecular weight of 85,000 daltons as determined by gel filtration and, in contrast with the work of Stanley et al., is active on both human and mouse marrow yielding granulocytic colonies.

Two other CSFs from a human source have been purified to apparent homogeneity (36,165). An established human pancreatic carcinoma cell line (MIA PaCa-2) (165) was found to secrete abundant CSF activity into the medium. Serum-free conditioned medium prepared from MIA PaCa-2 cells was concentrated by Amicon ultrafiltration and fractionated by flat-bed IEF. Two distinctly separable activities were identified, a high-molecular-weight CSF (type I) with low pI exhibiting greater activity in mouse marrow, and a low-molecular-weight CSF (type II) with high pI having greater activity in human marrow. Type-I CSF has been purified 1000-fold to apparent homogeneity by a two-step method of IEF followed by gel-filtration chromatography on Ultrogel AcA 44. Type-I CSF activity shows a polydisperse pattern on IEF with pI in the range of 3.6–4.7. After treatment with neuraminidase it emerges as a single activity peak with a pI of 4.7. When analyzed on microgel electrophoresis, purified type-I CSF shows a single activity peak coincident with a single band stained by Coomassie blue or PAS. The homogeneity of purified type-I CSF was also confirmed by microgel electrophoresis in SDS. It has a molecular weight of 50,000 daltons as determined by gel filtration and SDS-gel electrophoresis. Unlike mouse L-cell CSF, type-I CSF appears to be a single polypeptide, and the biological activity is not affected by mercaptoethanol or dithiothreitol. Similar to urinary CSF purified by Stanley, the purified type-I CSF stimulates CFU-GM growth in mouse marrow with very little activity in human marrow. However, both macrophage and granulocyte colonies are observed.

Type-II CSF was also recently purified to apparent homogeneity by similar methods including IEF, gel filtration, and preparative gel electrophoresis (178). The specific activity of the purified type-II CSF was in the range of 4×10^7–10×10^7 colonies/mg in human marrow depending on the CFU-GM content of the marrow sample used. On microgel electrophoresis it migrates as a single band as stained by Coomassie blue and a somewhat diffuse band as stained by PAS. The molecular weight of Type-II CSF is 27,000 daltons as determined by gel filtration on Ultrogel AcA 44. It has a pI of 5.7, which shifts to 6.2 after neuraminidase treatment. Thus both type-I and type-II CSF are sialic-acid-containing glycoproteins. Purified type-II CSF is active for both human and mouse marrow (human activity greater than mouse activity) yielding both granulocyte and macrophage colonies.

Another CSF from human-placenta-conditioned medium has been purified to apparent homogeneity by Wu and Fischer (36). Conditioned medium was prepared as described previously and first fractionated by IEF. As with MIA PaCa-2 CSF, two distinct types of CSF activities appear on IEF. Type-I CSF has been further purified by gel filtration, neuraminidase treatment, IEF, and preparative gel electrophoresis to apparent homogeneity as shown in microgel electrophoresis. The purified Type-I CSF has a molecular weight of 41,000 daltons and shares all the properties of Type-I CSF from MIA PaCa-2.

10. CHARACTERIZATION OF CSF

The general properties of highly purified CSF from both murine and human sources are summarized in Table 1. Some of the other characteristics are described below.

10.1. Molecular Heterogeneity

Heterogeneity of CSF exists between species, within the same species, and even in the same tissue. There are differences in size, charge, and biological specificities. It may be generalized that two types of CSF are produced in murine tissues, and both have been purified and partially characterized. One type is exemplified by mouse lung CSF, has a molecular weight of 23,000 daltons and stimulates granulocyte-macrophage colony formation. Another type is derived from mouse L cells, has a molecular weight of 70,000 daltons, consists of two subunits of 35,000 daltons each, and stimulates only macrophage colonies. Although crude mouse lung CSF shows heterogeneity on IEF and several molecular species on gel filtration, treatment with neuraminidase and fractionation on Sepharose CL-6B in 6 M guanidine hydrochloride reveals a single CSF activity band with a molecular weight of 23,000 daltons. When a variety of conditioned media from mouse tissue cell lines are similarly treated, CSF activity also appears as a single peak of 23,000 daltons as determined by gel filtration (160). An exception to this pattern is endotoxin serum, which contains two types of CSF activities separable on a ConA-Sepharose column, a nonadherent fraction with a molecular weight of 23,000 daltons that stimulates the growth of granulocyte-

Table 1. Properties of Highly Purified CSF From Various Sources

CSF Source	Molecular Weight	Specific Activity	Marrow Specificity	Colony Morphology	Reference
Mouse lung CM	23,000	7×10^7	Mouse	GM	55
Mouse L-cell CM	70,000	3.5×10^8	Mouse	M	52
	70,000	5×10^7	Mouse	M	53
Cloned mouse cell	68,000	1.8×10^6	Mouse	GM	172
Human urine	45,000	1.8×10^8	Mouse	M	175
	85,000	6.7×10^5	Human	G	177
		1×10^6	Mouse		
Mo-Cell	35,000	3.5×10^6	Human	GM	171
Human lung	41,000	2.7×10^6	Mouse	GM	32
Human placenta	41,000	7.5×10^7	Mouse	GM	36
	30,000	2.5×10^5	Human	GME	35
Human MIA PaCa-2	50,000	7×10^7	Mouse	GM	165
	27,000	$4\text{--}10 \times 10^7$	Human	GM	178
Human GCT	30,000	0.6×10^6	Mouse	GM	170
	30,000	1.1×10^6	Human	GMEos	170

macrophage colonies, and an adherent fraction with a molecular weight of 33,000 daltons yielding largely macrophage colonies (179). Heterogeneity has also been reported in conditioned medium of mouse peritoneum (180) and that of the WEHI-3 cell line (56). The L-cell type CSF has also been found in the extracts of uterus from pregnant mice and conditioned medium of mouse embryonic yolk sac (181).

Although the pattern of CSF in human tissue appears to be more complex, generally a similar pattern of two types of CSF has been encountered (13). Type-I CSF has a higher molecular weight, reported in the range of 40,000–150,000 daltons, and exhibits activity primarily in mouse marrow with little or no activity in unfractionated human marrow. It shows a polydisperse pattern of activity on IEF with a pI in the range of 3.6–4.7. Human urinary CSF and type-I CSF from human placenta-, lung-, and leukocyte-conditioned medium and conditioned media of MIA PaCa-2 cells and squamous cell carcinoma all share similar properties, with a molecular weight of 50,000 daltons. Human peripheral blood monocytes and mitogen-stimulated lymphocytes produce two types of CSF activities separable by gel filtration, a mouse-active CSF of molecular weight 150,000, and a human/mouse-active CSF of molecular weight 35,000 daltons (42). A similar pattern of two types of CSF was observed in a cultured GCT monocyte cell line (170); however, an additional mouse-active CSF of around 35,000 daltons and separable from the human-active CSF by IEF and gel electrophoresis was observed. Early reports by Price et al. (168) indicated four human-active species of CSF from leukocyte-conditioned medium, but no strictly mouse-active CSF was observed.

The high apparent molecular weight determined by gel filtration of type-I CSF could be the result of aggregation or charge interaction between sialic acid residues of the oligosaccharide side chain of CSF. Thus urinary CSF in its crude state also appears as a high-molecular-weight peak ($>$100,000 daltons) on gel filtration (175).

The second type of CSF from human sources is Type II of molecular weight 30,000 daltons and a much higher activity in human than in mouse marrow. It has a pI of 5.7 and usually appears as a single activity peak on IEF. Type-II CSFs from placenta (13, 36), lung (13), MIA PaCa-2 cells (13,165), GCT cells (170), Mo cells (171), squamous cell carcinoma (13), and peripheral blood leukocytes (13) all seem to share similar properties. However, with this type of CSF at least two biological activities can be separated on a phenyl-Sepharose column (169). One of these stimulates granulocyte-macrophage colony formation, and the other stimulates, in addition, the growth of eosinophilic colonies.

10.2. Biological Significance of Two Types of CSF

It has been known for some time that various CSFs exhibit differences in their activities when assayed in mouse compared with human bone marrow (14). Thus human urinary CSF is active in mouse marrow, but shows only ''cluster'' activity in human marrow. Also, crude CSF preparations generally exhibit higher activity in human marrow than purified preparations. These discrepancies have been a source of both confusion and controversy in this area. The recent finding by Wu and Yunis (13) of a common pattern of two distinct types of CSF in human tissues has helped clarify this problem. Using IEF as an initial step in CSF fractionation from various human sources, these researchers found two separable CSF activities. Type-I CSF is active in mouse marrow but exhibits little or no activity in human marrow, whereas type-II CSF exhibits greater activity in human marrow. Furthermore, type-I CSF is relatively stable, but type II is labile, losing much of its activity

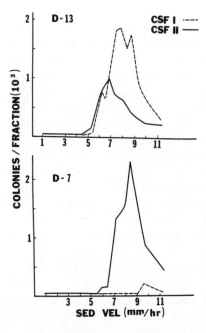

Figure 1. Heterogeneity of CFU-GM in response to types I and II CSF. Human bone marrow cells were fractionated by sedimentation velocity at unit gravity. Fractions were assayed for colony formation with CSFs I and II separately. Plates were read at days 7 (*bottom*) and 13 (*top*). The activity of the CSFs I and II in unfractionated marrow was, respectively, as follows: day 7, 4.5 and 74.5 colonies/10^5 cells; day 13, 30 and 13 colonies/10^5 cells. From *J. Clin. Invest.*, **67**, 1588 (1981) with publisher's permission.

upon purification. Type-I CSF appears to be both biologically and immunologically similar to human urinary CSF. There remained a major question regarding the significance of this so-called strictly mouse activity of type-I CSF. Because of this limited activity, its role as a stimulator of human CFU-GM growth has been neglected. If human CSF I has any role *in vivo*, it must have CFU-GM-growth promoting activity. Recent studies by Wu et al. have clearly shown that CSF I is indeed active in human marrow. When human marrow cells are fractionated by sedimentation velocity at unit gravity and the various fractions are cultured in the presence of crude human CSF (158), two CFU-GM peaks are observed (16,182) (*vide supra*), a fast-sedimenting peak forming colonies by day 7 of culture, and a slow-sedimenting peak not forming colonies until day 11–13 of culture. A similar CFU-GM profile is obtained when using purified CSF II (Figure 1). In contrast, when CSF I is used, essentially one CFU-GM peak is observed, exhibiting colonies on day 13 and having a sedimentation velocity different from that of the 13-day peak seen with CSF II. The virtual absence of 7-day colonies with CSF I offers a good explanation why "human activity" of CSF I has not been detected in the routine 7-day assay in the past. It is now clear that the so-called mouse-active CSF I is also human active and should be looked at in different perspective.

From these data it appears that the activity of CSF I is directed specifically at a CFU-GM subpopulation that forms colonies after 13 days of culture, an earlier, less-differentiated CFU-GM that is probably the immediate precursor of the 7-day CFU-GM (157). This pattern is reminiscent of the burst-forming unit (BFU-E) of erythroid precursors and their requirement for a burst-promoting activity (BPA) that is distinct from EP (183):

$$\text{CFU-S} \xrightarrow{\text{BPA}} \text{BFU-E} \xrightarrow{\text{EP}} \text{CFU-E} \rightarrow \text{erythroblasts.}$$

Thus one may postulate the following scheme for granulopoiesis:

$$\text{CFU-S} \xrightarrow{\text{CSF I?}} \text{CFU-D} \xrightarrow{\text{CSF I}} \text{CFU-GM}_{13d} \xrightarrow{\text{CSF II}} \text{CFU-GM}_{7d} \rightarrow \text{granulocytes-macrophages}$$

Whether CSF I and BPA are related has yet to be determined.

10.3. Chemical Properties of CSF

None of the purified CSFs have been fully characterized and none have been obtained in quantities sufficient for determining amino acid sequence. Most published reports indicate that CSFs are acidic glycoproteins containing sialic acid in various amounts. Evidence for this conclusion includes binding of CSFs to ConA-Sepharose columns, sensitivity to periodate oxidation, changes in pI upon treatment with neuraminidase (32,36), and, in some cases, direct PAS staining of carbohydrate in polyacrylamide gel (53, 165,175). The oligosaccharide side chain does not seem to be required for *in vitro* biological activity; treatment with neuraminidase and other glycosidases has little or no effect on the *in vitro* activity of CSF (32). In general CSFs are very sensitive to proteolytic enzymes such as pronase, chymotrypsin, and trypsin. Human type-I CSF, like urinary CSF, is quite resistant to papain digestion, and this property has been utilized in the purification procedure to remove contaminating proteins (175). Type-I CSF is relatively thermostable (30 minutes at 60°C), whereas type-II CSF is much more labile (36). Except for mouse L-cell CSF, which has two apparently identical subunits, most of the CSFs studied appear to be single polypeptides. The biological activity is unaffected by mercaptoethanol or dithiothreitol. These agents do not affect the size of type-I CSF from MIA PaCa-2 (Wu, unpublished).

10.4. Immunological Properties of CSF

Antibodies have been produced in rabbits against several CSFs including human urinary CSF (184), mouse lung CSF (185), mouse L-cell CSF (186), human pancreatic carcinoma CSFs I and II, and human lung CSF (16,32). All of the antibodies exhibit certain degrees of specificity. Thus anti-L-cell-CSF cross-inhibits human urinary CSF and endotoxin-induced mouse serum CSF, but does not cross-react with either mouse spleen or lung CSF (186). Antibody against human urinary CSF cross-inhibits type-I CSF of GCT cell but does not cross-inhibit CSF from mouse lung or L cells (184). Anti-human-lung-CSF cross-inhibits CSF from human placenta and urine but has no inhibitory effect on mouse lung CSF (32). Wu et al. (16) produced antibody in rabbits against purified type-I and type-II CSF from MIA PaCa-2. Anti-CSF-I cross-inhibits urinary CSF and CSF I from human placenta, lung, leukocytes, and human squamous cell carcinoma, but does not inhibit CSF from mouse lung or L cells. Anti-CSF-I does not inhibit CSF II. Antibody against CSF II of MIA PaCa-2 cells inhibits CSF II from all other human sources tested, but does not inhibit CSF I from the same sources. The immunological relationship between type-I and type-II CSF was also studied by competitive-binding assay (16). Type-I CSF from MIA PaCa-2 cells was found to be immunologically identical to type-I CSF from human lung and placenta, and human urine, but distinct from type II from these same sources. Thus human types I and II are immunologically distinct. Radioimmunoassay (RIA) for human type-I CSF was recently reported (16). The immunological relationship between murine CSFs has also been studied by the RIA (187,188) and competitive-receptor-binding assay (189). When anti-mouse-L-cell-CSF and radioiodinated CSF are used, no cross-binding is found between L-cell CSF and mouse lung or spleen CSF, and only partial cross-binding with WEHI-3 CSF. Further studies indicated that anti-L-cell-CSF binds to purified human urinary CSF and rat liver fibroblast CSF only at about 0.1% efficacy compared with L-cell CSF and does not bind at all to CSF from rat endotoxin-induced serum, human placenta, human embryonic kidney, GCT cells, human fetal fibroblasts, or human bone marrow fibroblasts (187).

Although human type-I CSF and mouse L-cell CSF are antigenically distinct as determined by the RIA method, recent studies by Das et al. (189) demonstrate that both CSFs compete for binding to a receptor site in a cultured macrophage cell line. The results of these radioreceptor-assay studies lend strong support to our generalization on the existence of two types of CSF in both human and mouse tissue.

11.   BIOSYNTHESIS OF CSF

Although many tissues and cell lines synthesize and secrete CSF, work on the biosynthesis of CSF has been very limited. Endotoxins and lectins stimulate CSF production in a number of CSF-producing cells, whereas lactoferrin inhibits it. The mechanisms involved in the regulation of CSF synthesis are as yet unknown. Since CSF is a secretory product and a gly-coprotein, chances are it is an N-glycosidic-linkage type of sialic-acid-containing glycoprotein, but concrete evidence for this is lacking. The antibiotic tunicamycin (TM) has been shown to specifically inhibit the syn-thesis of the N-glycosidic type of glycoproteins by blocking the transfer of sugar nucleotide to the lipid intermediate (190). In MIA PaCa-2 cells, the addition of TM at a concentration of 0.05 μg/ml inhibits [^{3}H]ᴅ-glucosamine incorporation up to 80% but does not inhibit the appearance of CSF activity in the medium (Reuben and Wu, unpublished). With fractionation of serum-free conditioned medium of TM-treated cells by IEF, CSF-I activity appears as a single peak of pI 4.75, in contrast with the control, which shows the normal multiple-peak pattern (pI 3.6–4.7) described previously (165). Further fractionation by gel filtration in phosphate buffer containing 6 M guanidine hydrochloride (162) shows a molecular weight of 50,000 daltons and 47,000 daltons for CSF I from control and TM-treated cells, respectively. Gel electrophoresis in SDS further confirmed the small molecular-weight dif-ference observed from gel filtration. Ayusawa et al. (191) have reported two types of CSF with molecular weights of 80,000 daltons and 35,000 daltons from cultured mouse mammary carcinoma FM$_3$A cells. In the presence of TM there was no reduction in total biological activity; however, only a single activity peak with molecular weight 30,000 daltons was observed in gel filtration. On the other hand, it is likely that the high molecular weight of 80,000 daltons observed in the untreated cell cultures was due to aggre-gation. Recently, Yamamoto et al. (192) have also reported the effects of TM on differentiation factors (D-factor) from mouse L cells. In the presence of TM (0.5 μg/ml), the molecular weight of D-factor is reduced from 67,000 to 25,000 daltons.

Subcellular fractionation of a CSF-producing GCT cell by DiPersio et al. (170) revealed a small pool of CSF in the cytoplasmic component with a molecular weight similar to that of the secreted CSF, but only a small amount of CSF was found in the membrane fraction. This is in contrast with the results reported by Price et al. (168), who found a strong association of CSF with membrane.

Further studies on the biosynthesis of CSF will be very important for a clear understanding of the regulation of CSF synthesis, the effect of mod-ulators, the influence of cell–cell interactions, and genetic control. For ex-ample, is the heterogeneity of CSF due to multiple-gene products or a function of post-translational modifications? If there are multiple genes, how many are there? How are they organized and regulated? If heterogeneity is a result of post-translational events, is there a pre-CSF product? How are the sugar moieties attached to the peptide? How are they synthesized and secreted?

12. PURIFICATION OF CFU-GM

In order to study the molecular mechanisms involved in CSF–CFU-GM interaction, highly purified preparations of both the hormone and its target cell are needed. In the marrow the CFU-GM constitute only about 0.05% of the total cell population. Many attempts at CFU-GM purification to date have met with only partial success. Utilizing a high-resolution density-gradient separation of rhesus monkey bone marrow cells, Moore et al. (131) obtained cell fractions containing up to 33% of CSF-responsive cells and 23% colony-forming cells (>50 cells/aggregate). The density of these cells was in the range of 1.05–1.059, and morphologically they resembled transitional lymphocytes (*vide supra*). Recent advances in flow cytometric techniques have provided new tools that are being utilized for CFU-GM purification and characterization. The flow cytometric instruments using laser optics can analyze and sort cells based on both light scattering and fluorescence. Nicola et al. obtained 50-fold enrichment of murine CFU-GM by cell sorting after tagging with fluorescently labeled lectins (193). Using similar techniques with the fucose-binding protein, Morstyn et al. have obtained populations consisting of up to 23% colony- and cluster-forming cells from human marrow (194). Selective removal of non-CFU-GM populations by monoclonal antibodies followed by sorting resulted in preparations containing 11% myeloid colony- and cluster-forming cells and 20% erythroid precursors from human marrow (195). Miller et al. (196) have utilized the binding of CSF to its target cell in attempting to purify CFU-GM. Thus incubation of bone marrow cells sequentially with highly purified CSF, anti-CSF, and fluorescent goat antirabbit γ globulin followed by sorting yielded up to 90-fold enrichment with preparations containing 11% colony- and cluster-forming cells (196,197) and 80–100% CFU-GM recovery (196). Clearly, cell sorting using a combination of parameters offers a potentially powerful tool for CFU-GM purification. For example, combining positive markers such as CSF or lectin that bind to CFU-GM with negative markers, for example, monoclonal antibodies or L-fucose binding protein, which remove or label non-CFU-GM cell populations, may yield much better results. Sorters are currently available that can discriminate between two different fluorochromes in such a way that the use of markers with different cell specificity becomes a potentially powerful approach for CFU-GM purification.

13. MECHANISM OF ACTION OF CSF

Although the absolute dependence of *in vitro* CFU-GM growth on CSF has been established beyond doubt, the mechanism(s) of CSF action remains poorly understood. Strong evidence exists that CSFs bind to myeloid cells including CFU-GM (189, 196–199). Utilizing radioiodinated CSF from L cells and human urine, known to preferentially stimulate macrophage colonies, Das et al. (189) demonstrated selective binding to a murine macrophage cell line, J 744. Shadduck et al. (198) observed that the binding of CSF to CFU-GM required 6–16 hours of incubation at 37°C but did not occur at 4°C. However, if marrow was first preincubated in medium at 37°C, rapid CSF binding could subsequently be demonstrated at 4°C. It was concluded from these studies that CSF receptors are normally occupied *in vivo*, and binding cannot occur until these receptors are freed or new receptors synthesized.

Our group has utilized indirect immunofluorescence to study CSF binding to CFU-GM (196,197). Human marrow cells preincubated with CSF and then treated with anti-CSF followed by fluorescein-labeled goat anti-rabbit-globulin (GARG) retained their ability to grow and form fluorescent aggregates in the presence of additional CSF. Thus bound CSF–anti-CSF complex appears to remain on CFU-GM membrane through at least five to six cell divisions. The relative fluorescence of marrow cells treated with CSF, its antibody, and fluorescent GARG, as determined by flow photometry, is dependent on both the length of incubation and the concentration of CSF in the incubates. These studies and those of Shadduck further suggest that new CSF receptors on CFU-GM are constantly being synthesized or made available.

Van Zant and Goldwasser have proposed that the effects of CSF and EP are antagonistic, possibly because they compete for the same receptor sites (200,201). However, Metcalf and Johnson have recently provided evidence against this postulate (202). Utilizing purified CSF and EP, they detected no competitive inhibition of CFU-GM growth. They further demonstrated that CSF will temporarily support the maintenance and limited proliferation of cells that will form erythroid, eosinophilic, and megakaryocytic colonies when subsequently exposed to their specific regulators. This observation suggested that CSF may act on an earlier multipotent progenitor cell (202).

Although it is certain that binding of CSF to CFU-GM is the initial event, the postbinding molecular events leading to CFU-GM proliferation and differentiation are poorly understood. Until recently, the unavailability of highly purified CFU-GM preparations has been a major limiting factor in these studies. Burgess and Metcalf studied the effect of CSF on RNA synthesis in mouse marrow cells *in vitro* (203,204). Significant stimulation of RNA synthesis was detected within 10 minutes, reaching a maximum at 9–11 hours. The magnitude of RNA synthesis was dependent on CSF levels. Stimulation of protein and DNA synthesis occurred at 9 and 19 hours, respectively. It is of interest that mature neutrophils contributed most to the increased RNA synthesis, indicating that in differentiated cells CSF stimulates biosynthetic processes (*vide supra*) unrelated to cell division. Wu et al. (33) have similarly noted stimulation by CSF of RNA synthesis in CFU-GM-enriched rat marrow cell preparations. The prior treatment of marrow cells with trypsin resulted in loss of response to CSF both in colony formation and stimulation of RNA synthesis.

Recent work from this laboratory (205,206) indicates that arachidonic acid metabolism may be intimately related to CSF action. Colony-stimulating factor stimulates the release of arachidonic acid from membrane phospholipids of rat peritoneal macrophages, and the released arachidonic acid is further transformed to products of cyclooxygenation and lipoxygenation (205). Furthermore, inhibitors of lipoxygenase, but not cyclooxygenase, block CSF-induced colony growth, and the block can be partially reversed by crude products of lipoxygenation (206). These results strongly suggest that lipoxygenation is an obligatory intermediary pathway for CSF action, but further studies are needed before a definite conclusion can be made.

14. ACTION OF CSF ON LEUKEMIC CFU-GM

One of the earlier observations made in the application of the clonogenic bone marrow assay system to the study of acute myelogenous leukemia (AML) was that the growth of leukemic CFU-GM is not autonomous, but instead is also dependent on CSF (8,39,207–211). However, marrow from patients with AML has a markedly reduced capacity for colony formation *in vitro* (37,174,212). Further *in vitro* marrow-culture studies coupled with karyotype and glucose 6-phosphate dehydrogenase analysis of individual colonies have clearly demonstrated the clonal origin of AML and the coexistence of normal and leukemic clones (209–213). The proliferative advantage of the leukemic clone coupled with decreased response to CSF *in vitro* and limited differentiation have raised a number of intriguing questions relevant to the pathogenesis of leukemia. For example, does leukemia cell proliferation *in vivo* occur in response to a specific growth factor distinct from normal CSF, perhaps an autostimulator? Does the leukemia cell lack responsiveness to normal differentiation factors, or is there a deficiency of these factors in leukemia?

Although factors have been found in various underlayers and conditioned media that stimulate the proliferation and differentiation of certain leukemia cell lines (214–217), there is no conclusive evidence to indicate that these factors are distinct from normal.

Recently the production of an autostimulator by a human promyelocytic cell line, HL-60, has been described (218). Its exact nature and relationship to CSF, however, have not been determined. At present it remains uncertain what growth factors the leukemic cell is responding to *in vivo*. On the other hand, the proliferative advantage of the leukemic clone may be due to cell–cell interaction, for example, suppression of the normal stem cell clone by leukemia cell products such as acidic isoferritins (121,122).

The block in cell differentiation in leukemia may be entirely a function of the leukemia cell. In support of this possibility is the work of Sachs et al. (219). These workers tested the action of a macrophage-granulocyte–inducer protein (MGI) (220–221) on a mouse leukemia cell line (214) and were able to distinguish between two leukemic cell populations, those cells responding to MGI by undergoing proliferation and differentiation into macrophages and/or granulocytes (D +) and those undergoing proliferation without differentiation (D −) (219). They further showed in genetic-segregation studies that D + gives D + and D − gives D − progeny. This pattern could be demonstrated in myeloid leukemia cells of both mouse and man. Since some leukemic cells can be induced to differentiate by certain factors *in vitro*, the possibility still exists that such factors are either altered or deficient *in vivo*. Unfortunately, data on the level of CSF in sera from patients with leukemia including AML are conflicting and have to be reassessed in the light of the recent observations by Wu et al. on two functionally and immunologically distinct types of CSF in human tissues (13,16). For example, CSF I appears to act on an earlier stage of CFU-GM and may act primarily to stimulate proliferation. The CSF II, on the other hand, may act primarily as a differentiation factor. The question must then be asked whether an imbalance between CSF I and CSF II exists in AML. Although this remains largely speculative at present, it is clear that one must specifically assay for CSFs I and II to answer this question.

Elucidation of the factors that induce proliferation and/or differentiation of leukemic cells could have a considerable impact on the therapy of AML. Many of the pathologic effects of the disease could be reversed if one could force leukemic cells to differentiate. When cells from a mouse leukemic cell line are induced to differentiate and then injected into syngeneic mice, a higher percentage of those mice survive than control mice injected with untreated cells (215,222). On the other hand, inducing leukemic cells from the resting phase into cycle by CSF renders them more vulnerable to cycle-specific chemotherapeutic agents. Clearly there is need to constantly search for and define new CSF species as well as to prepare large amounts of highly purified material in order to explore their therapeutic potential.

15. ALTERATION IN CSF, CFU-GM, AND THEIR INTERACTIONS: CLINICAL APPLICATION

Although our understanding of the regulatory control of granulopoiesis is currently far too imcomplete, the application of the CFU-GM assay system to various hematopoietic disorders has provided new and useful information concerning pathogenetic mechanisms and approaches to diagnosis and therapy. Accordingly, it has found wide clinical utility. Unfortunately, this area has been beset by considerable confusion and inconsistency resulting from variations in technique among laboratories, lack of a standard source of CSF, use of various crude CSF preparations probably with varied inhibitor activity, use of mouse versus human marrow, fractionated versus whole marrow cell suspensions, and so forth. Nevertheless, there is sufficient agreement in a number of clinical settings to warrant serious consideration. These are summarized below.

15.1. Neutropenia

In view of the inherent difficulties in quantitating granulocyte production and destruction, a detailed classification of the neutropenias according to increased destruction compared with decreased production has not been possible. The CFU-GM assay has been found useful in this regard. In general, neutropenias resulting from increased granulocyte destruction are characterized by increased numbers of bone marrow CFU-GM and the percentage in S phase, indicating rapid neutrophil turnover (223–225). The serum and urine CSF levels are usually increased. Examples of these neutropenias include the immune neutropenias, hypersplenism, and overwhelming infections. Decreased numbers of bone marrow CFU-GMs characterize neutropenias resulting from decreased production such as myeloid hypoplasia, Felty's syndrome, and some cases of idiopathic neutropenia (223, 226–230). Other cases of idiopathic neutropenia have increased CFU-GM, suggesting the heterogeneity of this disorder (231–234).

15.2. Aplastic Anemia

As expected, the bone marrow CFU-GMs are decreased to absent in aplastic anemia. More importantly, the CFU-GM assay has, in some cases, proved useful in clarifying pathogenetic mechanisms. Thus cell-mediated inhibition of granulopoiesis has been demonstrated in a significant number of cases (235–238). In such cases removal of lymphocytes from the marrow or pretreatment of marrow cells with anti-thymocyte globulin (ATG) and complement results in restoration of CFU-GM growth. Some of these patients show hematological response to ATG. Other patients with aplastic anemia have serum inhibitory factors. In a recent study by Abdou et al. (239) 3 of 21 patients with aplastic anemia had serum immunoglobulins directed against their marrow CFU-GM; plasmapheresis resulted in recovery of marrow function. Three others had suppressor T cells; one of these responded to ATG and one recovered spontaneously. In 12 of the 21 patients no pathogenetic mechanism was suggested by the study.

In spite of technical pitfalls and possible errors in interpretation in some of the studies reported, the CFU-GM assay has added new dimensions to the evaluation and management of patients with aplastic anemia. Perhaps more importantly, it has uncovered the heterogeneity of pathogenetic mechanisms in this disease.

15.3. Acute Myelogenous Leukemia

The leukemic CFU-GM, like the normal, is dependent on CSF for *in vitro* growth. However, it exhibits a characteristic defect of impaired proliferation and differentiation even in the presence of optimal or supraoptimal CSF levels (240–244). This defective growth pattern ranges from nongrowing, or cluster formation only, to small colonies with an excess of clusters. There is agreement among many workers that the identification of the growth pattern is of predictive value in determining patient response to therapy and remission rate (242,244–247). Patients in whom microcluster formation (3–20 cells) predominates and those with a normal growth pattern are said to have a more favorable prognosis. Patients with macrocluster formation (up to 40 cells) and those whose cells form small colonies with an abnormal cluster:colony ratio have an unfavorable prognosis (248). In addition to the abnormal growth pattern, the leukemic CFU-GMs can be distinguished from the normal CFU-GMs by their lighter density (<1.062 g/cm^3). Remission of the disease is often heralded by a return of the growth pattern and the CFU-GM density distribution to normal.

15.4. Chronic Myelogenous Leukemia

The expanded myeloid mass in this disease is reflected by a 15-fold increase in the number of CFU-GM in the marrow and up to 500-fold increase in the number of CFU-GM in the peripheral circulation (248). Colony size is normal, as is the colony:cluster ratio. As in AML, the CFU-GM exhibits a shift to light density. This CFU-GM is similar to the CFU-GM of human fetal liver between 9 and 14 weeks of gestation, suggesting an oncofetal transformation. Blastic transformation in this disease is often heralded by a change to a proliferation pattern similar to that seen in AML.

15.5. Myeloproliferative Disorders and Preleukemic States

Myeloproliferative disorders such as chronic myelogenous leukemia, myeloid metaplasia with myelofibrosis, and polycythemia vera are known to undergo transformation to acute myelocytic or myelomonocytic leukemia (preleukemic states). A sequential study of the CFU-GM in such patients has been of value in predicting this terminal event. Thus the appearance of an abnormal or "leukemic" growth pattern (similar to that in AML) along with elevations in serum and urinary CSF often precede blastic transformation by 3–14 months (239,248). Similar observations have been made in certain refractory anemias, including sideroblastic anemia, which also have a propensity for termination in acute leukemia (241,248–250).

16. CONCLUDING REMARKS

It is evident that our knowledge of the control of granulopoiesis is at present far too incomplete and uncertain to allow the construction of any definite and meaningful scheme. Clearly CSF plays a critical role in granulopoiesis *in vitro*, but the existing evidence for its *in vivo* role, although persuasive, cannot yet be considered conclusive. If CSF is a true granulopoietin *in vivo*, how might one explain its ubiquitous occurrence and the fact that so many tissues are capable of its production? The answer to this question now can only be speculative. The possibility that CSF might exert some other metabolic effects or functions independent of its action on granulopoiesis cannot be excluded.

Even less certain is the role of various modulators. Attractive postulates have been put forth regarding the role of substances such as lactoferrin, isoferritins, PGs, and so forth, in the feedback control of granulopoiesis. Unfortunately, these are based largely on *in vitro* observations, none of which can yet be safely assumed to apply *in vivo*.

It became apparent through the use of the standard mouse assay that CSF is a heterogeneous family of stimulator molecules exhibiting both interspecies and intraspecies differences. The finding that some human CSF preparations are active in mouse marrow, but show little or no activity in human marrow was until recently a source of confusion and controversy. The discovery in our laboratory of a common pattern of two distinct types of CSF in human tissues and cultured cells, one stable "mouse-active" factor (CSF I) and another labile human-active factor (CSF II), has largely resolved this problem. The CSF I, which exhibits little or no activity in unfractionated human marrow in the usual 7-day assay, is active on a subpopulation of human CFU-GM that form colonies after 13 days. Thus CSF I acts on a less-differentiated CFU-GM, probably the immediate precursor of the CSF-II-responsive 7-day CFU-GM. The CSFs I and II are also biochemically and immunologically distinct. The biological implications of these findings are very clear. Studies dealing with human granulopoiesis must now take into consideration these two distinct CSFs. For example, many of the results of previous studies involving CSF assays in human sera and conclusions derived from them have to be reexamined. A more meaningful determination of a "normal CSF profile" in serum and urine of a given patient might include (1) immunoassays for CSFs I and II, (2) biological 7- and 13-day assays in human marrow, and (3) biological assay in mouse marrow. One might then be able to assess deviations from this normal pattern in various disorders of granulopoiesis. The precise role of CSFs I and II in CFU-GM proliferation and differentiation and their differential actions on normal compared with leukemic CFU-GM should be of great interest.

Future research must deal with the basic questions of the exact biochemical differences between CSFs I and II, possible microheterogeneity, the genetic control of their production, the mechanism of synthesis and secretion, the intracellular distribution, the mechanism of action, the nature of CSF receptors, and the molecular interaction of CSF with normal and leukemic CFU-GM. Answers to these and other questions must ultimately come from studies with pure preparations of CSFs I and II and their target cells. Also, the preparation of specific monoclonal antibodies to CSFs I and II should facilitate many of these investigations. The availability of pure CSFs I and II and their antibodies will ultimately help clarify the role of CSF *in vivo*. A human pancreatic carcinoma cell line (MIA PaCa-2) established in our laboratory has proved to be an excellent source for CSF. Both CSFs I and II from MIA PaCa-2 have been purified to apparent homogeneity. However, the amounts of purified protein obtained have thus far been too limited to allow detailed biochemical studies. This limitation will likely continue to be a problem unless CSF is produced by gene-cloning techniques. The availability of cell lines such as MIA PaCa-2 that actively produce CSF should make this approach feasible.

ACKNOWLEDGMENTS

Work done by the authors was supported by USPHS grants AM 26218, CA 19182, AM 07114, AM 26207, and CA 00686, and by the Howard Hughes Medical Institute.

REFERENCES

1. Becker, A. J., McCulloch, E. A., and Till, J. E., *Nature*, **197**, 452 (1963).
2. Pluznik, D. H., and Sachs, L., *J. Cell. Comp. Physiol.*, **66**, 319 (1965).
3. Bradley, T. R., and Metcalf, D., *Aust. J. Exp. Biol. Med. Sci.*, **44**, 287 (1966).
4. Burgess, A. W., and Metcalf, D., *Blood*, **56**, 947 (1980).

5. Brennan, J. K., Lichtman, M. A., DiPersio, J. F., and Abboud, C. N., *Exp. Hematol.*, **8**, 441 (1980).
6. Quesenberry, P., and Levitt, L., *N. Engl. J. Med.*, **301**, 755 (1979).
7. Till, J. E., and McCulloch, E. A., *Biochim. Biophys. Acta*, **605**, 431 (1980).
8. Pike, B. L., and Robinson, W. A., *J. Cell. Physiol.*, **76**, 77 (1970).
9. Paran, M., and Sachs, L., *J. Cell. Physiol.*, **72**, 247 (1968).
10. Metcalf, D., *J. Cell. Physiol.*, **76**, 89 (1970).
11. Chan, S. H., *Aust. J. Exp. Biol. Med. Sci.*, **49**, 553 (1971).
12. Bol, S., and Williams, N., *J. Cell. Physiol.*, **102**, 233 (1980).
13. Wu, M.-C., and Yunis, A. A., *J. Clin. Invest.*, **65**, 722 (1980).
14. Lind, D. E., Bradley, M. L., Gunz, F. W., and Vincent, P. C., *J. Cell. Physiol.*, **83**, 35 (1974).
15. Inoue, S., and Ottenbreit, M. J., *Blood*, **51**, 195 (1978).
16. Wu, M.-C., Miller, A. M., and Yunis, A. A., *J. Clin. Invest.*, **67**, 1588 (1981).
17. Metcalf, D., *J. Cell. Physiol.*, **77**, 277 (1971).
18. Levi-Montalcini, R., and Angeletti, P. U., *Dev. Biol.*, **7**, 653 (1963).
19. Iscove, N. N., in C. F. Fox, Ed., *Hemopoietic Cell Differentiation*, Academic, New York, 1978, p. 37.
20. Handman, E., and Burgess, A. W., *J. Immunol.*, **122**, 1134 (1979).
21. Lin, H.-S., and Gordon, S., *J. Exp. Med.*, **150**, 231 (1979).
22. Kurland, J. I., Broxmeyer, H. E., Pelus, L. M., Bockman, R. S., and Moore, M. A. S., *Blood*, **52**, 388 (1978).
23. Kurland, J., and Moore, M. A. S., *Exp. Hematol.*, **5**, 357 (1977).
24. Kurland, J., and Moore, M. A. S., in S. Baum and D. Ledney, Eds., *Experimental Hematology Today*, Springer-Verlag, New York, 1977, p. 51.
25. Kurland, J. I., Bockman, R. S., Broxmeyer, H. E., and Moore, M. A. S., *Science*, **199**, 552 (1978).
26. Sheridan, J. W., and Stanley, E. R., *J. Cell. Physiol.*, **78**, 451 (1971).
27. Bradley, T. R., Stanley, E. R., and Sumner, M. A., *Aust. J. Exp. Biol. Med. Sci.*, **49**, 595 (1971).
28. Burgess, A. W., Metcalf, D., Russell, S. H. M., and Nicola, N. A., *Biochem. J.*, **185**, 301 (1980).
29. Stanley, E. R., Bradley, T. R., and Sumner, M. A., *J. Cell. Physiol.*, **78**, 301 (1971).
30. Sheridan, J. W., and Metcalf, D., *J. Cell. Physiol.*, **81**, 11 (1973).
31. Fojo, S. S., Wu, M.-C., Gross, M. A., and Yunis, A. A., *Biochim. Biophys. Acta*, **494**, 92 (1977).
32. Fojo, S. S., Wu, M.-C., Gross, M. A., Purcell, Y., and Yunis, A. A., *Biochemistry*, **17**, 3109.
33. Wu, M.-C., Fojo, S. S., and Yunis, A. A., in W. J. Whelan and J. Schultz, Eds., *Differentiation and Development*, Academic, New York, 1978, p. 93.
34. Ratzan, R. J., and Yunis, A. A., *Clin. Res.*, **22**, 402A (1974).
35. Burgess, A. W., Wilson, E. M. A., and Metcalf, D., *Blood*, **49**, 573 (1977).
36. Wu, M.-C., and Fischer, R. A., *Biochemistry*, **19**, 3846 (1980).
37. Brown, C. A., and Carbone, P. O., *J. Natl. Cancer Inst.*, **46**, 989 (1971).

38. Mintz, U., and Sachs, L., *Blood*, **41**, 745 (1973).

39. Paran, M., Sachs, L., Barak, Y., and Resnitzky, P., *Proc. Natl. Acad. Sci. USA*, **67**, 1542 (1970).

40. Golde, D. W., Finley, T. N., and Cline, M. J., *Lancet*, **2**, 1397 (1972).

41. Stanley, E. R., and Metcalf, D., *Aust. J. Exp. Biol. Med. Sci.*, **47**, 467 (1966).

42. Shah, R. G., Caporale, L. H., and Moore, M. A. S., *Blood*, **50**, 811 (1977).

43. Chervenick, P. A., and Lo Buglio, A. F., *Science*, **178**, 164 (1972).

44. Golde, D. W., and Cline, M. J., *J. Clin. Invest.*, **51**, 2981 (1972).

45. Parker, J. W., and Metcalf, D., *J. Immunol.*, **112**, 502 (1974).

46. Wu, A. M., *J. Cell. Physiol.*, **101**, 237 (1979).

47. Cline, M. J., and Golde, D. W., *Nature*, **248**, 703 (1974).

48. Ruscetti, F. W., and Chervenick, P. A., *J. Clin. Invest.*, **55**, 520 (1975).

49. Quesenberry, P. J., Gimbrone, M. A., and McDonald, M. J., *Exp. Hematol.*, **6**, 4 (1978).

50. Knudtzon, S., and Mortensen, B. T., *Blood*, **46**, 937 (1975).

51. Yunis, A. A., Arimura, G. K., Wu, M.-C., Gross, M. A., and Purcell, Y., *FEBS Lett.*, **90**, 279 (1978).

52. Stanley, E. R., and Heard, P. M., *J. Biol. Chem.*, **252**, 4305 (1977).

53. Waheed, A., and Shadduck, R. K., *J. Lab. Clin. Med.*, **94**, 180 (1979).

54. Howard, M., Burgess, A. W., McPhee, D., and Metcalf, D., *Cell*, **18**, 993 (1979).

55. Burgess, A. W., Camakaris, J., and Metcalf, D., *J. Biol. Chem.*, **252**, 1998 (1977).

56. Williams, N., Eger, R. R., Moore, M. A. S., and Mendelsohn, N., *Differentiation*, **11**, 59 (1978).

57. Ohno, T., Seki, M., and Shikita, M., *Blood*, **51**, 911 (1978).

58. Okabe, T., Sato, N., Kondo, Y., Asano, S., Ohsawa, N., Kosaka, K., and Ueyama, Y., *Cancer Res.*, **38**, 3910 (1978).

59. Golde, D. W., Quan, S. G., and Cline, M. J., *Blood*, **52**, 1068 (1978).

60. Svet-Moldavsky, G. J., Zinzar, S. N., Svet-Moldavskaya, I. A., Mann, P. E., Holland, J. F., Fogh, J., Arlin, Z., and Clarkson, B. D., *Exp. Hematol.*, **8** (Suppl. 7), 133 (1980).

61. Yunis, A. A., Arimura, G. K., and Russin, D. J., *Int. J. Cancer*, **19**, 128 (1977).

62. Lieber, M., Mazzetta, J., Nelson-Rees, W., Kaplan, M., and Todaro, G., *Int. J. Cancer*, **15**, 741 (1975).

63. Meck, R. A., Ingram, M., Meck, J. M., McCullough, J. L., Wu, M.-C., and Yunis, A. A., *Cancer Res.*, **41**, 1076 (1981).

64. Shadduck, R. K., and Nunna, N. G., *Proc. Soc. Exp. Biol. Med.*, **137**, 1479 (1971).

65. Shadduck, R. K., and Nagablushanam, N. G., *Blood*, **38**, 559 (1971).

66. Metcalf, D., *Immunology*, **21**, 427 (1971).

67. Niskanen, E., Quesenberry, P., Stohlman, F., Jr., Levin, J., and Ryan, M., *Proc. Soc. Exp. Biol. Med.*, **143**, 176 (1973).

68. Quesenberry, P., Morley, A., Stohlman, F., Jr., Rickard, K., Howard, D., and Smith, M., *N. Engl. J. Med.*, **286**, 227 (1972).

69. Quesenberry, P., Halperin, J., Ryan, M., and Stohlman, F., Jr., *Blood*, **45**, 789 (1975).

70. Metcalf, D., and Wilson, J. W., *J. Cell. Physiol.*, **89**, 381 (1976).

71. Zidar, B. L., and Shadduck, R. K., *J. Lab. Clin. Med.*, **91**, 584 (1978).

72. Hinterberger, W., Paukovits, W., and Mittermayer, K., *Scand. J. Hematol.*, **22**, 280 (1979).

73. Dale, D. C., Brown, C. H., Carbone, P., and Wolfe, S. M., *Science*, **173**, 152 (1971).

74. Moore, M. A. S., Spitzer, G., Metcalf, D., and Pennington, D. G., *Br. J. Hematol.*, **27**, 47 (1974).

75. Metcalf, D., Moore, M. A. S., and Warner, N. L., *J. Natl. Cancer Inst.*, **43**, 983 (1969).

76. Robinson, W. A., and Pike, B. L., *N. Engl. J. Med.*, **282**, 1291 (1970).

77. Sato, N., Asano, S., Ueyama, Y., Mori, M., Okabe, T., Kondo, Y., Ohsawa, N., and Kosaka, K., *Cancer*, **43**, 605 (1979).

78. Asano, S., Urabe, A., Okabe, T., Sato, N., Kondo, Y., Ueyama, Y., Chiba, S., Ohsawa, N., and Kosaka, K., *Blood*, **49**, 845 (1977).

79. Gordon, A. S., Zanjani, E. D., Gidari, A. S., and Kuna, R. A., in J. LoBue and A. S. Gordon, Eds., *Humoral Control of Growth and Differentiation*, Academic, New York, Vol. I, 1973, p. 25.

80. McGarry, M. P., Miller, A. M., and Colley, D. G., in S. J. Baum and G. D. Ledney, Eds., *Experimental Hemotology Today*, Springer-Verlag, New York, 1976, pp. 63–70.

81. Metcalf, D., and Stanley, E. R., *Br. J. Haematol.*, **20**, 549 (1971).

82. Metcalf, D., and Stanley, E. R., *Br. J. Haematol.*, **21**, 481 (1971).

83. Shadduck, R. K., Waheed, A., Porcellina, A., Rizzoli, V., and Pigoli, G., *Blood*, **54**, 894 (1979).

84. Shadduck, R. K., Carsten, A. L., Chikkappa, G., Cronkite, E. P., and Gerard, E., *Proc. Soc. Exp. Biol. Med.*, **158**, 542 (1978).

85. Burgess, A. W., and Metcalf, D., *Exp. Hematol.*, **5**, 456 (1977).

86. Tisman, G., and Herbert, V., *In Vitro*, **9**, 86 (1973).

87. Morley, A., Quesenberry, P., Garrity, M. and Stohlman, F., Jr., *Proc. Soc. Exp. Biol. Med.*, **138**, 57 (1971).

88. Oshita, A. K., Rothstein, G., and Lonngi, G., *Blood*, **49**, 585 (1977).

89. Pelus, L. M., Broxmeyer, H. E., Moore, M. A. S., *Cell Tissue Kinet.*, **14**, 515 (1981).

90. Moore, R. N., Urbascher, R., Wahl, L. M., and Mergenhagen, S. E., *Infect. Immun.*, **26**, 408 (1979).

91. Miller, A. M., Russell, T. R., Gross, M. A., and Yunis, A. A., *J. Lab. Clin. Med.*, **92**, 983 (1978).

92. Ziboh, V. A., Miller, A. M., Yunis, A. A., Jimenez, J. J., and Kursunoglu, I., *Cancer Res.*, **41**, 12 (1981).

93. Ziboh, V. A., Lord, J. I., Blick, G., Kursunuglu, I., Poietier, L., and Yunis, A. A., *Cancer Res.*, **37**, 3974 (1980).

94. Taetle, R., and Mendelsohn, J., *Blood Cells*, **6**, 679 (1980).

95. O'Connell, R. A., *Int. Pharmacopsychiat.*, **4**, 30 (1970).

96. Shopsin, B., and Gershon, S., *Clin. Pharmacol. Ther.*, **12**, 923 (1971).

97. Murphy, D. L., Goodwin, F. K., and Bunney, W. E., *Am. J. Psychiatry*, **127**, 1559 (1971).

98. Gupta, R., Robinson, W. A., and Albrecht, D., *Ann. Rheum. Dis.*, **34**, 156 (1975).

99. Tisman, G., Herbert, V., and Rosenblatt, S., *Br. J. Haematol.*, **24**, 767 (1973).

100. Barret, A. J., Longhurst, P. A., and Humbis, J. G., *Exp. Hematol.*, **4**, (Suppl) p. 43 (1976) (Abstract).

101. Rothstein, G., Clarkson, D. R., Larsen, W., Grosser, B. I., and Athens, J. W., *N. Engl. J. Med.*, **298**, 178 (1978).

102. Miller, A. M., and Yunis, A. A., *Exp. Hematol.*, **9**, 775 (1981).

103. Harker, W. G., Rothstein, G., Glarson, D., Athens, J. W., and McFarlane, J. L., *Blood*, **49**, 263 (1977).

104. Spitzer, G., Verma, D. S., Barlogie, B., Beran, M. A., and Dicke, K. A., *Cancer Res.*, **39**, 3215 (1979).

105. Richman, C. M., Kinnealey, A., and Hoffman, P. C., *Exp. Hematol.*, **9**, 449 (1981).

106. Yunis, A. A., and Adamson, J. W., *Am. J. Hematol.*, **2**, 355 (1977).

107. Levitt, L. J., and Quesenberry, P. J., *N. Engl. J. Med.*, **302**, 713 (1980).

108. Golde, D. W., Bersch, N., and Cline, M. J., *J. Clin. Invest.*, **57**, 57 (1976).

109. Gidari, A. S., and Levere, R. D., *J. Lab. Clin. Med.*, **93**, 872 (1979).

110. Zalman, F., Maloney, M., and Patt, H. M., *J. Exp. Med.*, **149**, 67 (1979).

111. Urabe, A., Hamilton, J., and Sassa, S., *Br. J. Haematol.*, **43**, 479 (1979).

112. Singer, J. W., Samuels, A. I., and Adamson, J. W., *J. Cell. Physiol.*, **88**, 127 (1976).

113. Golde, D. W., Bersch, N., Quan, S. G., and Cline, M. J., *Am. J. Hematol.*, **1**, 369 (1976).

114. Metcalf, D., *Proc. Soc. Exp. Biol. Med.*, **132**, 391 (1969).

115. Bagby, G. C., Jr., Goodnight, S. H., Mooney, W. M., and Richers-Boe, K., *Blood*, **54**, 322 (1980).

116. Broxmeyer, H. E., Moore, M. A. S., and Ralph, P., *Exp. Hematol.*, **5**, 87 (1976).

117. Broxmeyer, H. E., Smithyman, A., Eger, R. R., Meyers, P. A., and DeSousa, M., *J. Exp. Med.*, **148**, 1052 (1978).

118. Broxmeyer, H. E., DeSousa, M., Smithyman, A., Ralph, P., Hamilton, J., Kurland, J. I., and Bognacki, J., *Blood*, **55**, 324 (1980).

119. Gurney, C. W., and Fried, W., *Proc. Natl. Acad. Sci. USA*, **54**, 1148 (1965).

120. Bruce, W. R., and McCulloch, E. A., *Blood*, **23**, 216 (1964).

121. Broxmeyer, H. E., Jacobsen, N., Kurland, J., Mendelsohn, N., and Moore, M. A. S., *J. Natl. Cancer Inst.*, **60**, 497 (1978).

122. Broxmeyer, H. E., Bognacki, J., Dorner, M. H., and De Sousa, M., *J. Exp. Med.*, **153**, 1426 (1981).

123. Rytomaa, T., in P. Farnes, Ed., *Hemic Cells in Vitro*, Williams and Wilkins, Baltimore, 1969, p. 47.

124. Baker, F. L., and Galbraith, P. R., *Blood*, **52**, 241 (1978).

125. Bolin, R. W., and Robinson, W. H., *Am. J. Hematol.*, **6**, 1 (1979).

126. Baker, F. L., and Galbraith, P. R., *Blood*, **53**, 304 (1979).

127. Heit, W., Kern, P., Kubanek, B., and Heimpel, H., *Blood*, **44**, 511 (1974).

128. Greenberg, P. L., and Mosney, S. A., *Cancer Res.*, **37**, 1794 (1977).

129. McNeill, T. A., *Immunology*, **18**, 39 (1970).

130. Bradley, T. R., Telfer, P. A., and Fry, P., *Blood*, **38**, 353 (1971).

131. Moore, M. A. S., Williams, N., and Metcalf, D., *J. Cell. Physiol.*, **79**, 283 (1972).

132. Rickard, K. A., Shadduck, R. K., Howard, D. E., and Stohlman, F., Jr., *Proc. Soc. Exp. Biol. Med.*, **134**, 152 (1970).

133. Iscove, N. N., Till, J. E., and McCulloch, E. A., *Proc. Soc. Exp. Biol. Med.*, **134**, 33 (1970).

134. Worton, R. G., McCulloch, E. A., and Till, J. E., *J. Cell Physiol.*, **74**, 171 (1969).

135. Haskill, J. S., McNeil, T. A., and Moore, M. A. S., *J. Cell. Physiol.*, **75**, 167 (1970).

136. Metcalf, D., Moore, M. A. S., and Shortman, K., *J. Cell. Physiol.*, **78**, 441 (1971).

137. Lajtha, L. G., Pozzi, L. V., and Schofield, R., *Cell Tissue Kinet.*, **2**, 39 (1969).

138. Rickard, K. A., Morley, A., Howard, D., and Stohlman, F., Jr., *Blood*, **37**, 6 (1971).

139. Morley, A., Rickard, K. A., Howard, D., and Stohlman, F., Jr., *Blood*, **37**, 14 (1971).

140. Chen, M. G., and Schooley, J. C., *J. Cell. Physiol.*, **75**, 89 (1970).

141. Sumner, M. A., Bradley, T. R., and Hodgson, G. S., *Br. J. Haematol.*, **23**, 221 (1972).

142. Sutherland, D. J. A., Till, J. E., and McCulloch, E. A., *Cell Tissue Kinet.*, **4**, 479 (1971).

143. Moore, M. A. S., and Williams, N., in W. A. Robinson, Ed., *Hemopoiesis in Culture: Second International Workshop*, DHEW Publication NIH 74-205, U.S. Government Printing Office, Washington, D.C., 1973, p. 17.

144. Richman, C. M., Chess, L., and Yankee, R. A., *Blood*, **51**, 1 (1978).

145. Moore, M. A. S., *Clin. Hematol.*, **8**, 287 (1979).

146. Fitcher, J. H., and Cline, M. J., *Blood*, **53**, 794 (1979).

147. Fitcher, J. H., Ferrone, S., Quaranta, V., Molinaro, G. A., and Cline, M. J., *J. Immunol.*, **125**, 2004 (1980).

148. Foor, K. A., Fitcher, J. H., Billing, R., Belzer, M. B., Terasaki, P. I., and Cline, M. J., *Clin. Immunol. Immunopathol.*, **16**, 416 (1980).

149. Taetle, R., and Royston, I., *Blood*, **56**, 943 (1980).

150. Foor, K. A., Fitcher, J. H., Billing, R., Belzer, M. B., Terasaki, P. I., and Cline, M. J., in R. P. Gale and C. F. Fox, Eds., *ICN-UCLA Symposium on Molecular and Cellular Biology*, Academic, New York, Vol. 16, 1980, p. 477.

151. Fitcher, J. H., Foor, K. A., and Cline M. J., *N. Engl. J. Med.*, **305**, 17 (1981).

152. Janoshwitz, H., Moore, M. A. S., and Metcalf, D., *Exp. Cell Res.*, **68**, 220 (1971).

153. Byrne, P., Heit, W., and Kubanek, B., *Cell Tissue Kinet.*, **10**, 341 (1977).

154. Das, C., Metcalf, D., and Bilski-Pasquier, G., *Blood*, **50**, 833 (1977).

155. Morley, A., Quesenberry, P., Garitty, M., and Stohlman, F., Jr., *Proc. Soc. Exp. Biol. Med.*, **138**, 57 (1971).

156. Johnson, G. R., Dresch, C., and Metcalf, D., *Blood*, **50**, 823 (1977).

157. Jacobsen, N., Broxmeyer, H. E., Grossbard, E., and Moore, M. A. S., *Blood*, **51**, 221 (1978).

158. Miller, A. M., Gross, M. A., and Yunis, A. A., *J. Lab. Clin. Med.*, **92**, 38 (1978).

159. Dresch, C., Faille, A., Poirier, O., Balitrand, N., and Nan Jean, Y., *Exp. Hematol.*, **7**, 337 (1979).

160. Miller, A. M., Gross, M. A., and Yunis, A. A., *Exp. Hematol.*, **8**, 236 (1980).

161. Jacobsen, N., Broxmeyer, H. E., Grossbard, E., and Moore, M. A. S., *Cell Tissue Kinet.*, **12**, 213 (1979).

162. Nicola, N. A., Burgess, A. W., and Metcalf, D., *J. Biol. Chem.*, **254**, 5290 (1979).

163. Nicola, N. A., Metcalf, D., Johnson, G. R., and Burgess, A. W., *Leuk. Res.*, **2**, 313 (1978).

164. DiPersio, J., Brennan, J. K., Lichtman, M. A., and Speise, B. L., *Blood*, **51**, 507 (1978).

165. Wu, M.-C., Cini, J. K., and Yunis, A. A., *J. Biol. Chem.*, **254**, 6226 (1979).

166. Wu, M.-C., Arimura, G. K., and Yunis, A. A., *Biochemistry*, **16**, 1908 (1977).

167. Iscove, N. N., Senn, J. S., Till, J. E., and McCulloch, E. A., *Blood*, **37**, 1 (1971).

168. Price, G. B., Senn, J. S., McCulloch, E. A., and Till, J. E., *Biochem. J.*, **148**, 209 (1975).

169. Nicola, N. A., Metcalf, D., Johnson, G. R., and Burgess, A. W., *Blood*, **54**, 614 (1979).

170. DiPersio, J. F., Brennan, J. K., Lichtman, M. A., Abboud, C. N., and Kirkpatrick, F. H., *Blood*, **56**, 717 (1980).

171. Lusis, A. J., Quon, D. H., and Golde, D., *Blood*, **57**, 13 (1981).

172. Guez, M., and Sachs, L., *FEBS Lett.*, **37**, 149 (1973).

173. Landau, T., and Sachs, L., *FEBS Lett.*, **17**, 339 (1971).

174. Robinson, W. A., Stanley, E. R., and Metcalf, D., *Blood*, **33**, 396 (1969).

175. Stanley, E. R., Hansen, G., Woodcock, J., and Metcalf, D., *Fed. Proc.*, **34**, 2272 (1975).

176. Metcalf, D., *Exp. Hematol.*, **2**, 157 (1974).

177. Motoyoshi, K., Takaku, F., Mizoguchi, H., and Miura, Y., *Blood*, **52**, 1012 (1978).

178. Wu, M.-C., Miller, A. M., and Yunis, A. A., *Exp. Hematol.*, **8**, (Suppl. 7) 9 (1980).

179. Burgess, A. W., and Staber, F. G., *J. Cell. Physiol.*, **102**, 1 (1980).

180. Horiuchi, M., and Ichikawa, Y., *Exp. Cell Res.*, **110**, 79 (1977).

181. Johnson, G. R., and Burgess, A. W., *J. Cell. Physiol.*, **102**, 1 (1980).

182. Wu, M.-C., Miller, A. M., and Yunis, A. A., in W. A. Scott, R. Werner, J. Schultz, and L. W. Mozes, Eds., *Cellular Response to Molecular Modulators*, Academic, New York, 1981, p. 219.

183. Peschle, C., *Annu. Rev. Med.*, **31**, 303 (1980).

184. Stanley, E. R., McNeill, T. A., and Chan, S. H., *Br. J. Haematol.*, **18**, 585 (1969).

185. Sheridan, J. W., Metcalf, D., and Stanley, E. R., *J. Cell. Physiol.*, **84**, 147 (1974).

186. Shadduck, R. K., and Metcalf, D., *J. Cell. Physiol.*, **86**, 247 (1975).

187. Stanley, E. R., *Proc. Natl. Acad. Sci. USA*, **76**, 2969 (1979).

188. Shadduck, R. K., and Waheed, A., *Blood Cells*, **5**, 421 (1979).

189. Das, S. K., Stanley, E. R., Guilbert, L. J., and Forman, L. W., *J. Cell. Physiol.*, **104**, 359 (1980).

190. Heath, E. C., Brinkley, S. A., Haugen, T. H., Das, R. C., and Oeltman, T. N., in T. R. Russell, K. Brew, J. Schultz, and H. Faber, Eds., *From Gene to Protein: Information Transfer in Normal and Abnormal Cells*, Academic, New York, 1979, p. 379.

191. Ayusawa, D., Isaka, K., Seno, T., Tomida, M., Yamamoto, Y., Hozumi, M., Takatsuki, A., and Tamura, G., *Biochem. Biophys. Res. Commun.*, **90**, 783 (1979).

192. Yamamoto, Y., Tomida, M., Hozumi, M., Ayusawa, D., Seno, T., and Tamura, G., *Cancer Res.*, **41**, 2534 (1981).

193. Nicola, N. A., Burgess, A. W., Staber, G., Johnson, G. K., Metcalf, D., and Battye, T. L., *J. Cell. Physiol.*, **103**, 217 (1980).

194. Morstyn, G., Nicola, N. A., and Metcalf, D., *Blood*, **56**, 798 (1980).

195. Beverly, P. C. L., Linch, D., and Delia, D., *Nature*, **287**, 332 (1980).

196. Miller, A. M., Wu, M.-C., Files, N., Ingram, M., and Yunis, A. A., *Stem Cell.*, **1**, 193 (1981).

197. Yunis, A. A., Wu, M.-C., Miller, A. M., Ingram, M., and Files, N., *Blood Cells*, **679** (1980).

198. Shadduck, R. K., Waheed, A., and Caramatti, C., *Clin. Res.*, **29**, 522A (1981).

199. Metcalf, D., Johnson, G. R., and Burgess, A. W., *Blood*, **55**, 138 (1980).

200. Van Zant, G., and Goldwasser, E., *Science*, **198**, 733 (1977).

201. Van Zant, G., and Goldwasser, E., *Blood*, **53**, 946 (1979).

202. Metcalf, D., and Johnson, G. R., *J. Cell. Physiol.*, **99**, 159 (1979).

203. Burgess, A. W., and Metcalf, D., *J. Cell. Physiol.*, **90**, 471 (1976).

204. Burgess, A. W., and Metcalf, D., in S. J. Baum and G. D. Ledney, Eds., *Experimental Hematology Today*, Springer-Verlag, New York, 1977, p. 135.

205. Ziboh, V., Miller, A. M., Wu, M.-C., and Yunis, A. A., *Clin. Res.*, **29**, 354A (1981).

206. Miller, A. M., Ziboh, V., and Yunis, A. A. International Symposium on Prostaglandins and Cancer, Washington, D.C., A. R. Liss Inc., New York, 1982, p. 481.

207. Greenberg, P. L., Nichols, W. C., and Schrier, S. L., *N. Engl. J. Med.*, **284**, 1225 (1971).

208. Chervenick, P. A., Lawson, A. L., Ellis, L. D., and Pan, S. F., *J. Lab. Clin. Med.*, **78**, 838 (1971).

209. Moore, M. A. S., Williams, N., and Metcalf, D., *J. Natl. Cancer Inst.*, **50**, 603 (1973).

210. Moore, M. A. S., and Metcalf, D., *Int. J. Cancer*, **11**, 143 (1973).

211. Moore, M. A. S., Williams, N., and Metcalf, D., *J. Natl. Cancer Inst.*, **50**, 591 (1973).

212. Senn, J. S., McCulloch, E. A., and Till, J. E., *Lancet*, **2**, 597 (1967).

213. Fialkow, P., Singer, J., Adamson, J., Berkow, R., Freidman, J., Jacobson, R., and Moohr, J., *N. Engl. J. Med.*, **301**, 1 (1979).

214. Ichikawa, Y., *J. Cell. Physiol.*, **74**, 223 (1969).

215. Ichikawa, Y., *J. Cell. Physiol.*, **76**, 175 (1970).

216. Metcalf, D., *Int. J. Cancer*, **25**, 225 (1980).

217. Williams, N., and Van den Engh, G. J., *J. Cell. Physiol.*, **86**, 237 (1975).

218. Brennan, J. K., Nemchick, D., Luk, C., and Lichtman, M. A., *Blood*, **54** (Suppl. 1), 437 (1979).

219. Sachs, L., in B. Clarkson and R. Baserga, Eds., *Control of Proliferation in Animal Cells*, Cold Spring Harbor Conferences on Cell Proliferation, Vol. 1, Cold Spring Harbor, New York, 1974, p. 915.

220. Landau, T., and Sachs, L., *Proc. Natl. Acad. Sci. USA*, **68**, 2540 (1971).

221. Landau, T., and Sachs, L., *FEBS Lett.*, **17**, 229 (1971).

222. Honma, Y., Kasukabe, T., Okabi, J., and Hozumi, M., *Cancer Res.*, **39**, 3167 (1979).

223. Greenberg, P. L., and Selvier, S. L., *Blood*, **4**, 753 (1973).

224. Price, T. H., and Dale, D. C., *Clin. Hematol.*, **7**, 501 (1978).

225. Robinson, W. A., and Mangalic, A., *Semin. Hematol.*, **12**, 7 (1975).

226. Greenberg, P. L., *Scand. J. Hematol.*, **25**, 369 (1980).

227. Dicke, K. A., and Lowenberg, B., in T. M. Fliedner and S. Perry, Eds., *Workshop on Prognostic Factors in Human Acute Leukemia*, Pergamon, New York, 1975, p. 259.

228. Singer, J. W., and Brown, J. E., *Clin. Hematol.*, **7**, 487 (1978).

229. Abdou, N. I., Naponbejara, C., Balentine, L., and Abdou, N. L., *J. Clin. Invest.*, **61**, 738 (1978).

230. Bagby, G. C., and Gaboural, J. D., *J. Clin. Invest.*, **64**, 72 (1979).

231. Bishop, C. R., Rothstein, G., Ashenbrucker, H. E., and Athens, J. W., *J. Clin. Invest.*, **50**, 1678 (1971).

232. Price, T., Lee, M., Dale, D., and Finch, C., *Blood*, **54**, 581 (1979).

233. Dale, D., Guerry, D., and Wewerka, J., *Medicine*, **58**, 128 (1979).

234. Kurnick, J. E., Robinson, W. A., and Dickey, C. A., *Proc. Soc. Exp. Biol. Med.*, **137**, 917 (1971).

235. Richard, K., Brown, R., Wilkinson, T., and Kronenberg, H., *Scand. J. Hematol.*, **22**, 121 (1979).

236. Ascensao, J., Kagan, W., Moore, M. A. S., Pahwa, R., Hansen, J., and Good, R., *Lancet*, **1**, 669 (1976).

237. Singer, J. W., Brown, J. E., James, M. C., Doney, K., Warren, R., Storb, R., and Thomas, E. D., *Blood*, **52**, 37 (1978).

238. Singer, J., Doeny, K., and Thomas, E. D., *Blood*, **54**, 180 (1978).

239. Abdou, N. I., Verdirame, J. D., Amare, M., and Abdou, N., *Ann. Intern. Med.*, **95**, 43 (1981).

240. Pike, B. L., and Robinson, W. A., *J. Cell. Physiol.*, **76**, 77 (1970).

241. Greenberg, P. L., Nichols, W., and Schrier, S. L., *N. Engl. J. Med.*, **284**, 1225 (1971).

242. Moore, M., Spitzer, G., Williams, N., Metcalf, D., and Buckley, J., *Blood*, **44**, 1 (1974).

243. Bull, J. M., Duttera, M. J., Stashik, E. D., Northrup, J., Henderson, E., and Carbone, P. P., *Blood*, **42**, 679 (1973).

244. Spitzer, G., Dicke, K., Gehan, E., Smith, T., McCredie, K., Barlogie, B., and Freireich, E., *Blood*, **48**, 795 (1976).

245. Vincent, P. C., Sutherland, R., Bradley, M., Lind, D., and Gunz, F., *Blood*, **49**, 903 (1977).

246. Goldberg, J., Tice, D., Nelson, D., and Gottlieb, A., *Am. J. Med. Sci.*, **277**, 81 (1978).

247. Beran, M., Reizenstein, P., and Uden, A., *Br. J. Haematol.*, **44**, 39 (1980).

248. Moore, M. A. S., in R. Silber, J. LoBue, and A. Gordon, Eds., *The Year in Hematology*, Plenum, New York, 1978, p. 33.

249. Greenberg, P. L., Mara, B., Bax, I., Brossel, R., and Schrier, S., *Am. J. Med.*, **61**, 878 (1976).

250. Greenberg, P. L., and Mara, B., *Am. J. Med.*, **66**, 951 (1979).

9

DEFINED MEDIA AND STUDIES OF GROWTH FACTORS

Jane E. Bottenstein

CONTENTS

Abbreviation

MSA   Multiplication-stimulating activity

1. INTRODUCTION

The regulation of cell proliferation is a complex phenomenon, and identification of the factors involved and analyses of their mechanisms of action are of central importance in cell biology. Because of the complexities of *in vivo* experimentation, the ability to study proliferation of cells in culture provides a useful tool for the investigation of some aspects of this process. Ideally, proliferation of a specific cell type would be investigated in a rigorously defined and controlled environment, so that reproducibility of experiments would be maximized and interpretation of results would be simplified. The inclusion of serum in culture medium impairs these goals, since it is a complex biological fluid of variable and largely undefined nature (1–5). Although serum contains growth-stimulatory components, factors that inhibit growth are also present. It has been reported that sera from several species can effect transformation of cells and induce chromosomal damage (6–8). Furthermore, cells *in vivo* are not normally exposed to serum, so that serum-containing cultures are not the best approximation to *in vivo* conditions. Although serum has traditionally been used to sustain survival or division of cells *in vitro*, it is clearly not an ideal supplement for culture medium. This chapter reviews recent developments in serum-free culture methods that sustain proliferation of established cell lines and primary cultures. It also describes some of the benefits and novel uses of these media and discusses future directions in this rapidly expanding field.

2. BASIC GROWTH REQUIREMENTS OF CELLS IN CULTURE

The principal components of the earliest culture media were biological fluids, for example, lymph, embryonic extract, plasma, or serum. The disadvantages of using these undefined substances were recognized from the very beginning. Early attempts to determine the growth requirements of mammalian cells in culture focused on formulating synthetic media of defined constituents that would substitute for biological fluids (9,10). Since all cell types do not have the same requirements for optimal growth, a variety of different formulations have been devised. These basal media usually satisfy the general requirements of a number of cell types for a balanced salt solution of appropriate osmolarity, buffered pH, energy source, amino acids, vitamins, and some trace elements. The various synthetic media now available can support the survival of some cell types, but the continuous division of most cells still requires supplementation with serum or other undefined substances. This need for further supplementation may reflect a requirement for growth-promoting substances (including hormones), transport proteins, and/or other unknown factors. Although essential fatty acids are required for the growth of multicellular organisms, most cells in culture proliferate in the absence of essential fatty acids (11). Many established cell lines are able to synthesize fatty acids from nonlipid precursors; however, they will preferentially utilize exogenous sources of lipids if they are supplied in the culture medium (12).

In addition to the requirement for soluble factors, an appropriate substratum is essential for the proliferation of adherent cells. If serum is present in the medium, a layer of adsorbed serum molecules forms on the surface of the culture dish, and cells attach and spread on this layer (13). Some cells in addition require a collagen (14–16) or polylysine (17–19) precoating of culture dishes for good viability or proliferation. Two glycoproteins known to be components of extracellular matrices have also been used for similar purposes: fibronectin (19–21) and laminin (22). Although the molecular mechanisms involved in each case are not clear at the present time, modulation of ligand–receptor interaction or of the transduction of mitogenic signals may be involved. It may be that these various substratum modifiers substitute for and/or modulate production of the extracellular matrix of cells in culture. Alterations in cell–substratum interactions may then influence cell division via cytoskeletal perturbations or some other mechanism.

3. FORMULATION OF SERUM-FREE DEFINED MEDIA

3.1. Critical Factors in the Design of Defined Media

In a limited number of cases it has been possible to select serum-independent variants by adapting cells to grow in medium without serum (23–27). However, very long periods of time are often required for successful adaptation, growth rates and final cell densities are often markedly reduced, and loss of differentiated properties may occur. Others have attempted to fractionate serum and isolate its growth-modulating factors; however, this has not been the easiest or most fruitful approach to identifying serum constituents that influence survival or cell division. A different approach is to add purified substances singly or in combinations to basal media and determine the effects on cell proliferation without adapting cells, to minimize selection of subpopulations.

There are several critical factors in designing a defined medium: basal medium, supplements, and substratum (for adherent cells). In addition, high-purity water should be used in making the defined medium; water that has been triple-distilled or run through a reverse-osmosis unit followed by deionization is recommended for optimal results. The selection of basal medium can be extremely important; although a good starting point is to use the basal medium the cells have been maintained in when serum has been present, it has often been found that a mixture of media is preferable or that an entirely different one is optimal for this purpose. For example, we found an almost 10-fold increase in the incorporation of tritiated thymidine by U-251 Mg$_{sp}$ glioma cells after 4 days if Dulbecco-Vogt's modified Eagle's rather than Ham's F12 medium was used (28). The choice of supplements is a difficult task, and strategies vary. Since the effects of supplements are usually synergistic and single supplements often show no effect alone, they should be tested in various combinations and over a wide range of doses that includes physiological levels, if known, to find the optimal concentration. Dose–response curves for purified supplements are usually sigmoidal; inhibition of growth has been observed at higher concentrations for some of the supplements, for example, the trace element selenium (29). Although some cell types proliferate when plated in defined medium on tissue-culture surfaces, others show enhancement of growth (20) or an absolute requirement for a modified substratum (19,28). It has also been found that some defined media may support proliferation for days, but not for long term with serial subcultures. Cells may grow in the defined medium at high but not clonal densities. The ability to propagate cells serially in defined medium eliminates the problem of residual serum effects, and clonal assays eliminate significant medium conditioning by the cells that can influence proliferation. To attain these goals, further modifications of the specific defined medium may then be required.

3.2. Defined Media for Proliferation of Established Cell Lines

Lieberman and Ove (30) and Higuchi (31) both described the growth-stimulatory effects of insulin alone added to serum-free medium approximately 20 years ago. However, it was not until the 1970s that major advances were made in replacing serum with defined additives. Higuchi and Robinson (32) developed a defined medium that supports the serial propagation of a variety of established cell lines. However, they were unable to culture primary cells successfully in this medium. Supplements to their basal medium include insulin, hydrocortisone, thyroxine, cholesterol, oleic acid, lecithin, and methylcellulose. Although this serum-free supplemented medium has the virtue of sustaining the proliferation of 16 different cell lines, it is not optimal for each one and is not cell-type specific. Yamane (33) described the growth of 12 established cell lines, as well as various primary cultures, in basal medium supplemented with sodium pyruvate, insulin, putrescine, zinc sulfate, ferrous sulfate, various nucleotides, oleic acid, linoleic acid, and 1% fatty acid-free bovine serum albumin. The latter compound has no growth-stimulating effect by itself. This defined medium also does not show cell-type specificity.

The major contribution in the field of defined media has come from Gordon Sato and his colleagues (34,35). Other significant work has been done by Richard Ham who has stressed the importance of qualitative and quantitative optimization of the basal media (36). These and other investigators have formulated an assortment of serum-free defined media optimized for the proliferation of particular cell lines. Table 1 lists the cell lines that are able to proliferate in defined media without adaptation; those requiring a serum preincubation before switching to defined medium are not included. A variety of tissue sources and species are represented, and clearly there are unique complexes of growth factors and hormones that promote optimal proliferation of specific cell types. The most consistent requirements appear to be for the polypeptide hormone insulin and the iron-transport protein transferrin. Although transferrin preferentially binds two ferric ions, manganese- and zinc-transferrin complexes have been described (66). Other supplements include polypeptide and steroid hormones, thyroid hormone, prostaglandins, polypeptide growth factors, trace elements, reducing agents, diamines, vitamins, and albumin complexed with unsaturated fatty acids. Figure 1 shows an example of cell lines from three different species grown in one of these defined media (N2 medium): B104 rat neuroblastoma (19,29), LA-N-1 human neuroblastoma (45), and C17-S$_1$ mouse teratocarcinoma (46). All three cell lines exhibit neuronal characteristics in this medium.

There are two examples in Table 1 of a requirement for fatty acid-free albumin complexed with fatty acids (53,56). In these studies the fatty acid-

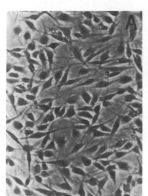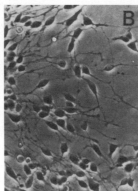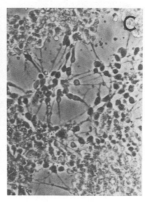

Figure 1. Phase-contrast micrographs of various cells in defined medium. (A) B104 rat neuroblastoma on day 3, (B) LA-N-1 human neuroblastoma on day 3, and (C) C17-S$_1$ (clone 1003) mouse teratocarcinoma on day 12. Culture medium consists of 1:1 mixture of Dulbecco-Vogt's modified Eagle's and Ham's F12 media supplemented with 5 μg of bovine insulin per milliliter, 100 μg of human transferrin per milliliter, 20 nM progesterone, 30 nM sodium selenite, 100 μM putrescine dihydrochloride, and 5 μg of human fibronectin per milliliter. Dishes are precoated with poly-D-lysine.

254

Table 1. Proliferation of Established Cell Lines in Defined Media

Cell Line	Source	Basal Medium	Supplements[a]	Substratum Modification[a]	Reference
GH$_3$	Rat pituitary carcinoma	F12	Ins, trf, T$_3$, TRH, PTH, som C, FGF	—	37
HeLa	Human cervical carcinoma	F12	Ins, trf, NIH-LH (or FGF), EGF, hc, trace elements	—	38
PCC.4aza-1	Mouse embryonal carcinoma	F12	Ins, trf, 2-mercaptoethanol, fetuin	—	39
M2R	Mouse melanoma	DMEM/F12	Ins, trf, test (or prog), FSH, NGF, LRH, sel	—	40
TM4	Mouse testes (Sertoli)	DMEM/F12	Ins, trf, FSH, som C, GH, retinoic acid	—	34
RF-1	Rat ovarian follicle	DMEM/F12	Ins, trf, hc	fn	20
M1	Mouse myeloid leukemia	F12	Ins, trf, trace elements	—	41
B104	Rat neuroblastoma	DMEM/F12	Ins, trf, prog, putr, sel	fn, polylysine	19, 29
C62BD	Rat glioma	DMEM/F12	Ins, trf, FGF	fn	42
MDCK	Dog renal epithelium	DMEM/F12	Ins, trf, T$_3$, hc, PGE$_1$, sel	—	43
MCF-7	Human mammary carcinoma	DMEM/F12	Ins, trf, EGF, PGF$_{2\alpha}$	fn	44
LA-N-1	Human neuroblastoma	DMEM/F12	Ins, trf, prog, putr, sel	polylysine	45
C17-S$_1$(1003)	Mouse embryonal carcinoma	DMEM/F12	Ins, trf, sel	fn	46
F$_9$	Mouse embryonal carcinoma	DMEM/F12	Ins, trf	fn	21

Cell line	Cell type	Medium	Supplements	Substrate	Ref.
OTT-6050	Mouse embryonal carcinoma	IMEM	Ins (or MSA), trf, EGF, FGF, fetuin, zinc	polylysine or collagen	47
BHK-21	Hamster kidney	DMEM/F12	Ins, trf, EGF, FGF, BSA	fn	48
Swiss 3T6	Mouse embryo fibroblasts	DMEM/Waymouth	Ins, $FeSO_4$, EGF	—	49
31A-F_2	Rat ovarian epithelium	Coon's modified F12	Ins, trf, OGF, EGF, FGF	—	50
1116NS-19 1116NS-33a 1083-17-1A	Mouse hybridoma	MEM (or RPMI 1640)	Ins, trf	—	51
OV1N	Rat ovarian carcinoma	Coon's modified F12	Trf, EGF	—	52
SV40-Balb/c3T3	Mouse embryo fibroblasts	DMEM/F12 (3:1)	Ins, trf, FAF-BSA, linoleic acid	fn	53
HC84S	Human colon carcinoma	DMEM/F12	Ins, trf, EGF, hc, glucagon, T_3, sel	collagen	54
HL-60	Human promyelocytic leukemia	DMEM/F12	Ins, trf, sel	—	55
C6BU-1	Rat glioma	DMEM/F12 (3:1)	Ins, trf, FGF, FAF-BSA, linoleic acid, trace elements	polylysine	56
NCI-H69	Human lung small cell carcinoma	RPMI 1640	Ins, trf, hc, sel, estradiol	—	57
CC1-39	Hamster lung fibroblasts	DMEM/F12	Ins, trf, EGF, thrombin	fn	58
MPC-11	Mouse plasmacytoma	DMEM/F12	Trf, NIH-LH, LRH, PGE, EGF, T_3, glucagon, NGF, $PGF_{2\alpha}$, sel	—	59
Flow 2000	Human embryo fibroblasts	MCDB 108	Ins, EGF, dex	polylysine	60

Table 1. *(continued)*

Cell Line	Source	Basal Medium	Supplements[a]	Substratum Modification[a]	Reference
NB41A3	Mouse neuroblastoma	MCDB 411	—	insulin	61
W138	Human embryo fibroblasts	MCDB 104	Ins, trf, EGF, dex, PDGF	—	62
W138 Flow 2000 MRC-5 IMR-90	Human embryo fibroblasts	MCDB 110	Ins, EGF, dex, PGE₁, PGF$_{2\alpha}$, DTT, glutathione, PEP, lipid mixture	polylysine	63
GM86-745 GM79-3TC1 K562(S)	Human erythroleukemia	RPMI 1640	Trf, sel, BSA	—	64
PC-G2	Rat pheochromocytoma	DMEM	Ins, trf, prog, putr, sel, EGF (or NGF)	—	65
U-251 MG$_{sp}$	Human glioma	DMEM	Trf, FGF, hc, sel, biotin	fn	28
C62BD	Rat glioma	DMEM	Trf, FGF, hc, sel, biotin	fn	28
RN-22	Rat schwannoma	DMEM	Trf, sel, biotin	fn	28

[a] Abbreviations: **ins**, insulin; **trf**, transferrin; **T₃**, triiodothyronine; **TRH**, thyrotropin-releasing hormone; **PTH**, parathyroid hormone; **som C**, somatomedin C; **FGF**, fibroblast growth factor; **LH**, luteinizing hormone; **EGF**, epidermal growth factor; **hc**, hydrocortisone; **test**, testosterone; **prog**, progesterone; **FSH**, follicle-stimulating hormone; **NGF**, nerve growth factor; **LRH**, LH-releasing hormone; **sel**, selenium; **GH**, growth hormone; **putr**, putrescine; **PGE₁**, prostaglandin E₁; **PGF$_{2\alpha}$**, prostaglandin$_{2\alpha}$; **MSA**, multiplication-stimulating activity; **BSA**, bovine serum albumin; **OGF**, ovarian growth factor; **FAF**, fatty acid-free; **dex**, dexamethasone; **PDGF**, platelet-derived growth factor; **DTT**, dithiothreitol; **PEP**, phosphoenolpyruvate; **fn**, fibronectin.

Table 2. Proliferation of Primary Cell Cultures in Defined Media

Source	Species	Basal Medium	Supplements[a]	Substratum Modification[a]	Reference
Bone	Rat	Fitton-Jackson modified BGJ	BSA, ascorbate, glutamine	—	81
B Lymphocytes	Mouse	IMDM	Trf, FAF-BSA, soybean lipid, LPS	—	82
T Lymphocytes	Human	RPMI 1640	Trf, leucoagglutinin	—	83
Testes (Sertoli)	Mouse	DMEM/F12	Ins, trf, EGF, FGF, som C, GH	—	73
Red cell precursors	Mouse	IMDM	Trf, $FeCl_3$, FAF-BSA, lecithin, cholesterol, linoleic acid, erythropoietin	—	84
Renal epithelium	Dog	DMEM/F12	Ins, trf, PGE_1, hc, T_3, sel	—	74
Renal epithelium	Mouse	DMEM/F12	Ins, trf, PGE_1, hc, T_3, sel	—	75
Kidney	Baboon	Modified M199	Ins, pyruvate, zinc	—	85
Chondrocytes	Rat	F12	MSA, ascorbate	—	86
Brain glia	Human	MCDB 105	PDGF (or EGF)	collagen	87
Renal glomeruli	Guinea pig	Waymouth MB752/1	Ins, trf, pyruvate, PGE_1, db-cAMP	fn	88
Arterial smooth muscle	Rat	DMEM/F12	Ins, trf, IGF-1, MSA, hc, α-thrombin, EGF, PDGF, ascorbate, trace elements, ovalbumin	fn	89

[a] Abbreviations: **BSA**, bovine serum albumin; **trf**, transferrin; **FAF**, fatty acid-free; **LPS**, lipopolysaccharide; **ins**, insulin; **EGF**, epidermal growth factor; **FGF**, fibroblast growth factor; **som** C, somatomedin C; **GH**, growth hormone; **PGE_1**, prostaglandin E_1; **hc**, hydrocortisone; **T_3**, triiodothyronine; **sel**, selenium; **MSA**, multiplication-stimulating activity; **PDGF**, platelet-derived growth factor; **db-cAMP**, dibutyryl cyclic AMP; **IGF**, insulin-like growth factor; **fn**, fibronectin.

free albumin has no effect by itself. On the other hand, DNA synthesis of lectin-activated human T lymphocytes is stimulated by fatty acid-free albumin alone (67), and Ham (68) reported that low levels of linoleic acid, but not oleic acid, can replace albumin for the clonal growth of CHD-3 cells. Other defined media listed in Table 1 contain native albumin, and its effect may be due to a bound contaminant when albumin is added in milligram-per-milliliter quantities. Albumin is known to bind many different molecules tightly, including, but not limited to, steroids, thyroid hormone, prostaglandins, ascorbic acid, proteases, alpha$_1$-acid glycoprotein, and various lipids (69–71). Since many growth-promoting substances are known to be active in the picogram to microgram-per-milliliter range, factors bound to albumin could account for the stimulation of proliferation.

3.3.   Defined Media for Proliferation of Primary Cultures

Information about the growth requirements of established cell lines, including tumorigenic ones, has proved useful for maintaining primary cultures of proliferating normal cells (72–75). In addition, a medium designed to sustain continuous division of neuroblastoma cells is also able to maintain postmitotic neurons with retention of differentiated properties (76–80). Table 2 lists different types of primary cells that proliferate in defined media, including adherent cells and those normally grown in suspension. As observed with established cell lines, these defined media illustrate the cell-type differences in growth requirements. As new serum-free defined media become available, this repertoire of cells will increase.

4.   BENEFITS AND NOVEL USES OF DEFINED MEDIA

4.1.   Identification of Growth-Promoting Factors for Specific Cell Types

The ability to replace serum with hormones and growth factors has led to the identification of unique sets of requirements for growth of specific cell types. In the past some of these requirements could be determined *in vitro* by using serum depleted of a particular substance or class of substances; endocrine ablation of serum donors and various extraction or immunoaffinity procedures applied to serum have been employed. The use of defined medium offers clear advantages in this respect. The importance of cell–substratum interactions in cell proliferation has also been highlighted in these defined systems, and cell-type differences have been demonstrated. When species differences in requirements for the division of the same cell type in defined medium have occurred, they have been more quantitative than qualitative.

Cells that can now grow in defined medium for short but not long periods can be used to identify soluble factors or substrata that will sustain continuous cell division and subculturing. Cells that require a serum preincubation or low levels of serum (<0.5%) will be useful in determining the residual requirements for serum-free growth of those cell types. Finally, cells that proliferate poorly even in conventional serum-containing medium may fare better in a serum-free defined medium.

The physiological role *in vivo* of many of the growth requirements determined for cells in culture needs to be evaluated in each case. It is likely that many of these play important roles during development and in various pathological states, including cancer. For example, transferrin receptors are present on the surface of various cultured human cells of embryonic and tumorigenic origin, but not on nonmitotic normal adult liver and kidney membranes (90). Furthermore, Larrick and Cresswell (91) reported that human transformed lymphoid cells have up to 1000 times more transferrin receptors than normal resting lymphocytes, and lectin stimulation of lymphocyte proliferation results in a 50-fold increase in the number of transferrin-binding sites.

Knowledge of specific growth requirements may be exploited in new forms of cancer therapy involving priming or targeting of cytotoxic agents. For example, hybrid toxins consisting of transferrin coupled to diphtheria fragment A exhibit potent cytotoxicity on rat neuroblastoma cells in culture (J. Bottenstein, unpublished data). Trowbridge and Domingo (92) reported recently that conjugates of a monoclonal antibody to the human transferrin receptor coupled to ricin A subunit or diphtheria fragment A specifically kill human tumor cells *in vitro*. These techniques may also be used for positive selection of variants useful in studies of growth regulation (93) and for negative selection against specific types of cells in developmental studies. The more restricted the distribution of the growth-related molecule is, the more specific the selection will be.

4.2. Selection for Specific Cell Types in Primary Cultures

Some of the defined media show cell-type specificity when tested on other cell lines (28,45), and this property has been used to advantage in primary cultures to select for postmitotic neurons with death of glial and fibroblast cells (78). Suppression of fibroblast proliferation in defined medium has also been noted by Mather and Sato (73) as well as by Jefferson et al. (74) in their primary cultures of dividing cells. The problem of fibroblast overgrowth has been dealt with in the past by treatment with antimitotic poisons or exploitation of differences in cell-substratum adhesion. Another example of the selective properties of a defined medium was described by

Mather and Sato (73). They injected metastatic M2R mouse melanoma cells into a syngeneic host, and after 2 weeks the lungs, spleen, lymph nodes, and liver were minced and plated in a defined medium. Even though metastases could not be detected at these sites initially, after 10 days of proliferation in defined medium only melanoma cells were evident, and all the normal cells had died.

Studies of cell proliferation often involve established cell lines, some of clonal origin, although primary cells have also been used. The ability to select for specific cell types in primary cultures would be a useful tool to further our knowledge of the proliferation of normal cells. Studies in defined medium of primary cells isolated from other cell types could be expanded in the future to investigate the influence of one cell type on the proliferation of another.

4.3.   Analysis of Cell-Produced Growth Factors

Both normal and tumorigenic cells in culture may provide alternatives to plasma or serum as sources for the isolation of growth factors. Identification and purification of cell-produced growth factors is enormously simplified when serum is absent, since the tremendous background of serum molecules is eliminated in defined medium. Furthermore, serum may inhibit the synthesis of some gene products. To circumvent these problems, many investigators have transferred cells in serum-containing medium to a basal medium without supplementation before analyzing cell-derived factors in the conditioned medium. Multiplication-stimulating activity (MSA) from normal Buffalo rat liver cells has been isolated in this way (94). Continued production of growth factors is only possible for cells that remain viable in serum-free basal medium, and maximal yields can be obtained only if they continue to divide. Neither is true for the majority of cells. The rate of total protein synthesis declines rapidly when serum is withdrawn from 3T6 mouse fibroblasts (95), for example, and presumably most cells, if they survive at all, would have lower yields of cell-derived growth factors in basal medium alone. Thus the improved viability and ability of cells to proliferate in basal medium supplemented with defined components will be obvious advantages in analyzing cell-produced growth factors.

Cells generally produce growth factors that affect other cell types; however, cells may also have receptors for the growth factors they produce. Examples of the latter include transforming growth factors, which are produced by sarcoma virus-transformed mouse fibroblasts (96), several human tumor cell lines (97), and chemically transformed mouse cell lines (98) (Chapter 7). Sarcoma growth factors stimulate DNA synthesis in normal fibroblast and epithelial cells (99). Moreover, a human fibrosarcoma cell line produces

MSA-related growth factors (100). All of these growth factors derived from tumor cell lines are obtained from the conditioned medium of cells maintained in serum-free basal medium. Although the cell-derived factors described here are related to known growth factors (epidermal growth factor and MSA), it is probable that new growth factors can be isolated in a similar way. Growth factors that are not stored in any tissue or gland *in vivo* are attractive candidates for this method. The availability of defined media should expand the number of possible producer cells of both normal and tumorigenic origin.

4.4. Study of Mechanisms of Growth Factor Action

It is generally agreed that polypeptide growth factors (including hormones) bind to cell surface receptors, followed by aggregation of the ligand–receptor complex and subsequent internalization (or down-regulation). Whether the effects of growth factors can be explained solely by their interaction with the plasma membrane is not clear at the present time. A number of early biological effects of growth factors have been described: increased nutrient and ion transport, stimulation of ornithine decarboxylase, modulation of adenylate cyclase activity, and/or changes in protein phosphorylation (101–105). The necessity of the molecular changes correlated with stimulation of cell proliferation by growth factors needs to be demonstrated in each case.

Of particular interest are recent studies indicating that tyrosine-specific protein kinases may be involved in growth regulation. Epidermal growth factor (106) (Chapter 5), platelet-derived growth factor (107) (Chapter 4), and human transforming growth factors (108) (Chapter 7) all induce phosphorylation of specific tyrosine residues. Moreover, the gene products of several, but not all, tumor viruses are protein kinases that also phosphorylate specific tyrosine residues (109–116). Both Rous sarcoma virus kinase and affinity-purified epidermal growth factor receptor-kinase phosphorylate antibodies against the viral kinase, suggesting their relatedness (117). A non-mitogenic analogue of epidermal growth factor, however, shows a pattern of membrane protein phosphorylation similar to that of unmodified epidermal growth factor; this suggests either that the phosphorylation is not related to cell proliferation or that it may be necessary, but not sufficient, for the induction of DNA synthesis (118). Another possible mechanism for epidermal growth factor action has been described by Das (119). Her results indicate that epidermal growth factor induces an intracellular protein messenger that stimulates DNA synthesis in isolated nuclei of frog spleen cells.

Cell proliferation is a complex process that may involve different pathways for initiation (120) and many different regulatory points. In addition, interaction of several growth factors, often synergistic or permissive, is frequently required for a maximal effect. The interpretation of the influence of a single growth factor on cells *in vitro* is further complicated when serum is present in the culture medium, since experimental variability may be introduced, and undefined components may enhance or mask the effect under study. These interactions can be studied best in a defined medium. It is known, for example, that in serum-free medium insulin can increase the number of membrane receptors for vasopressin in kidney epithelial cells (121), and this may account for the potentiation by insulin of vasopressin stimulation of DNA synthesis in mouse fibroblasts (122). It is also known that glucocorticoids enhance the binding and action of epidermal growth factor in human fibroblasts (123). When the binding of iodinated epidermal growth factor to HeLa cells proliferating in defined medium is compared with that of HeLa cells in serum-containing medium, a constant number of receptors is found in the former condition and a loss of receptors in the latter condition (124), suggesting, in contrast with a proposed model (125), that down-regulation may not be required for cell division to occur. The availability of defined media for a variety of cell types will facilitate the studies of molecular mechanisms of growth factor action that are important in understanding both malignant transformation and cell proliferation during normal development.

5.   FUTURE DIRECTIONS

The number of different cell types that can now proliferate in defined medium is substantial and can be expected to expand rapidly. Very significant progress has been made in the last few years, and several lines of investigation are beginning to converge in this area. New growth factors are being added to the list of potential supplements, basal media are being optimized for particular cell types, and there is increasing information about the biochemistry and the physiological effects of extracellular matrices that play a role in cell–substratum interactions. Extension of knowledge on all of these frontiers can be exploited in the modification of existing defined media as well as in the design of new media. The development and use of these various defined media will undoubtedly further our knowledge of the complex phenomenon of cell proliferation.

REFERENCES

1.   Olmsted, C. A., *Exp. Cell Res.*, **48**, 283 (1967).
2.   Esber, H. J., Payne, I. J., and Bogden, A. E., *J. Natl. Cancer Inst.*, **50**, 559 (1973).

3. Bittles, A. H., *Med. Lab. Technol.*, **31**, 253 (1974).

4. Honn, K. V., Singley, J. A., and Chavin, W., *Proc. Soc. Exp. Biol. Med.*, **149**, 344 (1975).

5. Pye, D., *J. Biol. Standard.*, **5**, 307 (1977).

6. Evans, V. J., and Andresen, W. F., *J. Natl. Cancer Inst.*, **37**, 247 (1966).

7. Sanford, K. K., Parshad, R., Handleman, S. L., Price, F. M., Gantt, R. R., and Evans, V. J., *In Vitro*, **15**, 488 (1979).

8. Chessebeuf, M., Exilie, M. F., Piard, G., Chatelain, P., and Padieu, P., *Cell Biol. Int. Rep.*, **5**, 399 (1981).

9. Swim, H. E., *Wistar Inst. Symp. Monogr.*, **6**, 1 (1967).

10. Waymouth, C., in G. H. Rothblat and V. J. Cristofalo, Eds., *Growth, Nutrition, and Metabolism of Cells in Culture*, Academic, New York, 1972, Vol. 1, pp. 11–47.

11. Bailey, J. M., and Dunbar, L. M., *Exp. Molec. Pathol.*, **18**, 142 (1973).

12. Spector, A. A., in G. H. Rothblat and V. J. Cristofalo, Eds., *Growth, Nutrition, and Metabolism of Cells in Culture*, Academic, New York, 1972, Vol. 1, pp. 257–296.

13. Culp, L., and Buniel, J., *J. Cell. Physiol.*, **88**, 89 (1976).

14. Ehrmann, R. L., and Gey, G. O., *J. Natl. Cancer Inst.*, **16**, 1375 (1956).

15. Liu, S. C., and Karasek, M., *Invest. Dermatol.*, **71**, 157 (1978).

16. Liotta, L. A., Vembu, D., Kleinman, H., Martin, G. R. and Boone, C., *Nature*, **272**, 622 (1978).

17. McKeehan, W. L., and Ham, R. G., *J. Cell Biol.*, **71**, 727 (1976).

18. Yavin, Z., and Yavin, E., *Dev. Biol.*, **75**, 454 (1980).

19. Bottenstein, J. E., and Sato, G. H., *Exp. Cell Res.*, **129**, 361 (1980).

20. Orly, J., and Sato, G., *Cell*, **17**, 295 (1979).

21. Rizzino, A., and Crowley, C., *Proc. Natl. Acad. Sci. USA*, **77**, 457 (1980).

22. Rizzino, A., Terranova, V., Rohrbach, D., Crowley, C., and Rizzino, H., *J. Supramol. Struct.*, **13**, 243 (1980).

23. Evans, V., Bryant, J., Fioramonti, M., McQuilkin, W., Sanford, K., and Earle, W., *Cancer Res.*, **16**, 77 (1956).

24. Waymouth, C., *J. Natl. Cancer Inst.*, **22**, 1003 (1959).

25. Evans, V. J., Bryant, J. C., Kerr, H. A., and Schilling, E. L., *Exp. Cell Res.*, **36**, 439 (1964).

26. Takaoka, T., and Katsuta, H., *Exp. Cell Res.*, **67**, 295 (1971).

27. Donta, S., *Exp. Cell Res.*, **82**, 119 (1973).

28. Michler-Stuke, A., and Bottenstein, J. E., *J. Neurosci. Res.*, **7**, 215 (1982).

29. Bottenstein, J. E., and Sato, G. H., *Proc. Natl. Acad. Sci. USA*, **76**, 514 (1979).

30. Lieberman, I., and Ove, P., *J. Biol. Chem.*, **234**, 2754 (1959).

31. Higuchi, K., *J. Infect. Dis.*, **112**, 213 (1963).

32. Higuchi, K., and Robinson, R. C., *In Vitro*, **9**, 114 (1973).

33. Yamane, I., *J. Natl. Cancer Inst. Monogr.*, **48**, 131 (1978).

34. Bottenstein, J., Hayashi, I., Hutchings, S., Masui, H., Mather, J., McClure, D., Ohasa, S., Rizzino, A., Sato, G., Serrero, G., Wolfe, R., and Wu, R., *Methods Enzymol.*, **58**, 94 (1979).

35. Barnes, D., and Sato, G., *Cell*, **22**, 649 (1980).

36. Ham, R. G., *Cold Spring Harbor Conf. Cell Prolif.*, **9**, 39 (1982).

37. Hayashi, I., and Sato, G., *Nature*, **259**, 132 (1976).

38. Hutchings, S. E., and Sato, G. H., *Proc. Natl. Acad. Sci. USA*, **75**, 901 (1978).

39. Rizzino, A., and Sato, G., *Proc. Natl. Acad. Sci. USA*, **75**, 1844 (1978).

40. Mather, J., and Sato, G., *Exp. Cell Res.*, **120**, 191 (1979).

41. Honma, Y., Kasukabe, T., Okabe, J., and Hozumi, M., *Exp. Cell Res.*, **124**, 421 (1979).

42. Bottenstein, J. E., *Cancer Treat. Reports*, **65** (Suppl. 2), 67 (1981).

43. Taub, M., Chuman, L. Saier, M. H., Jr., and Sato, G., *Proc. Natl. Acad. Sci. USA*, **76**, 3338 (1979).

44. Barnes, D., and Sato, G., *Nature*, **281**, 388 (1979).

45. Bottenstein, J. E., in A. E. Evans, Ed., *Advances in Neuroblastoma Research*, Raven, New York, 1980, pp. 161–170.

46. Darmon, M., Bottenstein, J., and Sato, G., *Dev. Biol.*, **85**, 463 (1981).

47. Salomon, D. S., *Exp. Cell Res.*, **128**, 311 (1980).

48. Maciag, T., Kelley, B., Cerundolo, J., Ilsley, S., Kelley, P. R., Gaudreau, J., and Forand, R., *Cell Biol. Intl. Rep.*, **4**, 43 (1980).

49. Dicker, P., Heppel, L. A., and Rozengurt, E., *Proc. Natl. Acad. Sci. USA*, **77**, 2103 (1980).

50. Johnson, C. C., Dawson, W. E., Turner, J. T., and Wyche, J. H., *J. Cell Biol.*, **86**, 483 (1980).

51. Chang, T. H., Steplewski, Z., and Koprowski, H., *J. Immunol. Methods*, **39**, 369 (1980).

52. Turner, J. T., and Wyche, J. H., *J. Cell. Physiol.*, **104**, 233 (1980).

53. Rockwell, G. A., Sato, G. H., and McClure, D. B., *J. Cell. Physiol.*, **103**, 323 (1980).

54. Murakami, H., and Masui, H., *Proc. Natl. Acad. Sci. USA*, **77**, 3464 (1980).

55. Breitman, T. R., Collins, S. J., and Keene, B. R., *Exp. Cell Res.*, **126**, 494 (1980).

56. Wolfe, R. A., Sato, G., and McClure, D. B., *J. Cell Biol.*, **87**, 434 (1980).

57. Simms, E., Gazdar, A. F., Abrams, P. G., and Minna, J. D., *Cancer Res.*, **40**, 4356 (1980).

58. Perez-Rodriguez, R., Franchi, A., and Pouyssegur, J., *Cell Biol. Intl. Rep.*, **5**, 347 (1981).

59. Murakami, H., Masui, H., Sato, G., and Raschke, W. C., *Anal. Biochem.*, **114**, 422 (1981).

60. Walthall, B. J., and Ham, R. G., *Exp. Cell Res.*, **134**, 301 (1981).

61. Agy, P. C., Shipley, G. D., and Ham, R. G., *In Vitro*, **17**, 671 (1981).

62. Phillips, P. D., and Cristofalo, V. J., *Exp. Cell Res.*, **134**, 297 (1981).

63. Bettger, W. J., Boyce, S. T., Walthall, B. J., and Ham, R. G., *Proc. Natl. Acad. Sci. USA*, **78**, 5588 (1981).

64. Pessano, S., McNab, A., and Rovera, G., *Cancer Res.*, **41**, 3592 (1981).

65. Goodman, R., *Cold Spring Harbor Conf. Cell Prolif.*, **9**, 1053 (1982).

66. Frieden, E., *Trends Biochem. Sci.*, **1**, 273 (1976).

67. Polet, H., and Spieker-Polet, H., *J. Exp. Med.*, **142**, 949 (1975).

68. Ham, R. G., *Science*, **140**, 802 (1963).

69. Wilson, W. D., and Foster, J. F., *Biochemistry*, **10**, 1772 (1971).

70. Allen, P. C., Hill, E. A., and Stokes, A. M., Eds., *Plasma Proteins: Analytical and Preparative Techniques*, Blackwell Scientific, Oxford, 1977, pp. 160–229.

71. Lima, J. J., and Salzer, L. B., *Biochem Pharmacol.*, **30**, 2633 (1981).

72. Yamane, I., in H. Katsuta, Ed., *Nutritional Requirements of Cultured Cells*, University Park Press, Baltimore, 1978, pp. 1–21.

73. Mather, J. P., and Sato, G. H., *Exp. Cell Res.*, **124**, 215 (1979).

74. Jefferson, D. M., Cobb, M. H., Gennaro, J. F., Jr., and Scott, W. N., *Science*, **210**, 912 (1980).

75. Taub, M., and Sato, G., *J. Cell. Physiol.*, **105**, 369 (1980).

76. Shoemaker, W., Bottenstein, J., Milner, R., Clark, B., and Bloom, F., *Soc. Neuroscience*, **5**, 758 (1979).

77. Varon, S., Skaper, S., Adler, R., Bottenstein, J., and Sato, G., *Soc. Neuroscience*, **5**, 761 (1979).

78. Bottenstein, J. E., Skaper, S. D., Varon, S. S., and Sato, G. H., *Exp. Cell Res.*, **125**, 183 (1980).

79. Bottenstein, J., in J. Barker and J. McKelvy, Eds., *Current Methods in Cellular Neurobiology*, in press.

80. Bottenstein, J., in S. Fedoroff and L. Hertz, Eds., *Advances in Cellular Neurobiology*, in press.

81. Peck, W. A., and Burks, J. K., in J. Horton, T. Tarpley, and W. Davis, Eds., *Mechanisms of Localized Bone Loss*, Information Retrieval, Washington, D.C., 1978, pp. 3–12.

82. Iscove, N. N., and Melchers, F., *J. Exp. Med.*, **147**, 923 (1978).

83. Dillner-Centerlind, M., Hammarstrom, S., and Perlmann, P., *Eur. J. Immunol.*, **9**, 942 (1979).

84. Iscove, N. N., Guilbert, L. J., and Weyman, C., *Exp. Cell Res.*, **126**, 121 (1980).

85. Weiss, S. A., Lester, T. L., Kalter, S. S., and Heberling, R. L., *In Vitro*, **16**, 616 (1980).

86. Kato, Y., Nasu, N., Takase, T., Daikuhara, Y., and Suzuki, F., *Exp. Cell Res.*, **125**, 167 (1980).

87. Heldin, C., Wasteson, A., and Westermark, B., *Proc. Natl. Acad. Sci. USA*, **77**, 6611 (1980).

88. Oberley, T. D., Murphy-Ullrich, J. E., Steinert, B. W., and Muth, J. V., *Am. J. Pathol.*, **104**, 181 (1981).

89. Weinstein, R., Stemerman, M. B., and Maciag, T., *Science*, **212**, 818 (1981).

90. Hamilton, T. A., Wada, H. G., and Sussman, H. H., *Proc. Natl. Acad. Sci. USA*, **76**, 6406 (1979).

91. Larrick, J. W., and Cresswell, P., *J. Supramol. Struct.*, **11**, 579 (1979).

92. Trowbridge, I. S., and Domingo, D. L., *Nature*, **294**, 171 (1981).

93. Miskimins, W. K., and Shimuzu, N., *Proc. Natl. Acad. Sci. USA*, **78**, 445 (1981).

94. Dulak, N. C., and Shing, Y. W., *J. Cell. Physiol.*, **90**, 127 (1976).

95. Mostafapour, M., and Green, H., *J. Cell. Physiol.*, **86**, 313 (1975).

96. De Larco, J. E., and Todaro, G. J., *Proc. Natl. Acad. Sci. USA*, **75**, 4001 (1978).

97. Todaro, G. J., Fryling, C., and De Larco, J. E., *Proc. Natl. Acad. Sci. USA*, **77**, 5258 (1980).

98. Moses, H. L., Branum, E. L., Proper, J. A., and Robinson, R. A., *Cancer Res.*, **41**, 2842 (1981).

99. Keski-Oja, J., De Larco, J. E., Rapp, U. R., and Todaro, G. J., *J. Cell. Physiol.*, **104**, 41 (1980).

100. De Larco, J. E., and Todaro, G. J., *Nature*, **272**, 356 (1978).

101. Bradshaw, R. A., and Rubin, J. S., *J. Supramol. Struct.*, **14**, 183 (1980).

102. Kaplan, J. G., *Annu. Rev. Physiol.*, **40**, 19 (1978).

103. Koch, K. S., and Leffert, H. L., *Cell*, **18**, 153 (1979).

104. Janne, J., Poso, H., and Raina, A., *Biochim. Biophys. Acta*, **473**, 241 (1978).

105. Goldfine, I. D., in G. L. Litwack, Ed., *Biochemical Actions of Hormones*, Academic, New York, 1981, Vol. 8, pp. 273–305.

106. Ushiro, H., and Cohen, S., *J. Biol. Chem.*, **255**, 8363 (1980).

107. Ek, B., Westermark, B., Wasteson, Å., and Heldin, C., *Nature*, **295**, 419 (1982).

108. Reynolds, F. H., Jr., Todaro, G. J., Fryling, C., and Stephenson, J. R., *Nature*, **292**, 259 (1981).

109. Hunter, T., and Sefton, B. M., *Proc. Natl. Acad. Sci. USA*, **77**, 1311 (1980).

110. Kawai, S., Yoshida, M., Segawa, K., Sugiyama, H., Ishizaki, R., and Toyoshima, K., *Proc. Natl. Acad. Sci. USA*, **77**, 6199 (1980).

111. Radke, K., Gilmore, T., and Martin, G. S., *Cell*, **21**, 821 (1980).

112. Collett, M. S., Purchio, A. F., and Erikson, R. L., *Nature*, **285**, 167 (1980).

113. Witte, O. N., Dasgupta, A., and Baltimore, D., *Nature*, **283**, 826 (1980).

114. Sefton, B. M., Hunter, T., Beemon, K., and Eckhart, W., *Cell*, **20**, 807 (1980).

115. Beemon, K., *Cell*, **24**, 145 (1981).

116. Sefton, B. M., Hunter, T., and Raschke, W. C., *Proc. Natl. Acad. Sci. USA*, **78**, 1552 (1981).

117. Chinkers, M., and Cohen, S., *Nature*, **290**, 516 (1981).

118. Schreiber, A. B., Yarden, Y., and Schlessinger, J., *Biochem. Biophys. Res. Commun.*, **101**, 517 (1981).

119. Das, M., *Proc. Natl. Acad. Sci. USA*, **77**, 112 (1980).

120. Jimenez de Asua, L., Richmond, K. M., and Otto, A. M., *Proc. Natl. Acad. Sci. USA*, **78**, 1004 (1981).

121. Roy, C., Preston, A. S., and Handler, J. S., *Proc. Natl. Acad. Sci. USA*, **77**, 5979 (1980).

122. Rozengurt, E., Legg, A., and Pettican, P., *Proc. Natl. Acad. Sci. USA*, **76**, 1284 (1979).

123. Baker, J. B., Barsh, G. S., Carney, D. H., and Cunningham, D. D., *Proc. Natl. Acad. Sci. USA*, **75**, 1882 (1978).

124. Wolfe, R. A., Wu, R., and Sato, G. H., *Proc. Natl. Acad. Sci. USA*, **77**, 2735 (1980).

125. Das, M., and Fox, C. F., *Proc. Natl. Acad. Sci. USA*, **75**, 2644 (1978).

10

CELL ATTACHMENT AND SPREADING FACTORS

Frederick Grinnell

CONTENTS

Abbreviations

BHK	Baby hamster kidney
PCF	Polycationic ferritin
WGA	Wheat germ agglutinin
ConA	Concanavalin A
RCA	Ricinus communis agglutinin
EDTA	Ethylene diamine tetraacetic acid
PBS	Phosphate-buffered saline
MEM	Minimal Eagle's medium

1. INTRODUCTION

The purpose of this review is to summarize recent studies on the problem of cell adhesion to substrata and to discuss certain interesting features of these interactions. The specific focus is on the extracellular factors that promote cell adhesion. These factors are the components isolated from the natural environment of cells (e.g., serum, connective tissue, cell microexudate) or added experimentally (e.g., lectins, polycations, antibodies) that constitute the substratum with which the cells interact. The review is divided into five sections. In the first section, an overview of the various endogenous and experimental factors that have been shown to promote cell adhesion is presented. In the second section, the mechanism of interaction between the cells and the factors is discussed, particularly in the context of a ligand–receptor bonding mechanism. In the third section, attention is directed toward one of the unifying features of ligand–receptor interactions in cell adhesion, namely, their multivalent characteristic. In the fourth section, the relationship between cell spreading and phagocytosis is considered. Finally, the last section deals specifically with a problem concerning cell adhesion under routine tissue-culture conditions, namely, is serum fibronectin responsible for cell spreading in this situation?

2. OVERVIEW OF CELL ATTACHMENT AND SPREADING FACTORS

Tables 1 and 2 present lists of factors that have been shown to promote cell attachment and spreading. In the usual experimental protocols, the factors are noncovalently or covalently bound to a material surface (e.g., plastic or glass). Cells are then permitted to interact with the factor-coated surfaces. Attachment is measured by quantitating the number of cells that

Table 1. Natural Cell-Attachment and Spreading Factors

FACTOR	REACTIVE CELL TYPES	REFERENCE
Fibronectin	Fibroblasts	1–3
	Mesoderm	4
	Hepatocytes	5, 6
	Carcinoma	7
	Other epithelial cells	8, 9
Fibronectin/denatured collagen	Fibroblasts	10–12
	Myoblasts	13
	Smooth muscle cells	14, 15
	Endothelial cells	14
	Neutrophils	16
	Platelets	17
Fibronectin/native collagen	Platelets	18, 19
Fibronectin/fibrin	Platelets	18
	Fibroblasts	20
Fibronectin/poly-L-lysine	Neuroblastoma	21
Serum α_1-protein	Fibroblasts	22–24
Native collagen	Fibroblasts	25, 26
	Hepatocytes	27
	Epithelial cells	8, 28–30
	Platelets	31, 32
Denatured collagen	Epidermal cells	33
	Fibrosarcoma	34
	Smooth muscle	15
Chondronectin	Chondrocytes	35
Laminin	Hepatocytes	36
Laminin/microexudate	Carcinoma	37
Laminin/denatured collagen	Epithelial cells	38
Ig complexes	Macrophages	39–40
	Monocytes	41
	Neutrophils	42
	Lymphocytes	43
Complement/Ig complexes	Macrophages	40
	Neutrophils	42
Von Willebrand factor/subendothelium	Platelets	44–45
Microexudate (conditioning factors, sub-stratum-adsorbed material)	Epithelial cells	46–48
	Neurons	49–50
	Fibroblasts	51–53
	Platelets	54

Table 2. Experimental Cell-Attachment and Spreading Factors

FACTOR	REACTIVE CELL TYPES	REFERENCES
Polycations	Fibroblasts	55–58
	Leukemia cells	55
	Glioma	59
	Carcinoma	60
	Hepatocytes	6
Lectins	Fibroblasts	58, 61, 62
	Glioma	59
	Hepatocytes	63
	Lymphocytes	64, 65
	Lymphosarcoma	66
	Carcinoma	66
Glycosidases	Fibroblasts	61
Anti-cell-surface antibodies	Fibroblasts	58, 67
	Lymphoma	59
Asialoglycoproteins	Hepatocytes	5, 6
Carbohydrate-derivatized gels	Hepatocytes	68, 69
	Cerebellar cells	70

bind to the surfaces in a given time period. Spreading is determined microscopically by observing the changes in cell morphology that accompany cell attachment. In most cases, the factors listed promote both attachment and spreading.

The lists of factors in Tables 1 and 2 are representative, but by no means inclusive. The natural factors listed in Table 1 are those that cells normally might be expected to encounter either in tissue culture or *in vivo*. The experimental factors are those that have been shown to promote cell–substratum interactions, but that cells normally would not be expected to encounter except under these limited experimental conditions.

More than 30 years ago, P. Weiss pointed out the possible significance of "conditioning" factors adsorbed to the culture-dish surface that might promote cell adhesion. Most of the specific adhesion factors listed in Tables 1 and 2, however, have been described during the past 5 years. In part, this reflects a change in focus of attention in experiments on cell–substratum interactions. In the past it was often assumed that the cells were interacting directly with the material surfaces used as culture supports. It has now become clear that proteins and other substances coat the material surfaces and constitute the biological substrata with which cells interact (for a review see 71). Thus the questions now under extensive investigation concern which substances that coat the material surfaces are able to promote cell adhesion and how they work. It should not be implied, however, that material surfaces are irrelevant. In fact, the extent of binding and conformation of adhesion-promoting substances can be controlled by the type of material surfaces used. In this way, the material surfaces exert considerable influence on the reactivity of specific adhesion factors. For instance, fibronectin has been shown to adsorb in different conformations on wettable and nonwettable surfaces, and the conformation on wettable surfaces is more biologically active (72).

The natural factor that has so far been shown to function with the widest variety of cell types is fibronectin. This high-molecular-weight plasma glycoprotein has been described extensively elsewhere with regard to its molecular properties (73–76) and its possible function in such diverse phenomena as embryogenesis (77), malignant cell invasion (78–80), reticuloendothelial function (81), thrombosis (74,75), and wound healing (74,82). As seen in Table 1, fibronectin has been shown to function as an attachment and spreading factor when adsorbed directly to material surfaces or when bound to denatured collagen, native collagen, fibrin, and poly-L-lysine. One significant problem associated with some of these studies is that it has not always been determined whether the effect of fibronectin is direct or indirect, that is, whether fibronectin itself is the adhesion factor or whether fibronectin acts indirectly by binding endogenous adhesion factors secreted by the cells. Although this problem is not limited to fibronectin, studies on this factor can serve as a good example of the more general situation.

Fibroblasts that secrete fibronectin can deposit their own adhesion factors on material surfaces (83) and on denatured collagen (25). The activity of the deposited material has been shown to be inhibited by anti-fibronectin (83). Also, if fibronectin secretion is inhibited, cell spreading is inhibited unless the surfaces are coated with fibronectin (84). In this case, therefore, it seems likely that fibronectin is acting directly as an adhesion factor. In studies on the interaction of certain epithelial cells with fibronectin, the situation is not so clear. For instance, fibronectin is probably not part of the basal lamina of epithelial cells, but may be necessary for basal lamina formation (85). Therefore, although it is possible that spreading of epithelial cells on fibronectin involves a direct interaction between fibronectin and a cell-surface fibronectin receptor (8,9), a more attractive hypothesis is that the fibronectin is necessary for binding epithelial-cell-secreted components (e.g., collagen IV or laminin) that form the "actual" sites involved in adhesion, that is, for which the cells have appropriate cell-surface receptors (33,38). In studying cell-adhesion factors, therefore, it is very important to determine whether the specific adhesion factors function in the absence of cell protein synthesis. Simply stopping protein synthesis at the time of the adhesion experiments, however, may not be sufficient, since large internal pools of adhesion proteins may be present. For instance, fibroblasts require 2–6 hours in cycloheximide to turn over their fibronectin pools (84,86).

That adhesion factors can act indirectly can also be inferred if the factors promote cell adhesion when present in the incubation medium, but have no effect if they are only used to precoat the material surface. Examples are chondronectin with chondrocytes (35) and epibolin with epidermal cells (87). The explanation can be quite complex. For instance, the factor may be required for cell viability or to reverse damage caused by trypsin or other treatments used to harvest the cells. Alternatively, the factor may promote the secretion of an endogenous cell-adhesion factor. Finally, the factor may work in combination with another component secreted by the cells such that both together constitute the adhesion factor. This latter possibility seems to be the case with chondronectin (88).

Several comments are pertinent concerning the research on collagen–cell interactions. Omitted from Table 1 are the numerous studies indicating that collagen substrata are useful in promoting cell growth (89) and differentiation (e.g., 90,91). In most of these cases, however, the effective factor in adhesion (e.g., collagen itself, fibronectin/collagen, etc.) has not been determined. Table 1 makes a distinction between native and denatured collagen. This refers to whether or not the collagen substrata are hydrated or have been air dried, respectively. The problems with air-dried gels are that they are at least partially denatured [based upon trypsin sensitivity (25)], and they present cells with a planar surface rather than a hydrated matrix (92). This changes the kinds of interactions that can occur between the cells and the substratum, as is discussed later in this review. Finally, with some cell types a preference for particular collagen types has been demonstrated. For instance, epidermal and fibrosarcoma cells prefer type-IV collagen (33,34); smooth muscle prefers type-V collagen (15). Hepatocytes, on the other hand, show no preference for a particular collagen type and will even react with collagen-related polypeptides (93).

Finally, although a large number of endogenous spreading factors have now been recognized, as indicated in Table 1, there are undoubtedly other factors that have yet to be discovered. This wide diversity of adhesion factors presumably reflects the different functions and physiological locations of cells and their requirements for specialized adhesive interactions under different circumstances.

3.   LIGAND–RECEPTOR MODEL FOR CELL ATTACHMENT AND SPREADING

There is a variety of evidence to suggest that the cell–substratum interactions promoted by the factors listed in Tables 1 and 2 involve ligand–

receptor interactions. The ligands are the adhesion factors that constitute the substratum, and the receptors are the ligand-binding sites on the cell surface. Among the endogenous factors, only the receptors for immune complexes (the Fc receptor) and complement-coated immune complexes (the C3 receptor) have been clearly identified. For the most part, the role of ligand–receptor interactions in adhesion has been worked out with the experimental adhesion factors.

The experimental ligands that have been shown to function as adhesion factors for the largest number of cell types are the polycationic proteins (see Table 2). The spreading of baby hamster kidney (BHK) cells on polycationic ferritin (PCF) is shown in Fig. 1. The model to explain what is occurring is presented in Fig. 2, in which it can be seen that the ligand on the substratum is proposed to interact with receptors on the cell surface. The reaction between PCF and anionic components of the cell surface would be expected to be electrostatic. Consistent with this view, addition of small amounts of the polyanionic polysaccharide heparin inhibits cell spreading on PCF-coated surfaces but not on surfaces coated by other ligands (i.e., concanavalin A, antibodies to BHK cell membranes, or fibronectin). Alternatively, specific inhibitors of cell spreading on surfaces coated by other

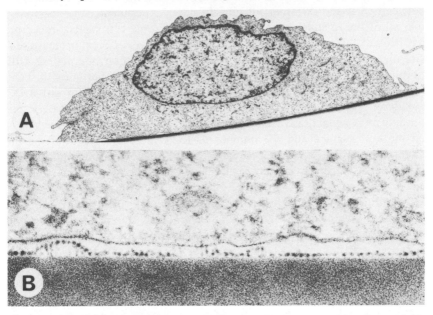

Figure 1. Appearance of BHK cells interacting with PCF-coated material surfaces. (A) The morphology of cells spread on PCF-coated surfaces is similar to that found with cells spread on serum- or fibronectin-coated surfaces. (B) Detail of the cell–material-surface interface, showing a monolayer of adsorbed PCF molecules and close interactions between cells and the PCF. (A) ×5000; (B) ×200,000. See references 58 and 94 for other details.

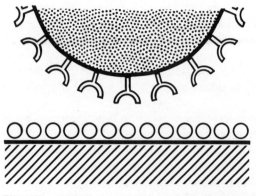

Figure 2. Ligand-receptor model for cell adhesion. Receptors on the cell surface interact with ligands adsorbed to the material surface. See text for additional discussion.

ligands (i.e., α-methylmannoside for ConA, anti-immunoglobulin for antibodies to BHK cells, and anti-fibronectin for fibronectin) have no effect on the interaction of BHK cells with PCF substrata (58).

These experiments indicate the specificity of the binding interactions between cells and different ligands. In other experiments, the possibility that all of the ligands are interacting with the same cell-surface receptors has been excluded. For instance, the receptors have different protease sensitivities. Pronase treatment of BHK cells inhibits their interactions with fibronectin or wheat germ agglutinin (WGA) substrata, but not with PCF, concanavalin A (ConA), ricinus communis agglutinin (RCA), or anti-BHK-membrane substrata (58,95). Also, as shown with several variant BHK cell lines, there is a quantitative relationship between the number of RCA receptors on the cell surface and the number of RCA molecules required on the material surface to promote cell adhesion (62). These results indicate that different cell-surface receptors on the same cell can mediate cell attachment and spreading.

In addition to the ligand–receptor interaction, cell spreading also appears to involve a cytoskeletal-reorganization process. This process appears to be independent of which ligand is used to promote cell spreading. For instance, addition of reagents like cytochalasin B or colchicine causes similar changes in the morphology of BHK cell spreading regardless of the ligand used to promote cell spreading (58). Also, treatment of BHK cells with WGA or with Fab fragments of antibodies directed against WGA receptors not only inhibits cell spreading on surfaces coated by different ligands, but also causes rounding up of cells previously spread on surfaces coated by different ligands (95,96). The situation appears to be similar to that which occurs in cell capping (e.g., antibody- or lectin-induced reorganization of cell-surface receptors to one pole of the cell), namely, different cell-surface receptors can be capped depending upon which ligand is added (97), but some sort of common cytoskeletal process is probably involved in every case (98,99).

In a previous review (71), the evidence was summarized that reagents such as trypsin and ethylene diamine tetraacetic acid (EDTA), which cause cell separation from the substratum, have their primary effect on the cell cytoskeleton and not on the ligand–receptor interactions that constitute the bonds of attachment per se. Recently, additional support for this view has been published (100–103). In related studies, several antibodies directed against cell-surface components have been reported to cause rounding of spread cells (104–107). Also, the rounding effect caused by either EDTA (103) or antibodies (96) requires cellular metabolic activity. These findings suggest the existence of a previously unrecognized *cell surface component* that apparently is involved in the linkage between ligand–receptor complexes and the cytoskeleton. The component appears to be trypsin sensitive and requires divalent cations and energy for continued function.

Thus, cell adhesion involves ligand-receptor interactions, cytoskeletal activity, and a coupling process between the ligand-receptor complexes and the cytoskeleton. This complicates the interpretation of studies attempting to analyze the ligand–receptor interactions. For instance, many investigators have suggested that divalent cations are required for activity of the fibroblast adhesion receptors for fibronectin because initial cell attachment does not occur in the absence of divalent cations (71). It should be emphasized, however, that initial cell attachment is preceded by a cytoskeleton-dependent initial contact process that requires divalent cations and can be inhibited by cytochalasin B or cold. These requirements can be overcome, however, if the necessity for the initial contact process is eliminated by centrifuging cells against the substratum (108). On the other hand, when small (0.76μm), fibronectin-coated latex beads are used to analyze the cell-surface fibronectin receptors directly, no requirement for an initial contact process such as described above is observed (109). Therefore, the fibronectin–receptor bonding mechanism per se is probably independent of divalent cations. The use of ligand-coated beads as probes for cell surface ligand-receptor sites may be generally useful.

A related problem in interpreting studies on ligand–receptor interactions occurs because cells continue to modulate the organization of their cytoskeletons even after initial cell spreading. With many types of fibroblasts, for example, initial cell spreading appears to be associated with close (15–30 nm) cell–substratum interactions that later mature to focal interactions (5–10 nm) (110–112). This is shown for early-passage human fibroblasts in Fig. 3 using an antibody-exclusion assay for focal adhesions (113). The

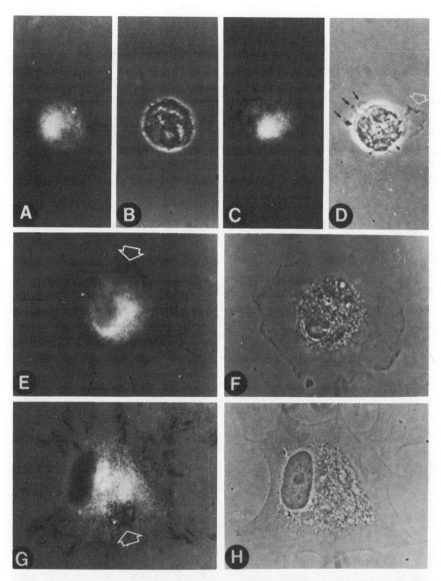

Figure 3. Appearance of marginal focal adhesions during spreading of human fibroblasts on fibronectin-coated surfaces. (A), (C), (E), (G) In indirect immunofluorescence analysis, focal adhesions are visualized as dark regions and spots from which antibody is excluded. (B), (D), (F), (H) Cell morphology is observed by phase-contrast microscopy. Cells attached for 15 minutes have focal adhesions beneath the cells (A), (C) and at the tips of filopodia (C), (D), (*small arrows*), but not beneath the region of the spreading lamellipodia (C), (D), (*large arrow*). After 30 minutes, complete cell spreading can be observed (F), but focal adhesions are either absent or very small (E), (*small arrows*). After 60 minutes, focal adhesions have formed all along the margins of the lamellipodia (G), (H). The region of focal adhesions beneath the center of the cells remains constant throughout spreading (E), (G), (*large arrows*). ×700. See reference 113 for other details.

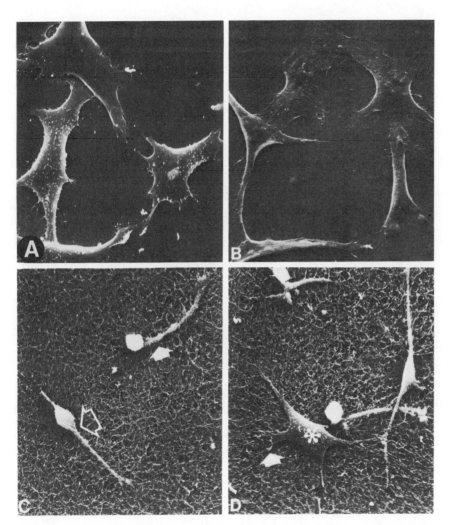

Figure 4. Adhesion of BHK cells on glass and collagen surfaces. (*A*) Glass. (*B*) Dried collagen. (*C*), (*D*) Hydrated collagen. Cells spread with lamellipodial extensions on glass (*A*) or dried collagen surfaces (*B*). In both cases, fibronectin is required. On hydrated collagen lattices, cells spread with pseudopodia and are usually monopolar [(*C*), *closed arrow*] or bipolar [(*C*), *open arrow*]. Fibronectin in not required. If, however, fibronectin is added, cell spreading is unchanged except for an increase in the number of well-spread cells [(*D*), *asterisk*] with lamillipodial extensions [(*D*), *arrow*]. ×750. See reference 92 for other details.

277

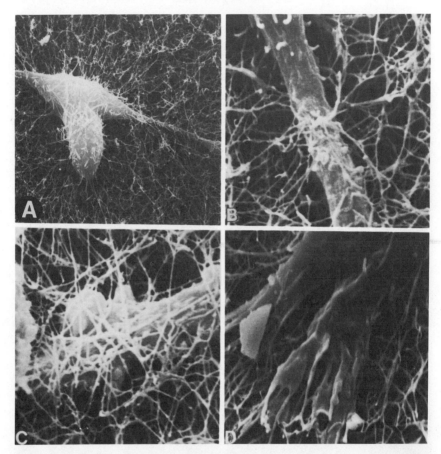

Figure 5. Adhesion of BHK cells on hydrated collagen lattices. (A) Cells can completely penetrate into the collagen lattice. (B), (C) Higher magnification of pseudopodia in Fig. 4C. Extensions from bipolar cell (B) and monopolar cell (C) penetrate into the lattice. (D) Higher magnification of lamellar extension in Fig. 4D, showing that the lamellipodium remains on top of the lattice. (A) ×2300; (B)–(D), ×7500. See reference 92 for other details.

formation of focal interactions at the cell margins occurs at a time well after cells are already spread. The parameters that control formation of focal contacts and the relationship of those contacts to ligand–receptor complexes are not well understood. There appears to be a strengthening of adhesions by changes in cytoskeletal organization (114) that result in the formation of stress fibers that insert into the focal contacts (115). Recently, studies of a mutant 3T3 fibroblast (AD6) that is unable to make focal adhesions have shown that fibronectin promotes the formation of close cell–substratum interactions (116). A relationship between fibronectin, focal interactions, and the cell cytoskeleton has also been demonstrated (117,118), although this point is controversial (119–121).

Before leaving the subject of the ligand–receptor model, it should be mentioned that physical-mechanical interactions, as well as specific chemical bonding, may also play a role in adhesion in situations where the cells can penetrate into the substratum. For instance, Figs. 4 and 5 present information on BHK cell spreading on hydrated and dried collagen matrices. As mentioned earlier, dried collagen substrata have a planar surface (92). The cells spread on top of the surface in a fibronectin-dependent interaction and appear similar to cells on other planar surfaces such as plastic or glass. With hydrated collagen lattices, the cells spread into the collagen matrix (i.e., they are invasive) in a fibronectin-independent interaction and have a more *in vivo*–like morphology (92). Although these cells may be interacting with the collagen through a cell-surface collagen receptor (122), it is also likely that the cell microvilli and filopodia that interweave with the collagen fibrils can provide a mechanical basis for stretching the cells. Since cells normally interact with hydrated matrices *in vivo*, the nature of cell interactions with matrices is of major concern, but so far has received little attention.

4.   MULTIVALENT CHARACTERISTIC OF CELL–SUBSTRATUM LIGAND–RECEPTOR INTERACTIONS

One of the important features of cell–substratum ligand–receptor interactions is their multivalency. That is, they involve both multiple ligand sites and multiple receptor sites. The multivalency of the interaction appears to be required for adhesion promoting activity, and in several instances specific threshold effects can be observed. Several systems in which multivalent interactions are important are described below.

4.1.   Fibroblast Spreading and Fibronectin

In order to promote spreading of fibroblasts on material surfaces (e.g., plastic, glass), fibronectin must adsorb onto the material surface. If protein adsorption sites on the material surfaces are blocked with nonfunctional proteins (e.g., albumin), then fibronectin cannot adsorb, and no cell spreading activity can be detected even with excess fibronectin in the medium (123). In addition, spreading of cells on fibronectin-coated surfaces demonstrates cooperative binding kinetics with respect to the amount of fibronectin adsorbed on the surfaces. That is, below a certain threshold concentration of fibronectin molecules adsorbed on the material surface, little cell spreading takes place.

Above the critical concentration (about 45,000 molecules beneath each cell), complete spreading occurs (67). Moreover, during spreading, most of the fibronectin receptors can no longer be detected on the upper cell surface and probably migrate around to interact with adsorbed fibronectin on the substratum (109).

Although fibronectin molecules adsorbed on the material surface promote cell adhesion, individual fibronectin molecules do not have a high affinity for the cells. Also, the presence of excess soluble fibronectin in the incubation medium does not affect the interaction of cells with substratum-bound fibronectin (67). Binding of radiolabeled fibronectin to cells in suspension cannot be detected at 37°C although it does occur at 4°C (124). If, on the other hand, multimeric fibronectin is produced by allowing individual fibronectin molecules to adsorb to latex beads, then binding with cells occurs readily at 37°C (109).

4.2. Hepatocyte Spreading on Collagen and Attachment to Immobilized Sugars

Spreading of hepatocytes on native collagen depends upon the concentration of collagen molecules on the substratum and occurs faster with intact collagen fibrils than with individual collagen chains (93). Although there is no detectable cell-surface binding of individual collagen molecules in solution (27), a weak interaction must occur, since the addition of soluble collagen molecules to the incubation medium slightly retards the initial rate of cell adhesion to substratum-bound collagen (93).

Hepatocytes also attach to substrata coated by asialoglycoproteins (5), presumably by the asialoglycoprotein receptor (125). This interaction has been studied using polyacrylamide gels that contain the individual carbohydrate molecules that constitute the recognition sites for asialoglycoproteins (68). There is a dramatic threshold effect in cell binding dependent upon the concentration of carbohydrate in the gels; a 10% increase above the threshold concentration results in complete cell attachment to the gels, whereas no attachment occurs below the threshold concentration (69). Moreover, during formation of the stable attachments, the cell-surface receptors undergo redistribution to the cell–substratum binding region (126).

4.3. Platelet Aggregation by Collagen and Adhesion Mediated by Von Willebrand Factor

Several types of molecules are able to cause platelet aggregation including collagen, immune complexes, aggregated immunoglobulin, fibrinogen derivatives, and high-molecular-weight poly-L-lysine. It has been noted that in all of these instances, the eliciting molecules are large and have a repeating structure (127). The relative abilities of tropocollagen and fibrillar collagen to promote platelet aggregation have been compared, and it has been found that there is a correlation between the amount of collagen-fibril formation and the extent of platelet aggregation (31). Individual tropocollagen molecules also can be formed into a random supermolecular structure by glutaraldehyde cross-linking. These molecules have been found to be almost as active in promoting platelet aggregation as normal collagen fibrils (32).

Platelets are also able to attach to and spread on the subendothelial basement membrane (54). This interaction is decreased in patients with von Willebrand deficiency but can be corrected by the addition of von Willebrand factor–containing cryoprecipitate (44). Recently, it has been found that von Willebrand factor binds to subendothelial basement membrane and forms the sites to which platelets attach (45); this attachment occurs even in the presence of excess soluble von Willebrand factor found in the plasma. Von Willebrand factor exhibits molecular heterogeneity (i.e., it exists as a series of multimers), and it is the high-molecular-weight polymers that are active (128). Also, a multimeric form prepared by coating gold particles with the low-molecular-weight species of von Willebrand factor is able to bind to platelets (129).

4.4. Macrophage Phagocytosis and Immunoglobulin

Spreading of macrophages on antigen-coated material surfaces is considered to be equivalent to the phagocytosis of a particle of infinite diameter (see Section 5). The system in which multivalent binding interactions were first studied was that of macrophage phagocytosis of antigen particles opsinized by immunoglobulins. In a study using small antigens with variable valencies, it has been found that there is a correlation between the degree of antigen valency and the ability of antigen–antibody complexes to bind to the cells (130). That is, conditions that favor the formation of a polyvalent antibody–antigen lattice promote binding. Also, the polyvalent complexes dissociate from the cells more slowly than the monovalent complexes. In other studies, analyses of γ globulins aggregated by heat (131) or chemical cross-linking (132) have shown that the higher-molecular-weight polymers are able to bind to the cells better than the monomers.

4.5. Multivalency, Strength of Interactions, and Threshold Effects

The first conclusion that can be drawn from the experiments described in Sections 4.1–4.4 is that multivalent interactions can result in cell binding to ligand-coated surfaces even if the individual ligand molecules in solution bind weakly to the cell-surface receptors. This is because the effective strength of binding between the cells and the ligand-coated surfaces is much stronger than would be predicted based upon the summation of the individual interactions that are occurring. Theoretical analysis indicates that for a multivalent interaction, the apparent affinity between multiple receptors and multiple ligands is a *multiplicative* function of the monomer affinities, not simply an *additive* function (133). This has been confirmed by measuring the affinities between antigen and antibody, comparing divalent immuno-globulins with monovalent F_{ab} fragments. With antibodies directed against red blood cells, the intact immunoglobulin has been found to have an affinity for the antigen 150–450 times greater than that of the F_{ab} fragments (134). In another study, with antibodies to dinitrophenol, the intact immunoglobulin has been found to have an affinity for the antigen 10,000 times greater than that of the F_{ab} fragments (135). When it is considered that cell interactions with ligand-coated surfaces may involve hundreds or thousands of ligand–receptor binding interactions, it becomes obvious that very large apparent binding affinities are possible.

The increased affinity resulting from multivalent ligand–receptor binding is also very important for cell interactions with adhesive surfaces *in vivo*. For example, the migration of fibroblasts into plasma clots during formation of the granulation tissue is in part dependent upon adhesion of the cells to fibronectin-coated fibrin and denatured collagen substrata (136). There is, however, excess soluble fibronectin found in the tissue fluid (137). Assuming that the affinity of the cell-surface fibronectin receptors is the same for soluble fibronectin molecules as for fibronectin molecules bound to fibrin and collagen, then there should be competiton for the fibroblast receptors. This competition could decrease or prevent the adhesion of cells to the fibronectin-coated matrix. Nevertheless, the cells do interact with, and move along, the matrix. Many of the other reactions mediated by the adhesion factors listed in Table 1 also must occur *in vivo* in the presence of excess soluble ligand molecules. Why, then, don't the soluble molecules prevent cell binding to ligand-coated surfaces? The reason is that multivalent in-teractions involve *simultaneous* binding between many ligands and receptors. The individual ligand molecules would have to reverse *all of the multivalent interactions at the same time* in order to prevent or reverse cell binding to the ligand-coated surfaces, which is very unlikely. Thus the multivalent interactions between cells and ligand-coated surfaces are probably an essential requirement for proper cell interaction with ligand-coated surfaces when excess soluble ligand is present.

Finally, attention has been drawn to the threshold levels of multivalency that are required for fibroblast spreading on fibronectin on RCA-coated material surfaces (62,67) and for hepatocyte binding to carbohydrate-linked gels (69). An attractive hypothesis is that a minimum number of ligand–

receptor interactions is required before some other cellular event involved in adhesion can occur, such as linkage of ligand–receptor complexes to the cytoskeleton (98,99). The explanation of the threshold effect is an important problem that requires further study.

5.   CELL SPREADING AND PHAGOCYTOSIS

The notion that spreading of macrophages on surfaces is an attempt by the cells to phagocytose a "particle" of infinite diameter was suggested by North a number of years ago (138). Some of the evidence favoring this idea was reviewed previously (71). In particular, similar ligand–receptor interactions, cytoskeletal requirements, and metabolic parameters appear to be

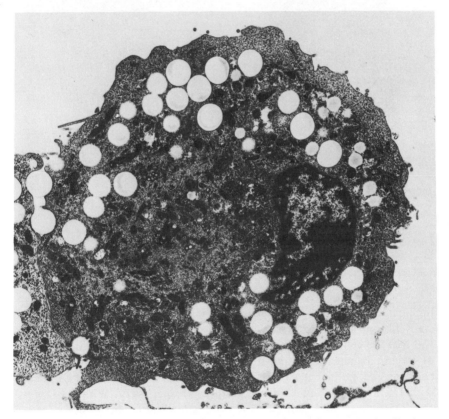

Figure 6.   Interaction of BHK cells with fibronectin-coated latex beads (1 μm). After 60 minutes, extensive phagocytosis has occurred. × 6500. See reference 109 for other details.

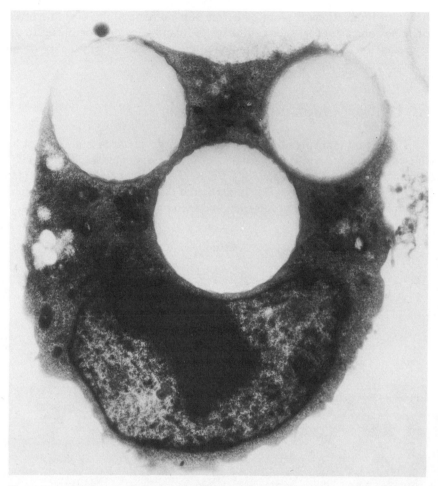

Figure 7.   Interaction of BHK cells with fibronectin-coated latex beads (5 μm). After 60 minutes, cells have phagocytosed several beads. ×6500. See reference 109 for other details.

implicated. Recently, latex particles coated with fibronectin were used to study fibronectin receptors on fibroblasts (109). A surprising observation was that the cells avidly phagocytose the particles at 37°C. Using particles of varying diameters, the transition between cell phagocytosis and spreading has been evaluated. Figures 6, 7, and 8 show the interactions of BHK cells with 1-μm, 5-μm, and 15.8-μm particles, respectively. With the largest-sized particle, what would be called cell spreading is observed.

Another interesting point relating cell spreading and phagocytosis concerns the "zipper" hypothesis. This hypothesis has been proposed based upon

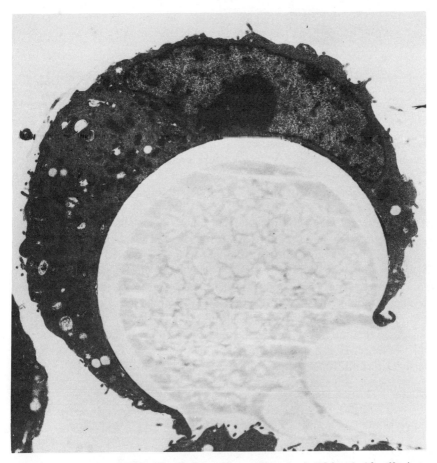

Figure 8.   Interaction of BHK cells with fibronectin-coated latex beads (15.8 μm). After 60 minutes, cells appear to spread around the bead surface but are unable to completely phagocytose the beads. ×6500. Compare with Fig. 1. See reference 109 for other details.

the finding with macrophages that particle phagocytosis required continuous ligand–receptor interactions between cell-surface receptors and ligands that form a coat around the entire particle circumference (139). Interactions between cell-surface receptors and ligands coating a small portion of the particle surface can promote particle attachment to the cells, but do not trigger the ingestion process. A variety of evidence also favors a zipper hypothesis for fibroblast spreading. Fibroblast spreading occurs by the extension of filopodia and other cell processes from the base of the cells along the ligand-coated material surface (140,141). If the ligand-coated surfaces have discontinuities in the ligand coating, then cell spreading does not occur beyond the regions where the ligand is present (83).

6.   INITIAL FIBROBLAST–SUBSTRATUM INTERACTIONS IN SERUM-CONTAINING MEDIUM

The last subject to be considered in this review concerns the problem of how fibroblasts spread on tissue-culture dishes in the presence of 10% serum-containing medium under routine culture conditions. The idea that cells interact initially with fibronectin adsorbed out of serum onto the surfaces of the culture dishes was favored by our laboratory (71). Several new experimental findings, however, have raised important questions about the previous interpretation of the data. Of particular significance is the observation that the spreading of fibroblasts on serum-coated dishes requires protein synthesis, whereas spreading of cells on fibronectin-coated dishes does not (24). Also, the divalent-cation requirements for fibroblast spreading on serum-coated dishes are somewhat different from those for spreading on fibronectin-coated dishes (123). Since other components of serum also have been reported to promote cell spreading (22–24), the possibility has to be considered that the interaction of the cells with culture dishes in the presence of 10% serum is not dependent upon an interaction of cells with serum fibronectin initially adsorbed on the dish surfaces.

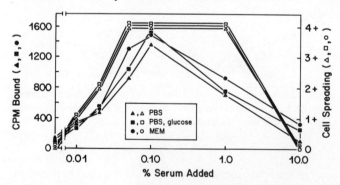

Figure 9.   Adsorption of fibronectin from serum solutions in relationship to cell-spreading activity. Pairs of tissue-culture dishes were treated with human serum at the concentrations indicated in several different buffers for 10 minutes at 22°C. The buffers were modified Dulbecco's phosphate-buffered saline *(PBS)*, PBS with 1 mg of glucose per milliliter *(PBS, glucose)*, or minimal essential growth medium *(MEM)*. At the end of the incubations, the dishes were rinsed with buffer and the cells fixed with formaldehyde. Subsequently, one dish from each of the pairs was used to determine the amount of fibronectin bound to the dish surfaces using an indirect radioactive-antibody assay. The other dish was used to determine BHK cell spreading in a 45-minute assay. Other details are found in reference 142.

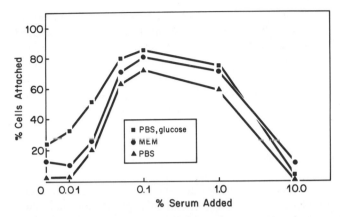

Figure 10. Attachment of BHK cells to tissue-culture dishes pretreated with serum solutions. The experiments were carried out as described in Fig. 9 except that the dishes were used to determine the extent of cell attachment with a radioactive cell-binding assay. Other details are found in reference 142.

Recent studies have been carried out to test this point directly (142). Figures 9 and 10 show experiments in which culture dishes were preincubated with various buffers or cell growth medium containing increasing levels of serum. Subsequently, the amount of fibronectin adsorbed onto the surfaces from the serum was quantitated using an indirect radiolabeled-antibody binding assay. In addition, the ability of BHK cells to spread (Fig. 9) and to attach to the surfaces (Fig. 10) was quantitated. The results show that there is a close correspondence between the extent of fibronectin adsorption and the degree of cell attachment and spreading under these assay conditions. Of particular importance, however, is the finding that above 1% serum there is a decrease in fibronectin adsorption and cell adhesion to the surfaces. The decrease in fibronectin adsorption can be attributed to the adsorption of serum albumin. Adsorption of albumin becomes dominant over adsorption of fibronectin when albumin is present at 5 mg/ml (72), which is the concentration found in 10% serum solutions. These findings indicate, therefore, that initial cell adhesion to 10%-serum-coated surfaces cannot be the result of cells attaching to adsorbed serum fibronectin.

Since the fibroblasts can eventually attach and spread on surfaces treated with 10%-serum-containing medium, to what are they binding? One possibility is that serum factors other than fibronectin immediately coat the dish surfaces (22–24). The requirement for protein synthesis, however, suggests that something more complex is going on. For instance, cells may bind to secreted extracellular matrix components by a fibronectin-independent mechanism (143). Alternatively, cells may deposit on the serum-coated surfaces proteoglycans to which endogenously secreted fibronectin or serum fibronectin can bind (144–146). This would result in a fibronectin-coated surface, albeit by an indirect route. Another possibility is that cells remove bound serum components from the culture-dish surfaces (121) and replace these with other substances (either fibronectin or some other extracellular matrix component) that function as cell-adhesion factors. In any event, the mechanism is clearly more complex than previously assumed.

7.   CONCLUDING COMMENTS

The idea that ligand–receptor interactions between extracellular components and cells could be a basic determinant of cell adhesive behavior was implied by Weiss and by Tyler more than 30 years ago (147,148). Now, as reviewed in this paper, there has been considerable success in isolating specific extracellular materials that function as cell attachment and spreading factors. Undoubtedly, additional factors will be described in the future. The problem now is to relate the adhesion factors to the *in vivo* situation and to determine which ones regulate cell adhesion and migration *in vivo* and under what circumstances they are active.

ACKNOWLEDGMENTS

The author's research has been supported by grants from the National Institutes of Health, CA 14609 and HL 24221. Drs. William Snell and Richard Anderson provided helpful criticism of the manuscript.

REFERENCES

1. Grinnell, F., Hays, D., and Minter, D., *Exp. Cell Res.*, **110**, 175 (1977).
2. Pena, S. D. J., and Hughes, R. S., *Cell Biol. Int. Rep.*, **2**, 339 (1978).
3. Thom, D., Powell, A. J., and Rees, D. A., *J. Cell Science*, **35**, 281 (1979).
4. Sanders, E. J., *J. Cell Science*, **44**, 225 (1980).
5. Hook, M., Rubin, K., Oldberg, A., Obrink, B., and Vaheri, A., *Biochem. Biophys. Res. Commun.*, **79**, 726 (1977).
6. Gjessing, R., and Seglen, P. O., *Exp. Cell Res.*, **129**, 239 (1980).
7. Rizzino, A., and Crowley, C., *Proc. Natl. Acad. Sci. USA*, **77**, 457 (1980).
8. Hughes, R. C., Mills, G., and Courtois, Y., *Biol. Cell.*, **36**, 321 (1979).
9. Gilchrest, B. A., Nemore, R. E., and Maciag, T., *Cell Biol. Int. Rep.*, **4**, 1009 (1980).
10. Klebe, R. J., *Nature*, **250**, 248 (1974).
11. Pearlstein, E., *Nature*, **262**, 497 (1976).

12. Kleinman, H. K., McGoodwin, E. B., and Klebe, R. J., *Biochem. Biophys. Res. Commun.*, **72**, 426 (1976).

13. Chiquet, M., Puri, E. C., and Turner, D. C., *J. Biol. Chem.*, **254**, 5475 (1979).

14. Gold, L. I., and Pearlstein, E., *Biochem. J.*, **186**, 551 (1980).

15. Grotendorst, G. R., Seppa, H. E., Kleinman, H. K., and Martin, G., *Proc. Natl. Acad. Sci. USA*, **78**, 3669 (1981).

16. Hoffstein, S. T., Weissman, G., and Pearlstein, E., *J. Cell Science*, **50**, 315 (1981).

17. Hynes, R. O., Ali, I. U., Destree, A. T., Mautner, V., Perkins, M. E., Senger, D. R., Warner, D. D., and Smith, K. K., *Ann. N.Y. Acad. Sci.*, **312**, 317 (1978).

18. Grinnell, F., Feld, M., and Snell, W. J., *Cell Biol. Int. Rep.*, **3**, 585 (1979).

19. Koteliansky, V. E., Leytin, V. L., Sviridov, D. D., Repin, V. S., and Smirnov, V. N., *FEBS Lett.*, **123**, 59 (1981).

20. Grinnell, F., Feld, M., and Minter, D., *Cell*, **19**, 517 (1980).

21. Bottenstein, J. E., and Sato, G. H., *Exp. Cell Res.*, **129**, 361 (1980).

22. Holmes, R., *J. Cell Biol.*, **32**, 297 (1967).

23. Barnes, D., Wolfe, R., Serrero, G., McClure, D., and Sato, G., *J. Supramol. Struct.*, **14**, 47 (1980).

24. Knox, P., and Griffiths, S., *J. Cell Science*, **46**, 97 (1980).

25. Grinnell, F., and Minter, D., *Proc. Natl. Acad. Sci. USA*, **75**, 4408 (1978).

26. Schor, S. L., and Court, J., *J. Cell Science*, **38**, 267 (1979).

27. Rubin, K., Oldberg, A., Hook, M., and Obrink, B., *Exp. Cell Res.*, **117**, 165 (1978).

28. Wicha, M. S., Liotta, L. A., Garbisa, S., and Kidwell, W. R., *Exp. Cell Res.*, **124**, 181 (1979).

29. Michalopoulos, G., Russell, F., and Biles, C., *In Vitro*, **15**, 796 (1979).

30. Emerman, J. T., Burwen, S. J., and Pitelka, D. R., *Tissue Cell*, **11**, 109 (1979).

31. Muggli, R., and Baumgartner, H. R., *Thromb. Res.*, **3**, 715 (1973).

32. Santoro, S. A., and Cunningham, L. W., *Thromb. Haemost.*, **43**, 158 (1980).

33. Murray, J. C., Stingl, G., Kleinman, H. K., Martin, G. R., and Katz, S. I., *J. Cell Biol.*, **80**, 197 (1979).

34. Murray, J. C., Liotta, L., Rennard, S. I., and Martin, G. R., *Cancer Res.*, **40**, 347 (1980).

35. Hewitt, A. T., Kleinman, H. K., Pennypacker, J. P., and Martin, G. R., *Proc. Natl. Acad. Sci. USA*, **77**, 385 (1980).

36. Johansson, S., Kjellen, L., Hook, M., and Timpl, R., *J. Cell Biol.*, **90**, 260 (1981).

37. Vlodavsky, I., and Gospodarowicz, D., *Nature*, **289**, 304 (1981).

38. Terranova, V. P., Rohrback, D. H., and Martin, G. R., *Cell*, **22**, 719 (1980).

39. Rabinovitch, M., Manijas, R. E., and Nussenzweig, V., *J. Exp. Med.*, **142**, 827 (1975).

40. Michl, J., Pieczonka, M. M., Unkeles, J. C., and Silverstein, S. C., *J. Exp. Med.*, **150**, 607 (1979).

41. Douglas, S. D., *Cell. Immunol.*, **21**, 344 (1976).

42. Henson, P. M., *J. Immunol.*, **107**, 1547 (1971).

43. Alexander, E., and Henkart, P., *J. Exp. Med.*, **143**, 329 (1976).

44. Weiss, H. J., Baumgartner, H. R., Tschopp, T. B., Turitto, V. T., and Cohen, D., *Blood*, **51**, 267 (1978).

45. Sakariassen, K. S., Bolhus, P. A., and Sixma, J. J., *Nature*, **279**, 636 (1979).
46. Rheinwald, J. G., and Green, H., *Cell*, **6**, 331 (1975).
47. Gospodarowicz, D., Greenburg, G., and Birdwell, C. R., *Cancer Res.*, **38**, 4155 (1978).
48. Reid, L. M., Gaitmaitan, Z., Arias, I., Ponce, P., and Rojkind, M., *Ann. N.Y. Acad. Sci.*, **349**, 70 (1980).
49. Weiss, P., *J. Exp. Zool.*, **100**, 353 (1945).
50. Collins, F., *Proc. Natl. Acad. Sci. USA*, **75**, 5210 (1978).
51. Rubin, H., *Symp. Soc. Dev. Biol.*, **25**, 315 (1966).
52. Culp, L. A., *J. Cell Biol.*, **63**, 71 (1974).
53. Yasuda, K., *J. Cell Science*, **15**, 269 (1974).
54. Booyse, F. M., Quarfoot, A. J., Bell, S., Fass, D. N., Lewis, J. C., Mann, K. G., and Bowie, E. J. W., *Proc. Natl. Acad. Sci. USA*, **74**, 5702 (1977).
55. Macieira-Coelho, A., and Avrameas, S., *Proc. Natl. Acad. Sci. USA*, **69**, 2469 (1972).
56. Letourneau, P. C., *Dev. Biol.*, **44**, 77 (1975).
57. McKeehan, W. L., and Ham, R. G., *J. Cell Biol.*, **71**, 727 (1976).
58. Grinnell, F., and Hays, D. G., *Exp. Cell Res.*, **116**, 275 (1978).
59. Carlsson, J., Gabel, D., Larsson, E., Ponten, J., and Westermark, B., *In Vitro*, **15**, 844 (1979).
60. Bases, R., Mendez, F., Mendez, L., and Anigstein, R., *Exp. Cell Res.*, **76**, 441 (1973).
61. Rauvala, H., Carter, W. G., and Makomori, S-I., *J. Cell Biol.*, **88**, 127 (1981).
62. Aplin, J. D., and Hughes, R. C., *J. Cell Science*, **50**, 89 (1981).
63. Seglen, P. O., and Fossa, J., *Exp. Cell Res.*, **116**, 199 (1978).
64. Edelman, G. M., Rutishauser, U., and Millette, C. F., *Proc. Natl. Acad. Sci. USA*, **68**, 2153 (1971).
65. Wong, S. Y., Longenecker, B. M., Pazderka, F., and Ruth, R. F., *Exp. Cell Res.*, **92**, 428 (1975).
66. Guy, D., Latner, A. L., and Turner, G. A., *Exp. Cell Biol.*, **47**, 312 (1979).
67. Hughes, R. C., Pena, S. D. J., Clark, J., and Dourmashkin, R. R., *Exp. Cell Res.*, **121**, 307 (1979).
68. Schnaar, R. L., Weigel, P. H., Kuhlenschmidt, M. S., Lee, Y. C., and Roseman, S., *J. Biol. Chem.*, **253**, 7940 (1978).
69. Weigel, P. H., Schnarr, R. L., Kuhlenschmidt, M. S., Schmell, E., Lee, R. T., Lee, Y. C., and Roseman, S., *J. Biol. Chem.*, **254**, 10830 (1979).
70. Hatten, M. E., *J. Cell Biol.*, **89**, 54 (1981).
71. Grinnell, F., *Int. Rev. Cytol.*, **53**, 65 (1978).
72. Grinnell, F., and Feld, M. K., *J. Biomed. Mat. Res.*, **15**, 363 (1981).
73. Yamada, K. M., and Olden, K., *Nature*, **275**, 179 (1978).
74. Mosher, D. F., *Prog. Hemostasis Thromb.*, **5**, 11 (1980).
75. Mossesson, M. W., and Amrani, D. L., *Blood*, **56**, 145 (1980).
76. Ruoslahti, E., Engvall, E., and Hayman, E. G., *Collagen Res.*, **1**, 95 (1981).
77. Wartiovaara, J., and Vaheri, A., *Dev. Mammals*, **4**, 233 (1980).
78. Hynes, R. O., *Biochim. Biophys. Acta*, **458**, 73 (1976).
79. Chen, L. B., Gallimore, P. H., and McDougall, J. K., *Proc. Natl. Acad. Sci. USA*, **73**, 3570 (1976).

80. Vaheri, A., and Mosher, D. F., *Biochim. Biophys. Acta*, **516**, 1 (1978).

81. Saba, T. M., and Jaffe, E., *Am. J. Med.*, **68**, 577 (1980).

82. Grinnell, F., *Am. J. Dermatopathol.*, **4**, 185 (1982).

83. Grinnell, F., and Feld, M. K., *Cell*, **17**, 117 (1979).

84. Grinnell, F., and Feld, M. K., *J. Cell. Physiol.*, **104**, 321 (1980).

85. Brownell, A. G., Bessem, C. C., and Slavkin, H. C., *Proc. Natl. Acad. Sci. USA*, **78**, 3711 (1981).

86. Yamada, K. M., *J. Cell Biol.*, **78**, 520 (1978).

87. Stenn, K. S., *J. Invest. Dermatol.*, **74**, 262 (1980)

88. Hewitt, A. T., Varber, H. H., and Martin, G. R., *J. Cell Biol.*, **91**, 154a (1981).

89. Ehrmann, R. L., and Gey, G. D., *J. Natl. Cancer Inst.*, **16**, 1375 (1956).

90. Dodson, J. W., *Exp. Cell Res.*, **31**, 233 (1963).

91. Hauschka, S. D., and Konegsberg, I. R., *Proc. Natl. Acad. Sci. USA*, **55**, 119 (1966).

92. Grinnell, F., and Bennett, M. H., *J. Cell Science*, **48**, 19 (1981).

93. Rubin, K., Hook, M., Obrink, B., and Timpl, R., *Cell*, **24**, 463 (1981).

94. Grinnell, F., Tobleman, M. Q., and Hackenbrock, C. R., *J. Cell Biol.*, **70**, 707 (1976).

95. Oppenheimer-Marks, N., and Grinnell, F., *Eur. J. Cell Biol.*, **23**, 286 (1981).

96. Oppenheimer-Marks, N., and Grinnell, F., *J. Cell Biol.*, **91**, 255a (1981).

97. Raff, M. C., and De Petris, S., *Fed. Proc.*, **32**, 48 (1973).

98. Edelman, G. M., *Science*, **192**, 218 (1976).

99. Singer, S. J., Ash, J. F., Bourguignon, Y. W., Heggeness, M. H., and Louvard, D., *J. Supramol. Struct.*, **9**, 373 (1978).

100. Whur, P., Koppel, H., Urguhart, C. M., and Williams, D. C., *J. Cell Science*, **24**, 265 (1977).

101. Vogel, K. G., *Exp. Cell Res.*, **113**, 345 (1978).

102. Furcht, L. T., and Wendelschafer-Crabb, G., *Exp. Cell Res.*, **114**, 1 (1978).

103. Britch, M., and Allen, T. D., *Exp. Cell Res.*, **125**, 221 (1980).

104. O'Neill, C. H., and Follett, E. A. C., *J. Cell Science*, 7, 695 (1970).

105. Yamada, K. M., Yamada, S. S., and Pastan, I., *Proc. Natl. Acad. Sci. USA*, **73**, 1217 (1976).

106. Wylie, D. E., Damsky, C. H., and Buck, C. A., *J. Cell Biol.*, **80**, 385 (1979).

107. Hsieh, P., and Sueoka, N., *J. Cell Biol.*, **86**, 866 (1980).

108. Grinnell, F., in V. T. Marchesi, Ed., *Membranes and Neoplasia: New Approaches and Strategies*, Alan R. Liss, New York, 1976, pp. 227–236.

109. Grinnell, F., *J. Cell Biol.*, **86**, 104 (1980).

110. Bragina, E. E., Vasiliev, J. M., and Gelfand, I. M., *Exp. Cell Res.*, **97**, 241 (1976).

111. Couchman, J. R., and Rees, D. A., *J. Cell Science*, **39**, 149 (1979).

112. Izzard, C. S., and Lochner, L. R., *J. Cell Science*, **42**, 81 (1980).

113. Grinnell, F., *Cell Biol. Int. Rep.*, **4**, 1031 (1980).

114. Rees, D. A., Lloyd, C. W., and Thom, D., *Nature*, **267**, 124 (1977).

115. Heath, J. P., and Dunn, G. A., *J. Cell Science*, **29**, 197 (1978).

116. Norton, E. K., and Izzard, C. S., *J. Cell Biol.*, **91**, 110a (1981).

117. Hynes, R. O., and Destree, A. T., *Cell*, **15**, 875 (1978).

118. Singer, I. I., *Cell*, **16**, 675 (1979).
119. Birchmeier, C., Kreis, T. E., Eppenberger, H. M., Winterhalter, K. H., and Birchmeier, W., *Proc. Natl. Acad. Sci. USA*, **77**, 4108 (1980).
120. Chen, W.-T., and Singer, S. J., *Proc. Natl. Acad. Sci. USA*, **77**, 7318 (1980).
121. Avnur, Z., and Geiger, B., *Cell*, **25**, 121 (1981).
122. Goldberg, B., *Cell*, **16**, 265 (1979).
123. Grinnell, F., *Exp. Cell Res.*, **102**, 51 (1976).
124. Grinnell, F., and Lang, B. S., *J. Cell Biol.*, **87**, 127a (1981).
125. Ashwell, G., and Morell, A. G., *Adv. Enzymol.*, **41**, 99 (1974).
126. Weigel, P. H., *J. Cell Biol.*, **87**, 855 (1980).
127. Luscher, E. F., Pfueller, S. L., and Massini, P., *Ser. Haemat.*, **6**, 382 (1973).
128. Pietu, G., Obert, B., Larrieu, M. J., and Meyer, D., *Thromb. Res.*, **19**, 671 (1980).
129. Furlan, M., Perret, B. A., and Beck, E. A., *Thromb. Haemost.*, **45**, 242 (1981).
130. Phillips-Quagliata, J. M., Levine, B. B., Quagliata, F., and Uhr, J. W., *J. Exp. Med.*, **133**, 5891 (1971).
131. Knutson, D. W., Kijlstra, A., and Van Es, L. A., *J. Exp. Med.*, **145**, 1368 (1977).
132. Segal, D. M., and Hurwitz, E., *J. Immunol.*, **118**, 1338 (1977).
133. Metzger, H., *Ann. N.Y. Acad. Sci.*, **190**, 322 (1971).
134. Greenburg, C. L., Moore, D., and Nunn, L. A. C., *Immunology*, **8**, 420 (1965).
135. Hornick, C. L. and Karush, F., in J. Sterzl and I. Riha, Eds., *Developmental Aspects of Antibody Formation and Structure*, Academic, London, 1970, pp. 433–443.
136. Grinnell, F., Billingham, R. E., and Burgess, L., *J. Invest. Dermatol.*, **76**, 181 (1981).
137. Robbins, A. B., Doran, J. E., Reese, A. C., and Mansberger, A. R., *Am. Surg.*, **46**, 663 (1980).
138. North, R. J., *J. Reticuloendthal. Soc.*, **5**, 203 (1968).
139. Griffin, F. M., Jr., Griffin, J. A., Leider, J. E., and Silverstein, S. C., *J. Exp. Med.*, **142**, 1263 (1975).
140. Witkowski, J. A., and Brighton, W. D., *Exp. Cell Res.*, **68**, 372 (1971).
141. Rajaraman, R., Rounds, D. E., Yen, S. P. S., and Rembaum, A., *Exp. Cell Res.*, **88**, 327 (1974).
142. Grinnell, F., and Feld, M. K., *J. Biol. Chem.*, **257**, 4888 (1982).
143. Harper, P. A., and Juliano, R. L., *Nature*, **290**, 136 (1981).
144. Culp, L., *Curr. Top. Membr. Transp.*, **11**, 327 (1978).
145. Culp, L. A., Rollins, B. J., Buniel, J., and Hitri, S., *J. Cell Biol.*, **79**, 788 (1978).
146. Laterra, J., Ansbacher, R., and Culp, L. A., *Proc. Natl. Acad. Sci. USA*, **77**, 6662 (1980).
147. Tyler, A., *Growth*, **10**, 7 (1946).
148. Weiss, P., *Yale J. Biol. Med.*, **19**, 235 (1946).

11

MULTIPLICATION-STIMULATING ACTIVITY AND THE ROLE OF CARRIER PROTEINS

Gary L. Smith

CONTENTS

Abbreviations

MSA	Multiplication-stimulating activity
NSILA	Nonsuppressible insulin-like activity
BRL-3A	Buffalo rat liver cells, line 3A
NSILA-S	Soluble nonsuppressible insulin-like activity
Sm	Somatomedin
Sm A	Somatomedin A
Sm C	Somatomedin C
IGF	Insulin-like growth factor
MCP	MSA carrier protein
NSILA-P	High molecular weight nonsuppressible insulin-like protein
NSILP	Nonsuppressible insulin-like protein
EGF	Epidermal growth factor
NGF	Nerve growth factor

Multiplication-stimulating activity (MSA) is a designation originally used by Dr. Howard M. Temin to describe activities present in serum that are required for the growth of animal cells in culture (1–4). Purification of these growth-promoting activities from serum proved to be a formidable task until it was observed that high concentrations of insulin partially replaced the serum requirement for the growth of cultured animal cells (1,5). Since there is not enough insulin in serum to account for its growth-promoting properties, Temin and his associates reasoned that the active components in serum might be related to other insulin-like polypeptides such as nonsuppressible insulin-like activity (NSILA). This term refers to serum components that have considerable insulin-like bioactivity but whose actions are not suppressible by antibody directed against the insulin molecule itself. These factors were known to exist in serum in relatively high concentrations (6–9). Using purification techniques previously described for the isolation of insulin-like activity, Pierson and Temin (10) succeeded in purifying MSA from calf serum approximately 6000-fold. The active fraction had an apparent molecular weight of 4000–5000 and was shown to possess nonsuppressible insulin-like activity.

Further work in Temin's laboratory led to the concept that although the growth of most cultured cells required the addition of a macromolecular supplement to the medium (traditionally supplied as serum), other cells that grew in low concentrations of serum or in its complete absence might satisfy this requirement by producing their own growth factors. To test this hypothesis, a cloned rat liver cell line originally established by Dr. Hayden Coon (11) that grew in serum-free medium was examined for its ability to produce factors that would support the growth of other serum-dependent cells. Indeed, serum-free medium conditioned by the growth of these Buffalo rat liver cells (BRL-3A) stimulated the growth of chicken embryo and rat embryo fibroblasts (12). Temin also referred to the growth-promoting components in BRL-3A conditioned medium as MSA. Dulak and Temin (12,13) and Smith and Temin (14) utilized rat-liver-cell-conditioned medium as a source for the purification of MSA. The assay used during this isolation was the ability of MSA to stimulate the incorporation of [³H]thymidine into the DNA of chicken embryo fibroblasts. The BRL-3A-conditioned medium proved to be a rich source for the purification of MSA, whose isolation from serum was tedious and inefficient.

The MSA purified from BRL-3A-conditioned medium, like its counterpart from serum, was of low molecular weight and also possessed NSILA (12). Further characterization revealed that MSA purified from the rat liver cell cultures actually consisted of a family of active polypeptides with molecular weights of approximately 10,000 (13).

It is now generally accepted in the scientific community that the term MSA refers exclusively to the family of small polypeptides produced by the BRL-3A rat liver cell line, and the relationship of these polypeptides to the partially purified fraction isolated by Pierson and Temin (10) from calf serum remains to be determined. This review examines the biological and biochemical properties of MSA from BRL-3A-conditioned medium as well as its interaction with cell-surface receptors and serum carrier proteins. The relationship of MSA to other members of the somatomedin family of polypeptide hormones is also detailed. In addition, a brief comparison of somatomedin carrier proteins to the binding proteins of other growth factor families is presented.

1. RELATIONSHIP TO THE SOMATOMEDINS

Based on Temin's rationale, which led to the purification of MSA, and on subsequent biochemical and biological characterization (12–14), it became apparent that MSA shared striking similarities to the insulin-like activities in serum. These activities, namely soluble nonsuppressible insulin-like activity (NSILA-S) and sulfation factor, a serum component that stimulates sulfate incorporation into cartilage tissue, had been shown to play a pervasive role in mediating the action of growth hormone (somatotropin) on skeletal tissue. This mounting evidence demonstrating a role of these factors in mediating somatic cell growth led to the proposal that the term somatomedin

(Sm) be used as the designation for all growth-hormone-dependent plasma factors that have sulfation factor activity on cartilage tissue and insulin-like effects on extraskeletal tissues (15). The somatomedins thus became one of the first groups of so-called growth factors to be recognized as a bona fide family of hormones. For a more detailed discussion of the somatomedins and their history see references 16, 17, and 18.

Based on the most widely accepted criteria for inclusion of a substance into the somatomedin family, MSA was recognized as a representative. These criteria include its biochemical properties, its ability to stimulate sulfate incorporation into cartilage, and its insulin-like activity (12). Although MSA produced by BRL-3A cells does not strictly satisfy the requirement that the somatomedins be growth-hormone dependent, this criterion may be futile in this instance since the cells may have lost this regulatory control during continuous growth in culture. However, Schalch et al. (19) showed that the presence of rat growth hormone in the medium caused a marked increase in the release of MSA into the medium after 4 hours, although the level in the medium at 24 hours was not significantly altered.

Extensively purified and characterized substances that fulfill the criteria of a somatomedin include NSILA-S, somatomedin A (Sm A), somatomedin C (Sm C), all isolated from human plasma, and MSA from BRL-3A rat liver cell cultures.

A significant advance in the characterization of NSILA-S was the isolation of two distinct polypeptides with insulin-like activity by Rinderknecht and Humbel (20). These investigators determined the amino acid sequences of the two polypeptides and revealed their striking structural homology to insulin and proinsulin (21–23). This suggested an evolutionary relationship between the somatomedins and the proinsulin molecule. Based on these revelations the operational term NSILA-S was replaced with the designation insulin-like growth factors I and II (IGF I and IGF II) to indicate the evolutionary relationship to insulin and the physiological function of these two polypeptides (21). Insulin-like growth factor I is a 70-amino-acid polypeptide with a molecular weight of 7649, and IGF II contains 67 amino acids (24).

Somatomedin A was initially purified from human plasma by Uthne (25) on the basis of its ability to stimulate sulfate incorporation into chick cartilage. This substance also has insulin-like activity on adipose tissue (26). Fryklund et al. (27,28) reported the isolation of two polypeptides called A1 and A2 having molecular weights of approximately 7000 and isoelectric points near neutrality.

Van Wyk's group, using the stimulation of sulfate and thymidine incorporation into cartilage explants of hypophysectomized rats as an assay for activity, purified from human plasma a basic polypeptide of approximately 7500 daltons, which they called somatomedin C (29). Extensive characterization of Sm C indicates that it shares structural and biological properties with IGF I, and these molecules may ultimately be shown to be identical when the complete amino acid sequence of Sm C is determined (30–32).

Using objective biochemical and biological criteria, the somatomedins thus far characterized can be placed into two recognizable classes. Both Sm C and IGF I, which may be identical or slightly different polypeptides, are referred to as the "basic" somatomedins. With isoelectric points of 8.1–8.5, these substances exhibit virtually identical biological properties as well as identical competitive-binding curves in immunoassays and receptor assays (31,32). These somatomedins also exhibit greater growth hormone dependence and less insulin-like activity than the other somatomedins. Both MSA and somatomedin A are "neutral" polypeptides, with isoelectric points ranging from 5.6 to 7.0 (27,33). And IGF II is clearly less basic than IGF I (22). Somatomedin A also differs from the other somatomedins by its lack of the disulfide bridges that are usually required for biological activity (27). Although the neutral somatomedins may show greater differences with each other than do the basic somatomedins, they appear to be closely related, as demonstrated by similarities in biological activity (34) and similar potencies in competitive immunoassays and receptor assays (31,32,34). In addition, the neutral somatomedins appear to be less dependent on growth hormone for their activity and are more insulin-like than the basic somatomedins.

2. PURIFICATION OF MSA FROM BRL-3A-CONDITIONED MEDIUM

As discussed earlier, serum-free medium conditioned by the BRL-3A line of Buffalo rat liver cells was shown to be a rich and convenient source from which MSA could be purified with relative ease (12–14). Subsequently, many laboratories successfully purified MSA for use in a wide variety of investigations into the role of these important growth-regulatory hormones (33,35–41). The MSA can routinely be isolated by first subjecting the conditioned medium to ion-exchange chromatography using Dowex-50 resin in the sodium form (12,33,35). The MSA, which is present in conditioned medium at neutral pH in a form bound to a larger carrier protein, absorbs to the resin. Following extensive washing with 0.15 M sodium chloride and 0.1 M sodium bicarbonate (pH 9.0), the MSA can be eluted with 0.1 M ammonium hydroxide (pH 11). Dulak and Shing (35) recognized from amino acid composition data that MSA probably does not bind to the Dowex resin directly but does so in association with other more basic proteins in the conditioned medium. It has now been established that this behavior of MSA is indeed due to its association with a specific carrier protein (42). The MSA carrier protein and the role it plays in the biological activity of MSA are discussed in a subsequent section.

Following neutralization of the ammonium hydroxide eluant, it is dialyzed against 2% acetic acid, lyophylized, dissolved in 1 M acetic acid, and centrifuged to remove insoluble material. This preparation, called Dowex MSA (12,33), is then applied to a column of Sephadex G-50 or G-75 equilibrated in 1 M acetic acid. The MSA elutes from this column in the retarded region as three peaks exhibiting biological activity assayed by the stimulation of [³H]thymidine incorporation into chicken embryo fibroblasts. Moses et al. (33) designated these peaks I, II, and III on the basis of decreasing molecular size. The three peaks of biological activity are clearly separated from the majority of the protein eluting in the void-volume region of the column. Under these strongly dissociating conditions, the MSA–carrier-protein complex is also dissociated, and the carrier protein elutes with the majority of the protein (42). After pooling the respective regions of the profile, Moses et al. (33) were able to separate the family of MSA polypeptides into at least seven components by preparative-scale disc acrylamide gel electrophoresis in an acetic acid–urea system. Sephadex G-50 Peak I was shown to contain a single active polypeptide with a molecular weight of 16,270. Peak II contained four active polypeptides of similar size (II-1, II-2, II-3, II-4), one of which (II-1) was purified to homogeneity and was shown to have a molecular weight of 8700. Peak III contained two biologically active species (III-1, III-2). The MSA polypeptide III-2 was also purified further and shown to have a molecular weight of 7100. Based on amino acid composition data and polypeptide-reduction experiments, it was suggested (33) that the smaller MSA polypeptides may be contained within those of higher molecular weight and may be generated by processing or cleavage. The possibility also exists that the larger peak-I MSA is a prohormone for the smaller MSA species.

In support of this hypothesis, Moses et al. (43) showed, using immunological cross-reactivities, that antigenic determinants present in the smaller MSA polypeptides are also present in larger species, whereas some antigenic determinants may be lost during the generation of the smaller fragments.

Recently, Marquardt et al. (44) purified an MSA polypeptide from BRL-3A-conditioned medium by gel-permeation chromatography on BioGel P-10 and by high-pressure liquid chromatography. The amino acid sequence of this 7484-dalton polypeptide displayed 93% homology with the amino acid sequence of human IGF II. Based on this homology, these authors proposed that this MSA polypeptide be designated rat IGF II.

3.   BIOLOGICAL ACTIVITY OF MSA

Of course, MSA was originally isolated from BRL-3A-conditioned medium based on its ability to stimulate the incorporation of [³H]thymidine into the

DNA of serum-starved chicken embryo fibroblasts (12). Dulak and Temin (12,13) also appreciated the significance of the sulfation factor and NSILA of MSA. Because of their relative abundance and facility of purification, MSA polypeptides have been purified by many laboratories as tools with which to examine the effects of somatomedins on a variety of cell types in culture. Numerous biochemical parameters of cell growth and differentiation have also been investigated in the presence of purified MSA.

Multiplication-stimulating activity also has been shown to stimulate [³H]thymidine incorporation into rat embryo fibroblasts (12), human fibroblasts (45), mouse 3T3 cells (46), and a rat muscle cell line (47). Induction of cell multiplication by MSA has been reported for chicken and rat embryo fibroblasts (12), mouse 3T3 cells (46), and rat muscle cells (47). In addition, MSA stimulates the following: glucose transport in chicken embryo fibroblasts (14); amino acid transport in chicken embryo fibroblasts (14,48), rat muscle cells (38), and rat hepatoma cells (49); ornithine decarboxylase activity in mouse 3T3 cells (46), chicken embryo fibroblasts (50), and porcine granulosa cells (39); tyrosine aminotransferase activity in rat hepatoma cells (49); ouabain-sensitive rubidium uptake in chicken embryo fibroblasts (40) and rat muscle cells (37); and proteoglycan biosynthesis in rat chondrocytes (51).

In confirmation of the sulfation factor and insulin-like activities of MSA originally reported by Dulak and Temin (12), Rechler et al. (52) reported that MSA stimulated glucose oxidation in rat adipocytes. Moreover, it has been reported that MSA polypeptide II-1 stimulates sulfate incorporation into rat costal cartilage and lipogenesis in rat epididymal fat cells (33).

4. MSA CELL-SURFACE RECEPTORS

The initial step in the biological action of a polypeptide hormone is presumably the interaction of the hormone with its specific receptor molecule on the surface of the target cell. The availability of well-characterized and homogeneous preparations of MSA has allowed investigations into this interaction through labeling of the purified polypeptide with iodine-125. Somatomedin or MSA receptors have been demonstrated in a variety of tissues and cultured cells. Radioimmunoassays and receptor-binding assays have been developed for this family of hormones and have been widely used in examinations of hormone–receptor interactions. Receptors have also been shown to discriminate between various members of the somatomedin family, reflecting biochemical and possibly functional differences. In addition, receptors from various species and tissues may exhibit a diversity equivalent to that seen in the somatomedins themselves.

A logical outgrowth of the observed insulin-like biological activities of the somatomedins, including MSA, was the demonstration that these hormones could effectively compete with [^{125}I]insulin for binding to specific insulin receptors (52–58). Specific receptors for the somatomedins have been demonstrated in a large number of tissues and cells (for reviews see references 16, 17, 59). In general, insulin is able to displace labeled somatomedins from all of these receptors, but only at high unphysiological concentrations. Unlabeled somatomedin preparations, however, displace their homologous labeled ligand at low concentrations. Relative potency in competition for respective receptors normally reflects the biological response of the tissue to insulin or the somatomedins. Insensitivity to competitive binding by insulin establishes the existence of a distinct receptor for the somatomedins (31,32,52,59,60).

Specific receptors for MSA have been described in normal chicken embryo fibroblasts (52,61–63), Rous sarcoma virus–transformed chicken embryo fibroblasts (64), human fibroblasts (34,45,63,65), rat liver cells (53,61,63), human placental membranes (36,66), the BRL-3A2 rat liver cell line (34,52,53,63), human arterial and venous endothelial cells (67), three human tumor cell lines (65), and rat hepatoma cells (49). Basically, these MSA receptors can be categorized into two types depending on relative cross-reactivity with insulin (53,59). Type-I MSA receptors, found in rat liver cells and membranes, BRL-3A2 cells, and human endothelial cells, are relatively insensitive to competition by insulin for [^{125}I]MSA binding (52,53,59,67). In type-II receptors, expressed in human and chicken embryo fibroblasts, insulin displays greater effectiveness in competing for [^{125}I]MSA binding (36,52,53,59,61,63). Although type-II receptors interact with insulin, they can be easily discerned from distinct insulin receptors in the same cells, since insulin is roughly half as potent as MSA in displacing [^{125}I]MSA from its receptor (59,63), and MSA is less than 1% as effective as insulin in competitive-binding experiments in which [^{125}I]insulin is used as the ligand (59). Similarly, kinetic analysis of competitive-binding data for MSA and insulin to chicken embryo (52) and human fibroblasts (45) is consistent with the existence of distinct insulin and MSA receptors. Strong evidence has been collected that implicates the MSA receptor as the growth receptor mediating the proliferative response of chicken embryo fibroblasts to MSA and related polypeptides (34,52,59,61,62).

Although MSA receptors in various cell types can be classified on the basis of sensitivity to insulin, both type-I and type-II receptors respond similarly to competition by MSA, human somatomedins, and other peptides. Although all of the related members of the somatomedin family will compete with [^{125}I]MSA for binding, their relative potencies may differ widely depending on the tissue or cell type used. A summary of the relative activities of the somatomedins in competing for [^{125}I]MSA binding to receptors on various cell types is presented in Table 1. Also shown is the effect of

Table 1. MSA-Cell-Surface Receptors[a] and Competitive Potency of Related Polypeptides[b]

Unlabeled Competing Polypeptide	Type I (Insulin Insensitive)			Type II (Insulin Sensitive)	
	Rat Liver Membranes (53,59,63)	BRL-3A2 Cells (53,59,61)	Human Endothelial Cells (67)	Chicken Embryo Fibroblasts (53,62,63)	Human Fibroblasts (53,59,63)
MSA	2	2	+	2	3
IGF I	3	2		1	1
IGF II	1	1		1	2
Sm A	2	3		2	3
Sm C					
Insulin	—	—	—	3	4
Proinsulin	—	—	—	4	4
Anti-insulin receptor antibody	—	—	—	—	+

[a] Identified utilizing [^{125}I]MSA as the radiolabeled ligand.
[b] Arabic numerals indicate the order of decreasing competitive potency of peptides tested. Plus and minus signs reflect whether inhibition of binding was observed. Values are intended to reflect relative potency for each receptor system and do not reflect quantitative differences.

antibodies directed against the human insulin receptor on [^{125}I]MSA binding as reported by Moses et al. (53). This antibody inhibited the binding of [^{125}I]insulin to chicken embryo fibroblasts but had no effect on [^{125}I]MSA binding. This observation confirms the hypothesis that distinct receptors exist in these cells for MSA and insulin. In contrast, binding of [^{125}I]MSA to human fibroblasts was inhibited by the antibody, suggesting an antigenic relationship between these two receptors in human cells.

In further investigations demonstrating differences in relative competitive potencies of MSA, Moses et al. (33) performed binding studies using [^{125}I]MSA polypeptides II-I and III-2 as ligands. Polypeptide III-2 was nine times more potent than MSA II-1 in competing for binding of both labeled species to rat liver cell membranes. Peak-I MSA was even less potent than either polypeptide.

In light of these various experiments, it is strikingly apparent that a close relationship exists between the various members of the somatomedin family. However, it is also clear that wide differences exist in the relative ability of these polypeptides to interact with cell-surface receptors in a variety of tissues and cell types. Equally significant are the observations demonstrating the existence of diversity among the receptors for these hormones. How these differences play a role in the biological function of the somatomedins remains to be elucidated. It is important to recognize that the identification of a specific MSA receptor in any given cell type is an operational definition based on the fact that radiolabeled MSA was used as the ligand to demonstrate its presence. The identification of the biologically authentic ligand in these systems has not yet been achieved. MSA will, of course, compete for the binding of radiolabeled IGFs I and II, Sm A, and Sm C to receptors in various cells (31,32,34,53,63). Vast differences were noted in these systems in the relative potencies of unlabeled polypeptides as competitive inhibitors of binding.

Recently, Massague et al. (68) reported the identification of the MSA receptor as a 255,000-dalton protein in membranes of rat adipocytes, rat liver, and human placenta using affinity-labeling techniques. Labeling of this protein was totally inhibited by unlabeled MSA, but not by insulin or proinsulin, in all three cell types. Using similar techniques, Kasuga et al. (69) identified an MSA–receptor complex in membranes of rat liver cells and in BRL-3A2 cells as a 260,000-dalton complex. Binding of [^{125}I]MSA to this receptor was inhibited by unlabeled MSA or IGF I, but not by insulin, identifying it as the Type-I receptor described in Table 1.

5. *IN VIVO* ROLE OF MSA

Since MSA is the only current representative of the somatomedin family that is not isolated from plasma or serum, its precise relationship to the other somatomedins remains uncertain. The recent determination of the amino acid sequence of one of the MSA polypeptides revealed close structural homology to human IGF II and logically led to the proposal that this MSA polypeptide be designated rat IGF II (44).

A radioimmunoassay has been developed by Moses et al. (43) that specifically recognizes MSA. Other related polypeptides do not cross-react with MSA to any appreciable extent. Using this MSA-specific radioimmunoassay, the group of Nissley and Rechler (70,71) found high levels of MSA in fetal rat serum compared with maternal serum. After birth there was a gradual decline in the serum level of MSA until maternal levels were reached after 25 days. The activity measured by the radioimmunoassay in rat serum was growth hormone dependent, since levels were significantly lower in the sera from hypophysectomized rats (53,71). These observations, coupled with the finding that organ cultures of fetal rat liver synthesized a somatomedin that closely resembled MSA in biochemical and immunological properties (71,72), led these investigators to conclude that MSA is a fetal somatomedin playing an important role in fetal growth; it is the major somatomedin in the fetal circulation. Following birth, and in adult rats, MSA plays a minor role, with other somatomedins accounting for the majority of the insulin-like activity in the blood of these animals.

This contention is in apparent conflict with the fact that the BRL-3A cells, which produce MSA, were originally cloned from the liver of an adult rat (11). However, these cells have been cultured *in vitro* for an extended period and no longer resemble adult liver cells in many respects. Extended life and selective pressure in culture may have led to loss of normal biological control and a reversion to fetal function.

6. SOMATOMEDIN CARRIER PROTEINS

During the initial attempts to purify NSILA-S from serum, it was recognized that there was an apparent discrepancy between the size of the purified molecule and its native state in plasma (73). The activity in serum had an apparent molecular weight determined by gel chromatography in excess of 60,000, whereas following purification using strongly dissociating conditions of acid-ethanol extraction, the molecular weight was approximately 7000. The nature of the association of the low-molecular-weight component with larger serum proteins was unclear. Similar observations were documented for sulfation factor by Daughaday and Kipnis (74) and Van den Brande et al. (75). In a preliminary report, Hintz et al. (76) first presented evidence for the existence in plasma of a specific carrier protein for the somatomedins and evidence that the association of the low-molecular-weight hormone with larger proteins was not due to simple nonspecific adsorption. Confirmation of these results accumulated rapidly for Sm C (77), Sm A (78), and NSILA-S (IGFs I and II) (57,79,80,81).

When [125I]NSILA-S was incubated with serum and subsequently fractionated by gel chromatography on Sephadex G-200 at neutral pH, two peaks of specific binding activity could be detected with molecular weights of approximately 50,000–60,000 and 200,000 (79). Kaufmann et al. (80) demonstrated, upon injection of labeled NSILA-S into normal rats, that radioactivity first appeared in the 50,000–60,000-dalton region, followed by an accumulation of the labeled hormone in the 200,000-dalton peak. These results suggested the possibility of a normal conversion of the small carrier-protein complex into the larger one. Although the biological role of these two forms of somatomedin-carrier-protein complexes remained speculative, the existence of such carrier proteins was unique among polypeptide hormones. Steroid and thyroid hormones are well known to bind to specific plasma carrier proteins and recently, Peeters and Friesen (82) have reported the presence of a growth-hormone-binding factor in pregnant mouse serum.

In an informative study, Cohen and Nissley (83) proposed that somatomedin carrier proteins extend the biological half-life of the somatomedins in the circulation. These investigators determined that the half-life of injected somatomedin activity in hypophysectomized rats was greatly extended if the somatomedin was recombined with proteins of high molecular weight from which it had previously been dissociated. They also showed that the carrier proteins were under the regulation of growth hormone. These studies have been confirmed by Draznin et al. (84).

The recognition of the presence of carrier-protein complexes of somatomedins emphasized the reality that the free form of the somatomedins is essentially nonexistent in native plasma. Although the total plasma or serum concentration of the somatomedins is very high compared with that of other protein hormones, more than 1 μg/ml, little if any is present in the circulation as the free hormone (16,17,24,85,86). If only the free hormone is biologically active, then the significance of the activity detected by most current assays for the somatomedins is questionable. A controversy exists regarding the requirement of dissociating the somatomedins from their carrier proteins prior to their assay in competitive receptor- and protein-binding studies (70,87–89).

It is obvious that in order to fully understand the physiological role of the somatomedins in the control of cell growth, it is imperative to gain a knowledge of both the physical nature of these carrier-protein complexes and the role they play in the biological activity of the somatomedins. There is little evidence to shed light on how the hormone escapes from its apparent sequestration within the vascular space and ultimately gains access to its specific receptor on its target cell.

7. MSA AND CARRIER PROTEINS

Using MSA as the radiolabeled ligand, Moses et al. (90) demonstrated the presence of specific carrier proteins for this somatomedin in normal and hypophysectomized rat serum. When [^{125}I]MSA was incubated with normal rat serum and then fractionated on Sephadex G-200 at neutral pH, radioactivity was detected in five regions of the effluent. Binding to the second (molecular weight >150,000) and third (molecular weight >50,000) peaks was specific and could be inhibited by the inclusion of an excess amount of unlabeled MSA in the incubation mixture. Radioactivity appearing in the void-volume region of the column was due to nonspecific adsorption, and the last two peaks corresponded to free MSA and free iodine-125, respectively. Growth-hormone dependency of this binding pattern was amply demonstrated using serum from hypophysectomized rats. Specific binding of MSA to the high-molecular-weight region was completely absent in this serum, and binding to the low-molecular-weight region was substantially increased. Treatment of hypophysectomized rats with growth hormone resulted in a restoration of the normal binding pattern. The specific binding of [125I]MSA to two distinct components in normal rat serum was later confirmed by Knauer et al. (42). Figure 1 depicts the specific MSA-binding components of rat serum, labeled peaks 2 and 3.

In a more extensive characterization of the interaction of MSA with rat serum carrier proteins, Moses et al. (91) showed that treatment of normal rat serum with 1 M acetic acid dissociated somatomedin activity from the

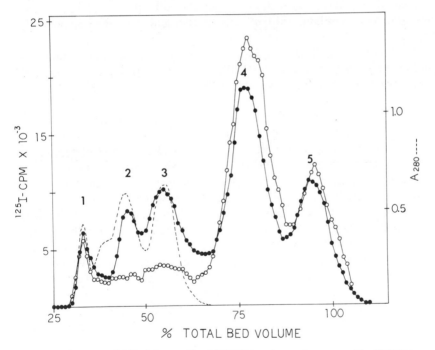

Figure 1. Sephadex G-200 elution profile of [125I]MSA and normal rat serum. The [125I]MSA was incubated with normal rat serum for 5 hours at 22°C. The reaction mixture was then applied to a 2.5 × 40 cm column of Sephadex G-200 equilibrated in phosphate-buffered saline, pH 7.4, at 4°C. Fractions were assayed for radioactivity (●). An identical reaction mixture contained an excess of unlabeled MSA for determination of specific binding (○). The dotted line represents the elution profile of a sample of calf serum used to calibrate the column by adsorbance at 280 nm. Reproduced by permission from reference 42.

carrier-protein complexes, and the carrier proteins could be separated from the low-molecular-weight hormone by Sephadex G-50 gel filtration under acidic conditions. However, when the dissociated carrier proteins in acid-treated serum were reincubated with [^{125}I]MSA and rechromatographed using Sephadex G-200 at neutral pH, only the smaller, peak 3, carrier-protein complex at 60,000–70,000 molecular weight was observed. All attempts to regenerate the high-molecular-weight, peak 2, carrier-protein complex following its dissociation by acid or milder treatments failed (91). The fact that the larger 150,000-dalton carrier-protein complex cannot be reformed following dissociation is very disappointing and suggests the presence of an acid-labile component that is required for its integrity. Furthermore, as documented earlier (90) the formation of the large complex is also dependent upon growth hormone, since only the 60,000–70,000-dalton carrier is seen in serum from hypophysectomized rats. The nature of the growth-hormone-dependent step in the formation of the 150,000-dalton complex remains obscure, and its relationship, if any, to the acid-sensitive component is unknown.

The binding of [^{125}I]MSA to rat serum somatomedin carrier proteins was inhibited by Sm A, IGF I, and IGF II (63,91). Insulin-like growth factor II was essentially equal to unlabeled MSA in competing for MSA binding, whereas IGF I was about 10 times less effective. Thus these human somatomedins appear to interact with the same carrier proteins as MSA in rat serum. Unlabeled MSA competes with labeled Sm A, IGF I, and IGF II for binding to rat serum carrier proteins as well (63,91). In striking contrast with the picture seen with somatomedin cell-surface receptors, the serum carrier proteins have no apparent affinity for insulin or proinsulin in spite of the close structural homology of these hormones (66,77,91).

Moses et al. (91) were the first to demonstrate that the BRL-3A rat liver cell line that produces MSA also synthesizes and secretes into the medium a specific carrier protein for MSA. This carrier protein exists in the conditioned medium complexed with an excess amount of MSA, much of which exists as the free hormone (42). In addition, a cell line cloned from the original BRL-3A cell line, known as BRL-3A2, also produces an MSA carrier protein but does not produce MSA (91,92). The size of this MSA–carrier-protein complex is similar to the low-molecular-weight, peak 3, complex seen in serum (91).

8. PURIFICATION OF SOMATOMEDIN CARRIER PROTEINS

Partially purified preparations of somatomedin carrier proteins can be readily obtained from serum by dissociating the complex under acidic conditions and separating the components by gel filtration using Sephadex G-50 in 1 M acetic acid. Under these conditions the carrier proteins elute in the void-volume region of the column, isolated from the free somatomedin polypeptides, which elute in the retarded fractions. Such carrier-protein preparations, free of contaminating somatomedins, have routinely been used in competitive-protein-binding assays for the somatomedins and for carrier protein itself (33,63,66,84,86,91,93–95). More extensive purification of somatomedin carrier protein from serum was reported by Fryklund et al. (78). Using polyethylene glycol precipitation, CM-Scphadcx chromatography, and gel filtration, a molecule was isolated that consisted of two distinct protein chains with molecular weights between 35,000 and 45,000. The amino acid composition of this component was given; however, the protein had low binding activity for Sm A and was not further characterized.

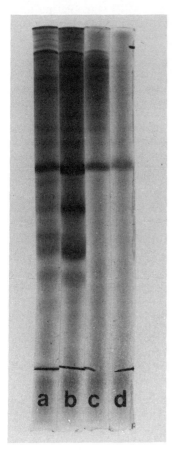

Figure 2. Acetic acid–urea gels of MCP at various stages of purification. Lanes: (*a*) BRL-3A-conditioned medium proteins; (*b*) Dowex MSA; (*c*) partially purified MCP following Sephadex G-50 chromatography in 1 M acetic acid; and (*d*) affinity-chromatography-purified MCP. Reproduced with permission from reference 100.

Draznin et al. (84) also partially purified from serum an IGF carrier protein that had a molecular weight of approximately 55,000–65,000. Gel chromatography revealed four peaks with binding activity, suggesting the presence of polymers or interacting molecules. The purified preparation yielded three bands upon polyacrylamide gel electrophoresis. In immuno-diffusion studies using specific antisera against known serum proteins, the preparation cross-reacted with only transferrin and α- and β-globulins. However, the purified carrier protein was judged to be only about 1% pure.

The first purification of a somatomedin carrier protein to homogeneity was accomplished in this laboratory by Knauer et al. (42), again taking advantage of the presence of MSA and its carrier protein in BRL-3A-con-ditioned medium and the relative ease of purification that this source affords. Following standard procedures, the MSA–carrier-protein complex was dis-sociated and the components separated by gel filtration using Sephadex G-50 in 1 M acetic acid. The MSA carrier protein (MCP) was then purified by affinity chromatography using Sepharose 4B to which MSA peptides had been covalently attached. At neutral pH, the MCP bound to the immobilized MSA, and after the column was carefully washed to remove inactive proteins, the carrier was eluted in 0.1 M acetic acid. The affinity-chromatography-purified MCP migrated as a single protein band in acetic acid–urea and sodium dodecyl sulfate (SDS) polyacrylamide gel systems, and [^{125}I]MSA-

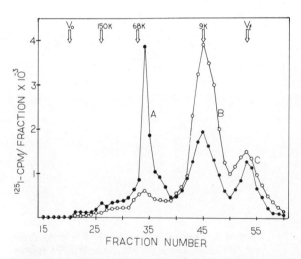

Figure 3. Sephadex G-200 elution profile of [^{125}I]MSA and purified MCP. The [^{125}I]MSA was incubated with purified MCP in the presence (○) or absence (●) of an excess of unlabeled MSA. The reaction mixtures were then applied to a column of Sephadex G-200. Conditions were similar to those described in Fig. 1.

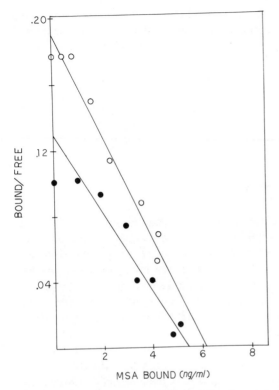

Figure 4. Scatchard analysis of MSA binding to purified MCP. Purified MCP (●) or BRL-3A2-conditioned medium (○) was incubated with [¹²⁵I]MSA and increasing concentrations of unlabeled MSA. Following separation of bound and free MSA, the amount of MSA bound to the MCP was determined. The slopes of the lines were determined by linear regression analysis. Reproduced with permission from reference 42.

binding activity was observed in gel slices corresponding to the observable protein band from the acetic acid–urea gels. Shown in Fig. 2 are acetic acid–urea gels of protein fractions from various stages in the purification of MCP from BRL-3A-conditioned medium. In SDS gels under reducing conditions, two bands were observed with molecular weights of 30,000 and 31,500. Purified MCP bound [¹²⁵I]MSA specifically, and the complex formed (Fig. 3, peak A) eluted from neutral Sephadex G-200 with a molecular weight between 60,000 and 70,000. The size of this complex is similar to the low-molecular-weight (Fig. 1, peak 3) somatomedin–carrier complex seen in serum and suggests that the composition of this complex includes each of the two subunits of MCP plus one MSA molecule. This apparent stoichiometry of one MCP molecule to one MSA polypeptide was confirmed through kinetic analysis of competitive-binding data (Fig. 4). Scatchard analysis revealed an affinity constant of $0.23 \times 10^9 \, M^{-1}$, and appropriate correction of the R_0 value to account for maximal bindability of the $[^{125}I]$MSA preparation used supported the claim of a 1:1 molar ratio of MCP to MSA in the complex. The binding of $[^{125}I]$MSA to affinity-chromatography-purified MCP was similar to its binding to unfractionated BRL-3A2 medium with regard to affinity and capacity, supporting the assertion that the purified carrier protein had not undergone major alteration during isolation.

9. ROLE OF CARRIER PROTEIN

The presence of serum carrier proteins for polypeptide hormones is unique and perhaps accounts for the high total concentrations of the somatomedins, which exceeds the levels of other protein hormones in plasma by several hundredfold. The demonstration of at least two forms of somatomedin–carrier-protein complexes and the fact that the generation of the larger form is regulated by growth hormone hint at the important role that the carrier proteins must play. The biological function of the carrier proteins in regulating the activity of the somatomedins is an area enjoying much recent speculation.

Using partially purified, acid-dissociated preparations of carrier proteins, many investigators have indeed demonstrated an effect of carrier protein on the biological activity of the somatomedins. Chochinov et al. (96) purified from human amniotic fluid a somatomedin-binding protein that prevented the binding of Sm C, but not insulin, to receptors in human placental membranes. This binding protein had a molecular weight of 33,000–35,000 and also inhibited the stimulation of thymidine incorporation into human fibroblasts by Sm C. Similarly, Drop et al. (97) isolated from amniotic fluid a binding protein of 34,500 molecular weight that inhibited the stimulatory effect of insulin-like activity on sulfate incorporation by rabbit chondrocytes and glucose incorporation into fatty acids in a rat epididymal fat pad assay. This protein also displaced labeled insulin-like activity, but not insulin, from receptors in human placental membranes.

Meuli et al. (98) demonstrated that partially purified carrier protein abolished the activity of NSILA-S on rat heart muscle using a perfusion system. In addition, the presence of carrier protein prevented the binding of $[^{125}I]$NSILA-S to its specific receptor site in this tissue.

Partially purified carrier protein has been shown by Zapf et al. (99) to inhibit the stimulation of glucose transport and lipogenesis by NSILA-S in isolated rat adipocytes. Association of $[^{125}I]$NSILA-S with its carrier protein

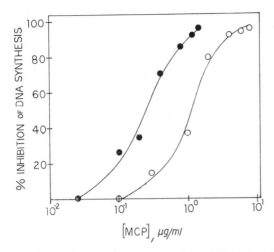

Figure 5. Inhibition by MCP of MSA-stimulated DNA synthesis in chicken embryo fibroblasts. Quiescent cultures of chicken fibroblasts were incubated with MSA and various concentrations of purified MCP (●) or partially purified MCP (○). Rates of DNA synthesis were determined 12 hours after stimulation. Reproduced with permission from reference 100.

prevented binding to both the NSILA-S receptor and the insulin receptor.

Knauer and Smith (100) showed that MCP purified by affinity chromatography from BRL-3A-conditioned medium completely inhibited the stimulation of DNA synthesis by MSA in chicken embryo fibroblasts (Fig. 5). Enhancement of the rate of glucose transport by MSA was also prevented in the presence of MCP, and the binding of [^{125}I]MSA to these cells was likewise precluded. As expected, the biological activity of insulin or [^{125}I]insulin binding in all of the studies just described was unaffected by the presence of somatomedin carrier protein (96–100). The association of [^{125}I]MSA with its receptor in human placenta membranes has also been shown to be inhibited by serum carrier proteins (66).

The documentation of the absence of biological activity and binding ability when the somatomedins are bound to their carrier protein offers a ready explanation of how these hormones can circulate in the plasma at concentrations far exceeding their biologically effective dose. These complexes have been hypothesized to represent the somatomedin storage component in the body where the hormone is sequestered, restricting its accessibility to tissues outside the vascular space (79,81). Somatomedin activity in rat lymph has been shown to be much lower than that in rat serum, consistent with this concept (101). However, the role of somatomedin–

carrier-protein complexes appears to be much more involved than simply providing physical inaccessibility of the hormone to the tissue. The evidence noted above clearly establishes that the complexing of the hormone with purified or partially purified carrier-protein preparations results in loss of metabolic activity as well as loss of capacity to interact with specific cell-surface receptors.

It is important to acknowledge that all of the investigations concerning the biological activity of somatomedin–carrier-protein complexes have been done using carrier-protein preparations that have first been dissociated from somatomedin activity by acid treatment. Reassociation of these carrier-protein preparations with the low-molecular-weight hormone, resulting in a biologically inactive complex (96–100), assumably involves the reconstruction of only the smaller complex (molecular weight 60,000–70,000) found in serum. Therefore, it is not clear from these studies whether the larger complex (molecular weight >150,000) is also metabolically inactive, since thus far it has not been possible to reconstruct this complex from purified components (91). The *in vivo* generation of the larger complex is known to be under the influence of growth hormone (83), and the smaller complex may be a precursor to the larger one (80). Hintz and Liu (85,102) have hypothesized the existence of another protein, or a process, necessary for the formation of the complete larger complex and have suggested that this complex will be shown to be active. They further suggest that one of the functions of this complex is to mask the insulin-like activity of the somatomedin molecule, making it more specific for its own receptor. Some evidence has been presented that is consistent with this concept (87).

It therefore seems plausible to speculate that the smaller carrier-protein complex represents a biologically inactive reservoir maintaining a large supply of somatomedin in the circulation. The larger complex may then be generated via a growth-hormone-dependent process using the components of the smaller complex, with the possible involvement of additional proteins or a protein (the acid-sensitive component). This large somatomedin–carrier-protein complex may be the biologically significant form effecting a delivery system for utilization of the hormone at the cell-surface receptor. To examine the biological activity of the large complex it will be necessary to isolate this component intact from serum in the absence of free hormone and test its bioactivity in a sensitive assay system. Alternately, when the composition of the large complex becomes defined, it may be possible to reconstruct the complex from purified components using gentler techniques to effect dissociation and reassembly.

In a recent report, Furlanetto (103) fractionated human serum using ammonium sulfate precipitation and DEAE-Sephadex A-50 chromatography and obtained a preparation containing the acid-labile, growth-hormone-dependent component of the large somatomedin–carrier-protein complex. When this preparation was incubated with [^{125}I]Sm C and acid-dissociated carrier protein, a complex was generated that was of the same size as the large endogenous somatomedin–carrier-protein complex observed in native serum by immunoassay. The acid-labile component was demonstrated to be a glycoprotein under growth-hormone control, since it was absent in serum from growth-hormone-deficient patients. This is the first study reporting the assembly of the high-molecular-weight endogenous somatomedin–carrier-protein complex from partially purified components and emphasizes the possibility that this complex may have different biological properties than the smaller complex constructed from acid-dissociated carrier protein and somatomedin by other workers. Furlanetto (103) also observed the presence of an additional, previously undescribed, somatomedin-binding protein in serum that is not identical to, and is smaller than, the carrier protein obtained by acid dissociation of the large endogenous complex. This component did not associate with the acid-labile component to form the large complex, was independent of growth hormone, and apparently circulates in a free form with little associated somatomedin.

In light of the experimental evidence establishing that the small (60,000–70,000 molecular weight) somatomedin–carrier-protein complex is metabolically inactive and is unable to recognize its specific cell-surface receptor, it appears paradoxical that somatomedin can be detected in native plasma or serum by bioactivity, radioreceptor assay, or immunoassay. It appears, therefore, that these various assays are capable of recognizing somatomedin complexed with its carrier, since little free hormone exists in plasma or serum. Following this rationale, it is reasonable to predict that the large somatomedin–carrier-protein complex (>150,000 molecular weight) is biologically active. Alternately, various cell types and hence various classes of receptors may exist that are able to preferentially recognize somatomedins in the bound form and respond differently from other tissue types that require that the hormone be present in the free form (24). The carrier proteins may consequently offer an additional level of regulation in the pervasive role of the somatomedins in cell growth by providing a discrimination system between possible responsive tissues.

A recent proposal by D'Ercole et al. (104) may require a reassessment of the current concepts regarding somatomedin action. Although the liver has long been recognized as the probable site of somatomedin biosynthesis (19,56,72), these investigators found that multiple tissues in the fetal mouse synthesize Sm C and suggested that the primary biological action of these hormones may be exerted locally near the source of production. The Sm C produced by these various tissues was present in a large form complexed with a carrier protein, and assayable Sm C increased severalfold upon dissociation of the complex. It is conceivable that locally produced somatomedin may be then bound by serum carrier proteins to inactivate it and to prevent its action on more-distant tissues.

Complicating the investigation of the biological activity of somatomedin–carrier-protein complexes is the presence of other high-molecular-weight insulin-like activities in serum. The original isolations of NSILA-S from serum involved the use of acid extraction, which separated these low-molecular-weight polypeptides from their specific carrier proteins. However, it was recognized that not all of the insulin-like activity present in the serum behaved in this manner. A significant amount, if not most, of this activity in serum remained in an insoluble high-molecular-weight form after acid extraction and was termed NSILA-P (105). Poffenberger et al. (106) isolated a high-molecular-weight nonsuppressible insulin-like protein (NSILP) that is a glycoprotein consisting of two protein chains of 42,000 and 46,000 daltons. The NSILP cross-reacted with various members of the somatomedin family in numerous assays, suggesting a structural relationship between the high- and low-molecular-weight insulin-like activities in serum. Suggestions that NSILA-P or NSILP are precursors to the smaller polypeptides or represent the low-molecular-weight hormone covalently attached to their carrier proteins (24,106) have not been substantiated. Clearly the ultimate purification and characterization of these activities is necessary before the nature of the relationship between NSILP or NSILA-P and the somatomedins can be known.

10. OTHER GROWTH FACTORS AND BINDING PROTEINS

Although the somatomedins appear to be unique among the polypeptide hormones in that they circulate in high concentration bound to specific carrier proteins, two other growth factors are also known to exist in association with specific binding proteins. Both epidermal growth factor (EGF) and nerve growth factor (NGF) resemble the somatomedins in this property, although it is not yet clear whether similarities exist in the function of the binding protein to suggest that a common mechanism can be broadly applied.

Epidermal growth factor is a protein originally isolated from male mouse submaxillary glands by Cohen (107) that accelerates eyelid opening and incisor eruption in newborn mice. The factor has been well characterized biochemically and biologically and is a potent stimulator of cell proliferation both *in vivo* and *in vitro* (for reviews of the action of EGF see references 108–110 and Chapter 5). Epidermal growth factor is a single polypeptide chain with a molecular weight of 6045, and its amino acid sequence has been determined (111,112). When EGF is isolated from crude homogenates of mouse submaxillary gland at neutral pH, a high-molecular-weight complex is observed with a molecular weight of approximately 74,000 (113,114). The high-molecular-weight complex was shown to consist of two molecules of mouse EGF and two molecules of a 29,000-dalton protein termed the EGF-binding protein. Interestingly, the binding protein was shown to have enzymatic activity in that it cleaved arginine esters with a high degree of specificity (113,115). It has been suggested that the arginine esteropeptidase activity is responsible for the production of EGF from a possible precursor protein, since EGF has a carboxy-terminal arginine residue (113,115). The effect of EGF-binding protein on the biological activity of EGF is in striking contrast with that discussed earlier in regard to the inhibition of somatomedin activity in the presence of carrier protein. The EGF-binding protein enhanced the stimulation of DNA synthesis and cell growth in human fibroblasts by EGF (116). A similar increase in EGF-stimulated glucose uptake in mouse fibroblasts was observed when EGF was added in association with the binding protein (117).

Nerve growth factor is a protein, also isolated from mouse submaxillary glands as well as many other sources, that stimulates neurite outgrowth in sensory and sympathetic ganglia in culture. The biological and biochemical effects of NGF on nervous tissue have been extensively documented (for review see references 118–120 and Chapters 1 and 2 in this book). The factor has been isolated in two different forms from mouse submaxillary glands. Bocchini and Angeletti (121) reported the isolation of a 2.5S NGF complex that was a dimer of two identical molecules of NGF protein (molecular weight 13,259) and had a molecular weight of about 26,000. The 2.5S form of NGF appears to be part of a larger complex, termed 7S NGF, which has a size of approximately 140,000 daltons (122). Murphy et al. (123) and Young et al. (124) have reported the separation of at least six distinct species of NGF by chromatographic techniques.

The 7S NGF complex is composed of three subunits, which are associated by noncovalent interactions (122,125). The β subunit is identical with the 2.5S NGF, except for some minor proteolytic alterations during purification, and is the biologically active dimer of two NGF molecules (126–128). The amino acid sequence of this subunit has been determined and, like EGF, has a carboxy-terminal arginine residue (129). In addition to the β subunit, 7S NGF contains an α subunit, with as yet unknown biological activity, and a γ subunit. The γ subunit has been shown to be a protease having arginine esteropeptidase activity (130,131). The enzymatic activity of the γ subunit is not expressed in the 7S NGF complex. The presence of a carboxy-terminal arginine residue on the NGF molecule and an associated arginine esterase led to the proposal that NGF is cleaved from a larger protein by the γ subunit (129,132). Direct evidence for the conversion of a pro-β NGF to β NGF by the γ subunit has been provided by Berger and Shooter (133).

In a comparison of the arginine esteropeptidases associated with NGF and EGF, Server and Shooter (134) found that they are similar in size, amino acid composition, and substrate specificity. The EGF-binding protein could not, however, replace the γ subunit in the formation of the 7S NGF complex, demonstrating the specificity of these two complexes. The fact that both NGF and EGF possess carboxy-terminal arginine residues and are associated with arginine-specific esteropeptidases strongly implies that the associated proteolytic enzymes are involved in the biosynthesis of the active component from a larger precursor. This, as mentioned above, has been demonstrated for NGF (133).

Enzymatic activity of the somatomedin carrier protein has not been reported. In our laboratory we have been unable to detect arginine esteropeptidase activity associated with purified MSA carrier protein (R. Lyons and G. L. Smith, unpublished observations). Neither IGF I nor IGF II has carboxy-terminal arginine residues (22,24), suggesting that the somatomedins are not derived in the same fashion as are EGF and NGF. However, a putative precursor to MSA has been described by Schalch et al. (19). The somatomedin carrier proteins and the NGF- and EGF-binding proteins may confer a protective element in their respective ligands. Association of somatomedin with its carrier protein increases its relative half-life in rat serum (83,84), and NGF is protected from proteolytic degradation in the 7S NGF complex (130,135). Furlanetto (103) pointed out the resemblance in the general subunit structure of the large endogenous somatomedin–carrier-protein complex and 7S NGF.

11. SUMMARY

Although considerable progress has been made during the last decade, research into the role of the somatomedins in mediating the action of growth hormone appears to be on the threshold of significant contributions toward our understanding of the regulatory events involved in the control of cell growth and development. All of the representatives of the somatomedin family, including MSA, appear to be closely related and cross-react with the same receptors on the surface of responsive cells. Differences in competitive-binding potency among the various somatomedins and an equally striking diversity among the somatomedin receptors found in various cell types suggest that the identification of the biologically authentic ligand for any given receptor or tissue and the mechanism responsible for maintaining fidelity will be a significant advance. Evidence establishing the existence of at least two classes of somatomedins, neutral and basic, supports the notion that individual members may have unique biological functions.

Current research efforts into the identification and characterization of somatomedin–carrier-protein complexes in serum are also progressing toward an understanding of what appears to be a unique and complex manner of intense physiological control. The precise relationship between the two major sizes of carrier-protein complexes and the function of the growth-hormone-dependent, acid-labile component remain to be established. It is also unclear whether some cell types are able to recognize and respond to bound somatomedin as it exists in the larger complex, or if it too is biologically inactive, as is the small complex. Indeed, the mechanism by which the low-molecular-weight hormone is processed or channeled into the circulating carrier complexes and then ultimately is delivered to its cell-surface receptor remains unclear. It may also be that a distinct carrier protein exists in the plasma as a scavenger to bind locally produced hormone that finds its way into the vascular space. Additional clarification is also needed regarding the relationship of the high-molecular-weight nonsuppressible insulin-like activities in serum to the somatomedins and their carrier proteins.

One of the exciting advantages offered by the somatomedins is their powerful mitogenicity in cell-culture systems as well as their documented *in vivo* physiological regulation. Investigations by endocrinologists into the physiological role of the somatomedins in regulating tissue growth and development is being paralleled by investigations by cell biologists interested in defining in biochemical terms the events initiated by the interaction of somatomedins with their cell-surface receptors. The inevitable convergence of these two fields of endeavor promises to generate significant contributions to our understanding of the control of cell proliferation.

REFERENCES

1. Temin, H. M., in V. Defendi and M. Stoker, Eds., *Growth Regulating Substances for Animal Cells in Culture*, Wistar Institute Symposium Monograph 7, Wistar Institute Press, Philadelphia, 1967, pp. 103–114.

2. Temin, H. M., *J. Cell. Physiol.*, **74**, 9 (1969).

3. Temin, H. M., Pierson, R. W., and Dulak, N. C., in G. H. Rothblat and V. J. Cristafalo, Eds., *Growth, Nutrition and Metabolism of Cells in Culture*, Academic, New York, 1972, pp. 49–81.

4. Temin, H. M., *J. Cell. Physiol.*, **78**, 161 (1971).

5. Temin, H. M., *J. Cell. Physiol.*, **69**, 377 (1967).

6. Antoniades, H. N., *Science*, **127**, 593 (1958).

7. Antoniades, H. N., and Gunderson, K., *Endocrinology*, **70**, 95 (1962).

8. Bürgi, H., Müller, W. A., Humbel, R. E., Labhart, A., and Froesch, E. R., *Biochim. Biophys. Acta*, **121**, 349 (1966).

9. Gliemann, J., *Diabetologia*, **3**, 382 (1967).
10. Pierson, R. W., and Temin, H. M., *J. Cell. Physiol.*, **79**, 319 (1972).
11. Coon, H. G., *J. Cell Biol.*, **39**, 29a (1968).
12. Dulak, N. C., and Temin, H. M., *J. Cell. Physiol.*, **81**, 153 (1973).
13. Dulak, N. C., and Temin, H. M., *J. Cell. Physiol.*, **81**, 161 (1973).
14. Smith, G. L., and Temin, H. M., *J. Cell. Physiol.*, **84**, 181 (1974).
15. Daughaday, W. H., Hall, K., Raben, M. L., Salmon, W. D., Van den Brande, J. L., and Van Wyk, J. J., *Nature*, **235**, 107 (1972).
16. Brinsmead, M. W., and Liggins, G. C., in E. M. Scarpelli and E. V. Cosmi, Eds., *Reviews in Perinatal Medicine*, Raven, New York, 1979, Vol. 3, pp. 207–242.
17. Van Wyk, J. J., Furlanetto, R. W., Plet, A. S., D'Ecole, A. J., and Underwood, L. E., *Natl. Cancer Inst. Monogr.*, **48**, 141 (1978).
18. Hall, K., Takano, K., Fryklund, L., and Sievertsson, H., in R. Luft and K. Hall, Eds., *Advances in Metabolic Disorders*, Academic, New York-San Francisco-London, 1975, Vol. 8, pp. 19–46.
19. Schalch, D. S., Mauer, K., Draznin, B., Emler, C. A., and Müller, L. L., in A. Pecile and E. E. Muller, Eds., *Growth Hormone and Other Biologically Active Peptides*, Excerpta Medica, Amsterdam-Oxford-Princeton, 1980, pp. 144–160.
20. Rinderknecht, E., and Humbel, R. E., *Proc. Natl. Acad. Sci. USA*, **73**, 2365 (1976).
21. Rinderknecht, E., and Humbel, R. E., *Proc. Natl. Acad. Sci. USA*, **73**, 4379 (1976).
22. Rinderknecht, E., and Humbel, R. E., *J. Biol. Chem.*, **253**, 2769 (1978).
23. Blundell, T. L., Bedarkar, S., Rinderknecht, E., and Humbel, R. E., *Proc. Natl. Acad. Sci. USA*, **75**, 180 (1978).
24. Froesch, E. R., Zapf, J., Walter, H., Schoenle, E., Rinderknecht, E., and Humbel, R. E., in J. Dumont and J. Nunez, Eds., *Hormones and Cell Regulation*, Elsevier/North-Holland, New York, 1979, Vol. 3, pp. 149–167.
25. Uthne, K., *Acta Endocrinol.*, **175** (Suppl.), 1 (1973).
26. Werner, S., Hall, K., and Low, H., *Horm. Metab. Res.*, **6**, 319 (1974).
27. Fryklund, L., Uthne, K., and Sievertsson, H., *Biochem. Biophys. Res. Commun.*, **61**, 957 (1974).
28. Sievertsson, H., Fryklund, L., Uthne, K., Hall, K., and Westermark, B., in R. Luft and K. Hall, Eds., *Advances in Metabolic Disorders*, Academic Press, New York-San Francisco-London, 1975, Vol. 8, pp. 47–60.
29. Van Wyk, J. J., Underwood, L. E., Hintz, R. L., Clemmons, D. R., Voina, S. J., and Weaver, R. R., *Recent Prog. Horm. Res.*, **30**, 259 (1974).
30. Hintz, R. L., Liu, F., and Rinderknecht, E., *J. Clin. Endocrinol. Metab.*, **51**, 672 (1980).
31. Van Wyk, J. J., Svoboda, M. E., and Underwood, L. E., *J. Clin. Endocrinol. Metab.*, **50**, 206 (1980).
32. Svoboda, M. E., Van Wyk, J. J., Klapper, O. G., Fellows, R. E., Grissom, F. E., and Schleuter, R. D., *Biochemistry*, **19**, 790 (1980).
33. Moses, A. C., Nissley, S. P., Short, P. A., Rechler, M. M., and Podskalny, J. M., *Eur. J. Biochem.*, **103**, 387 (1980).
34. Rechler, M. M., Fryklund, L., Nissley, S. P., Hall, K., Podskalny, J. M., Skottner, A., and Moses, A. C., *Eur. J. Biochem.*, **82**, 5 (1978).

35. Dulak, N. C., and Shing, Y. W., *J. Cell. Physiol.*, **90**, 127 (1977).
36. Brinsmead, M. W., and Liggins, G. C., *Aust. J. Exp. Biol. Med. Sci.*, **56**, 513 (1978).
37. Merrill, G. F., Dulak, N. C., and Florini, J. R., *J. Cell. Physiol.*, **100**, 343 (1979).
38. Merrill, G. F., Florini, J. F., and Dulak, N. C., *J. Cell. Physiol.*, **93**, 173 (1977).
39. Veldhuis, J. D., and Hammond, J. M., *Endocrine Res. Commun.*, **6**, 299 (1979).
40. Smith, G. L., *J. Cell Biol.*, **73**, 761 (1977).
41. Bolen, J. B., and Smith, G. L., *J. Cell. Physiol.*, **91**, 441 (1977).
42. Knauer, D. J., Wagner, F. W., and Smith, G. L., *J. Supramol. Struct. Cell. Biochem.*, **15**, 177 (1981).
43. Moses, A. C., Nissley, S. P., Short, P. A., and Rechler, M. M., *Eur. J. Biochem.*, **103**, 401 (1980).
44. Marquardt, H., Todaro, G. J., Henderson, L. E., and Oroszlan, S., *J. Biol. Chem.*, **256**, 6859 (1981).
45. Rechler, M. M., Nissley, S. P., Podskalny, J. M., Moses, A. C., and Fryklund, L., *J. Clin. Endocrinol. Metab.*, **44**, 820 (1977).
46. Nissley, S. P., Passamoni, J., and Short, P., *J. Cell. Physiol.*, **89**, 393 (1976).
47. Florini, J. R., Nickolson, M. L., and Dulak, N. C., *Endocrinology*, **101**, 32 (1977).
48. Derr, J. T., and Smith, G. L., *J. Cell. Physiol.*, **102**, 55 (1980).
49. Heaton, J. H., Schilling, E. E., Gelehrter, T. D., Rechler, M. M., Spencer, E. J., and Nissley, S. P., *Biochim. Biophys. Acta*, **632**, 192 (1980).
50. Smith, G. L., and Stange, A. W., *Life Sci.*, **23**, 1871 (1978).
51. Stevens, R. L., Nissley, S. P., Kimura, J. H., Rechler, M. M., Caplan, A. J., and Hascell, V. C., *J. Biol. Chem.*, **256**, 2045 (1981).
52. Rechler, M. M., Podskalny, J. M., and Nissley, S. P., *J. Biol. Chem.*, **252**, 3898 (1977).
53. Moses, A. C., Nissley, S. P., Rechler, M. M., Short, P. A., and Podskalny, J. M., in G. Giordano, J. J. Van Wyk, and F. Minuto, Eds., *Somatomedins and Growth*, Academic, London-New York-San Francisco, 1979, pp. 45–57.
54. Hintz, R. L., Clemmons, D. R., Underwood, L. E., and Van Wyk, J. J., *Proc. Natl. Acad. Sci. USA*, **69**, 2351 (1972).
55. Marshall, R. N., Underwood, L. E., Voina, S. J., Foushee, D. B., and Van Wyk, J. J., *J. Clin. Endocrinol. Metab.*, **39**, 283 (1974).
56. Van Wyk, J. J., Underwood, L. E., Hintz, R. L., Voina, S. J., and Weaver, R. P., *Recent Prog. Horm. Res.*, **30**, 259 (1974).
57. Froesch, E. R., Zapf, J., Meuli, C., Mader, M., Waldvogel, M., Kaufmann, U., and Morell, B., in R. Luft and K. Hall, Eds., *Advances in Metabolic Disorders*, Academic Press, New York-San Francisco-London, 1975, Vol. 8, pp. 211–235.
58. Takano, K., Hall, K., Fryklund, L., Holmgren, A., Sievertsson, H., and Uthne, K., *Acta Endocrinol.*, **80**, 14 (1975).
59. Nissley, S. P., and Rechler, M. M., *Natl. Cancer Inst. Monogr.*, **48**, 167 (1978).
60. Megyesi, K., Kahn, C. R., Roth, J., Neville, D. M., Nissley, S. P., Humbel, R. E., and Froesch, E. R., *J. Biol. Chem.*, **250**, 8990 (1975).
61. Rechler, M. M., Podskalny, J. M., and Nissley, S. P., *Nature*, **259**, 134 (1976).
62. Nissley, S. P., Rechler, M. M., Moses, A. C., Short, P. A., and Podskalny, J. M., *Endocrinology*, **101**, 708 (1977).

63. Rechler, M. M., Zapf, J., Nissley, S. P., Froesch, E. R., Moses, A. C., Podskalny, J. M., Schilling, E. E., and Humbel, R. E., *Endocrinology*, **107**, 1451 (1980).

64. Knauer, D. J., and Smith, G. L., *J. Cell. Physiol.*, **100**, 311 (1979).

65. Todaro, G. J., and DeLarco, J. E., *Cancer Res.*, **38**, 4147 (1978).

66. Brinsmead, M. W., and Liggins, G. C., *Austr. J. Exp. Biol. Med. Sci.*, **56**, 527 (1978).

67. Bar, R. S., Peacock, M. L., Rechler, M. M., and Nissley, S. P., *J. Clin. Endocrinol. Metab.*, **52**, 814 (1981).

68. Massague, J., Guilette, B. J., and Czech, M. P., *J. Biol. Chem.*, **256**, 2122 (1981).

69. Kasuga, M., Obberghen, E. V., Nissley, S. P., and Rechler, M. M., *J. Biol. Chem.*, **256**, 5305 (1981).

70. Moses, A. C., Nissley, S. P., Short, P. A., Rechler, M. M., White, R. M., Knight, A. B., and Higa, O. Z., *Proc. Natl. Acad. Sci. USA*, **77**, 3649 (1980).

71. Nissley, S. P., Rechler, M. M., Moses, A. C., Eisen, H. J., Higa, O. Z., Short, P. A., Fennoy, I., Bruni, C. B., and White, R. M., in G. H. Sato and R. Ross, Eds., *Hormones and Cell Culture*, Cold Spring Harbor Laboratory, Cold Spring Harbor, N.Y., 1979, pp. 79–94.

72. Rechler, M. M., Eisen, H. J., Higa, O. Z., Nissley, S. P., Moses, A. C., Schilling, E. E., Fennoy, I., Bruni, C. B., Phillips, L. S., and Baird, K. L., *J. Biol. Chem.*, **254**, 7942 (1979).

73. Froesch, E. R., Bürgi, H., Muller, W. A., Humbel, R. E., Jacob, A., and Labhart, A., *Recent Prog. Hormone Res.*, **23**, 565 (1967).

74. Daughaday, W. H., and Kipnis, D. M., *Recent Prog. Hormone Res.*, **22**, 49 (1966).

75. Van den Brande, J. L., Van Wyk, J. J., Weaver, R. P., and Mayberry, H. E., *Acta Endocrinol.*, **66**, 65 (1971).

76. Hintz, R. L., Orsini, E. M., and Van Camp, M. G., *Endocrinol.*, **94** (Suppl.), A-71 (1974).

77. Hintz, R. L., and Liu, F., *J. Clin. Endocrinol. Metab.*, **45**, 988 (1977).

78. Fryklund, L., Skottner, A., Forsman, A., Coasensson, S., and Hall, K., in G. Sato and R. Ross, Eds., *Hormones and Cell Culture*, Cold Spring Harbor Laboratory, Cold Spring Harbor, N.Y., 1979, p. 49.

79. Zapf, J., Waldvogel, M., and Froesch, E. R., *Arch. Biochem. Biophys.*, **168**, 638 (1975).

80. Kaufmann, U., Zapf, J., Torrett, B., and Froesch, E. R., *J. Clin. Endocrinol. Metab.*, **44**, 160 (1977).

81. Megyesi, K., Kahn, C. R., Roth, J., and Gorden, P., *J. Clin. Endocrinol. Metab.*, **41**, 475 (1975).

82. Peeters, S., and Friesen, H. G., *Endocrinology*, **101**, 1164 (1977).

83. Cohen, K. L., and Nissley, S. P., *Acta Endocrinol.*, **83**, 243 (1976).

84. Draznin, B., Schalch, D. S., Heinrich, U. E., and Schlueter, R. J., in G. Giordano, J. J. Van Wyk, and F. Minuto, Eds., *Somatomedins and Growth*, Academic, London-New York-San Francisco, 1979, pp. 149–160.

85. Hintz, R. L., and Liu, L., in A. Pecile and E. E. Müller, Eds., *Growth Hormone and Other Biologically Active Peptides*, Excerpta Medica, Amsterdam-Oxford-Princeton, 1980, pp. 133–143.

86. Heinrich, U. E., Schalch, D. S., Koch, J. G., and Johnson, C. J., *J. Clin. Endocrinol. Metab.*, **46**, 672 (1978).

87. Horner, J. M., and Hintz, R. L., in G. Giordano, J. J. Van Wyk, and F. Minuto, Eds., *Somatomedins and Growth*, Academic, London-New York-San Francisco, 1979, pp. 177–183.

88. Daughaday, W. H., Mariz, I. K., and Blethen, S. L., *J. Clin. Endocrinol. Metab.*, **51**, 781 (1980).

89. D'Ercole, A. S., and Underwood, L. E., *Dev. Biol.*, **79**, 33 (1980).

90. Moses, A. C., Nissley, S. P., Cohen, K. L., and Rechler, M. M., *Nature*, **263**, 137 (1976).

91. Moses, A. C., Nissley, S. P., Passamani, J., White, R. M., and Rechler, M. M., *Endocrinology*, **104**, 536 (1979).

92. Nissley, S. P., Short, P. A., Rechler, M. M., Podskalny, J. M., and Coon, H. G., *Cell*, **11**, 441 (1977).

93. Burstein, P. J., Draznin, B., Johnson, C. J., and Schalch, D. S., *Endocrinology*, **104**, 1107 (1979).

94. Schalch, D. S., Heinrich, U. E., Koch, J. G., Johnson, C. J., and Schlueter, R. J., *J. Clin. Endocrinol. Metab.*, **46**, 664 (1978).

95. Zapf, J., and Froesch, E. R., in G. Giordano, J. J. Van Wyk, and F. Minuto, Eds., *Somatomedins and Growth*, Academic, London-New York-San Francisco, 1979, pp. 137–141.

96. Chochinov, R. H., Mariz, I. K., Hajek, A. S., and Daughaday, W. H., *J. Clin. Endocrinol. Metab.*, **44**, 902 (1977).

97. Drop, S. L., Valiquette, G., Guyda, H. I., Corval, M. T., and Posner, B. I., *Acta Endocrinol.*, **90**, 505 (1979).

98. Meuli, C., Zapfand, J., and Froesch, E. R., *Diabetologica*, **14**, 255 (1978).

99. Zapf, J., Schoenle, E., Jagars, G., Sard, I., Grunwald, J., and Froesch, E. R., *J. Clin. Invest.*, **63**, 1077 (1979).

100. Knauer, D. J., and Smith, G. L., *Proc. Natl. Acad. Sci. USA*, **77**, 7252 (1980).

101. Cohen, K. L., and Nissley, S. P., *Endocrinology*, **97**, 654 (1975).

102. Hintz, R. L., and Liu, F., in G. Giordano, J. J. Van Wyk, and F. Minuto, Eds., *Somatomedins and Growth*, Academic, London-New York-San Francisco, 1979, pp. 143–147.

103. Furlanetto, R. W., *J. Clin. Endocrinol. Metab.*, **51**, 12 (1980).

104. D'Ercole, A. J., Applewhite, G. T., and Underwood, L. E., *Dev. Biol.*, **75**, 315 (1980).

105. Jacob, A., Hauri, C., and Froesch, E. R., *J. Clin. Invest.*, **47**, 2678 (1968).

106. Poffenberger, P. L., Stuart, C. A., Prince, M. J., and Medina, A. T., in G. Giordano, J. J. Van Wyk, and F. Minuto, Eds., *Somatomedins and Growth*, Academic, London-New York-San Francisco, 1979, pp. 67–83.

107. Cohen, S., *J. Biol. Chem.*, **237**, 1555 (1962).

108. Carpenter, G., *J. Invest. Derm.*, **71**, 283 (1978).

109. Cohen, S., Carpenter, G., and Lemback, K. J., in R. Luft and K. Hall, Eds., *Advances in Metabolic Disorders*, Academic, London-New York-San Francisco, 1975, Vol. 8, pp. 265–284.

110. Carpenter, G., and Cohen, S., *Annu. Rev. Biochem.*, **48**, 193 (1979).

111. Savage, C. R., Inagami, T., and Cohen, S., *J. Biol. Chem.*, **247**, 7612 (1972).

112. Savage, C. R., Hash, J. H., and Cohen, S., *J. Biol. Chem.*, **248**, 7669 (1973).

113. Taylor, J. M., Cohen, S., and Mitchell, W. M., *Proc. Natl. Acad. Sci. USA*, **67**, 164 (1970).

114. Taylor, J. M., Mitchell, W. M., and Cohen, S., *J. Biol. Chem.*, **249**, 3198 (1974).

115. Taylor, J. M., Mitchell, W. M., and Cohen, S., *J. Biol. Chem.*, **249**, 2188 (1974).

116. Lembach, K. J., *Proc. Natl. Acad. Sci. USA*, **73**, 183 (1976).

117. Barnes, D., and Colowick, S. P., *J. Cell. Physiol.*, **89**, 633 (1976).

118. Levi-Montalcini, R., and Angeletti, P. U., *Physiol. Rev.*, **48**, 534 (1968).

119. Hogue-Angeletti, R. A., Bradshaw, R. A., and Frazier, W. A., in R. Luft and K. Hall, Eds., *Advances in Metabolic Disorders*, Academic, London-New York-San Francisco, 1975, Vol. 8, pp. 285–299.

120. Bradshaw, R. A., *Annu. Rev. Biochem.*, **47**, 191 (1978).

121. Bocchini, V., and Angeletti, P. U., *Proc. Natl. Acad. Sci. USA*, **64**, 787 (1969).

122. Varon, S., Nomura, J., and Shooter, E. M., *Biochemistry*, **6**, 2202 (1967).

123. Murphy, R. A., Saide, J. D., Blanchard, M. H., and Young, M., *Proc. Natl. Acad. Sci. USA*, **74**, 2672 (1977).

124. Young, M., Saide, J. D., Murphy, R. A., and Blanchard, M. H., *Biochemistry*, **17**, 1490 (1978).

125. Varon, S., Nomura, S., and Shooter, E. M., *Biochemistry*, **7**, 1296 (1968).

126. Greene, L. A., Varon, S., Pilth, A., and Shooter, E. M., Neurobiology, **1**, 37 (1971).

127. Angeletti, R. H., Bradshaw, R. A., and Wade, R. D., *Biochemistry*, **10**, 463 (1971).

128. Angeletti, R. H., Hermodson, M. A., and Bradshaw, R. A., *Biochemistry*, **12**, 100 (1973).

129. Angeletti, R. H., and Bradshaw, R. A., *Proc. Natl. Acad. Sci. USA*, **68**, 2417 (1971).

130. Greene, L. A., Shooter, E. M., and Varon, S., *Proc. Natl. Acad. Sci. USA*, **60**, 1383 (1968).

131. Greene, L. A., Shooter, E. M., and Varon, S., *Biochemistry*, **8**, 3735 (1969).

132. Moore, J. B., Mobley, W. C., and Shooter, E. M., *Biochemistry*, **13**, 833 (1974).

133. Berger, E. A., and Shooter, E. M., *Proc. Natl. Acad. Sci. USA*, **74**, 3647 (1977).

134. Server, A. C., and Shooter, E. M., *J. Biol. Chem.*, **251**, 165 (1976).

135. Mobley, W. C., Schenker, A., and Shooter, E. M., *Biochemistry*, **15**, 5543 (1976).

NOTE ADDED IN PROOF

Recently, Massague and Czech (6) further examined the structure of somatomedin receptors in several cell types. Confirming an earlier report by Kasuga et al. (3) there appear to be two structural types of somatomedin receptors. Massague and Czech have proposed that the insulin-sensitive receptor which shows a greater affinity for IGF I, is a tetrameric structure composed of two 130,000 dalton subunits and two 98,000 dalton subunits joined by interchain disulfide bridges. The structure of this receptor resembles that of the insulin receptor itself (8). The IGF receptors of chicken embryo fibroblasts (4) and human placenta (2) have also recently been shown to possess a similar subunit structure. In contrast, the insulin-insensitive receptor which exhibits greater affinity for IGF II and MSA is composed of a single protein chain containing intrachain disulfide bridges and has a molecular weight of approximately 260,000 daltons (6,3,7).

Morris and Schalch (9) provided additional evidence that the somatomedin binding protein of human plasma exists in two or more forms possessing a common 30,000 dalton component. These results are similar to those published by Knauer et al. (5) regarding the structure of MCP from BRL-3A conditioned medium.

Using an *in vitro* protein synthesizing system and RNA from BRL-3A cells, Acquaviva et al. (1) have identified a 22,200 dalton protein which may represent "pre-pro-MSA." The availability of this system will provide the opportunity to investigate the synthesis of MSA as well as the possible cloning of this rat gene in bacteria.

The writing of this review and investigations in the author's laboratory were supported by USPHS grant #CA 17620 from the National Cancer Institute.

1. Acquaviva, A. M., Bruni, C. R., Nissley, S. P., and Rechler, M. M., *Fed. Proc.*, **41**, 1086 (Abstract 4766), (1982).

2. Bhaumick, B., Bala, R. M., and Hollenberg, M. D., *Proc. Natl. Acad. Sci. USA*, **78**, 4279 (1981).

3. Kasuga, M., Van Obberghen, E., Nissley, S. P., and Rechler, M. M., *J. Biol. Chem.*, **256**, 5305 (1981).

4. Kasuga, M., Van Obberghen, E., Nissley, S. P., and Rechler, M. M., *Proc. Natl. Acad. Sci. USA*, **79**, 1864 (1982).

5. Knauer, D. J., Wagner, F. W., and Smith, G. L., *J. Supramol. Struct. Cell Biochem.*, **15**, 177 (1981).

6. Massague, J., and Czech, M. P., *J. Biol. Chem.*, **257**, 5038 (1982).

7. Massague, J., Guilette, B. J., and Czech, M. P., *J. Biol. Chem.*, **256**, 2122 (1981).

8. Massague, J., Pilch, P. F., and Czech, M. P., *Proc. Natl. Acad. Sci. USA*, **77**, 7137 (1980).

9. Morris, D. H., and Schalch, D. S., *Endocrinology*, **111**, 801 (1982).

AUTHOR INDEX

Numbers in parentheses are reference numbers and indicate that the author's work is referred to although his name is not mentioned in the text. Numbers in *italics* show the pages on which the complete references are listed.

SUBJECT INDEX